ADVANCED PRAISE

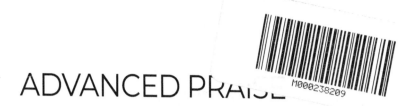

"I encourage everyone to take the time to read this thoughtful and inspiring book!"
Jim Treliving (Boston Pizza Co-Owner, *Dragons' Den* Investor)

"Dr. Chapin and I have won two Grey Cup Championships together. He exudes energy and is passionate about the well-being of his community. As the Argos Team Chiropractor, I've seen him inspire players with his care and motivate them to do the work necessary to realize their potential. I, too, am encouraged to learn that I can feel better, move better, think better, and do better at any stage of life. In *Take Good Care*, he thoughtfully explains how your body is as good to you as you are to it. We can all become champions of our lives. If you need a coach to show you the way, Dr. Chapin will teach you how to win. He's done it before!"
Michael "Pinball" Clemons (GM of the Toronto Argonauts
& Co-Founder of Pinball Clemons Foundation)

"Do NOT wait. Pick up this book NOW. Regardless of where you are in your wellness journey, Dr. Chapin will guide you with compassion, science, and actionable steps toward better health. Literally, add years to your life by reading this book."
Khamica Bingham (Olympic Track and Field Athlete
for Team Canada, Motivational Speaker)

"Dwight Chapin helped support my health and athletic performance toward the end of my career as a Toronto Argonaut, including our 2017 Grey Cup Championship season. He is a gifted clinician and someone you can trust."
Ricky Ray (Former Professional Football QB,
Class of 2022 - CFL Hall of Fame, 4x Grey Cup Champion)

"This is essential reading! Dr. Chapin has written a wellness manifesto and it's FOR YOU. You will absorb the advice and guidance in this book and when you do, it'll change everything for your benefit."
Herbie Kuhn (Toronto Raptors Public Address Announcer, Team Chaplain to the Toronto Argonauts, Toronto Raptors, and Athletics Canada)

"Staff at *The Globe and Mail* know Dwight as the go-to-guy for effective, pragmatic advice and treatment. He has helped me recover from two hip replacements and sundry other ailments that come with the aging process, delivering guidance with great good humor and confidence-inspiring wisdom. *Take Good Care* is a reflection of the bond he creates with people, whether they be pro athletes or an oldie with sore knees, like me. The stories he tells are an excellent roadmap for staying active and positive."

Phillip Crawley C.M., C.B.E. (Publisher and CEO of *The Globe and Mail*)

"Mastering the art of managing one's health and energy is what the very best leaders do differently. It requires dedication and discipline to prioritize self-care, and for those seeking a roadmap to success, Dr. Dwight Chapin's *Take Good Care* offers a robust and reliable framework for optimal health and peak performance."

Jim Reid (Executive Coach and Author of *Leading to Greatness*)

"We learned from Maya Angelou that people who know better, do better. In *Take Good Care*, Dr. Chapin has curated a phenomenal blueprint that helps us do better... and live fuller."

Claudette McGowan (CEO of Protexxa, Former Global Executive Officer of Cyber Security for TD Bank)

"The key is "storytelling" - by recounting real-life stories of real people, Dwight keeps you engaged and brings his seven wellness rituals alive and relatable."

Jim Leech (Chancellor Emeritus, Queen's University, Former President of the Ontario Teachers' Pension Plan)

"There is no one-size-fits-all approach to sleep, nutrition, exercise, or mental fitness. *Take Good Care* reveals the wellness rituals that are the essential building blocks to good health, but it is Dr. Chapin's guidance and the stories he shares that will help you craft an approach that works for you."

Jennifer Sygo (Team Dietitian for the Toronto Raptors, Athletics Canada, Swim Canada, and Gymnastics Canada)

"On our journey to be the best possible version of ourselves and find the greatest joy in our lives, it is important to listen to wise people and learn from their journeys. *Take Good Care* has just that. It will help you 'fall in love with the life you already have' and arm you with more tools to accept the things you cannot change, and courage to change the things you can."

Jeffrey Latimer (CEO of Canada's Walk of Fame, Owner of JL Entertainment)

"What we practice improves. Whether it is in physical fitness, mental fitness, or our overall wellness, in these profiles of 21 prominent Canadians, Dr. Chapin underlines the simple, straightforward but critical steps that we must intentionally take to be at the top of our games at work and in life. Bravo; this is a needed contribution to an important conversation."

Dr. Ian Dawe, MHSc, MD, FRCPC (Psychiatrist at Trillium Health Partners; Associate Professor of Psychiatry at UofT)

"If you have been searching for ways to live your best life, *Take Good Care* is the book for you. It is a step-by-step guide to taking back control of your life. Dr. Dwight captures the rituals and habits essential to living not only a good life, but shares the elements that are key to living a great life. It is a must-read if you are looking to make positive changes, and are ready to take back control of your life today."

Pattie Lovett Reid (Best-Selling Author, Financial Commentator)

"*Take Good Care* offers an inspiring look at the influence our daily habits have on health, performance, and longevity. It is a must-read for anyone looking to leverage their healing potential. Dr. Chapin shows us how to make meaningful, realistic changes to accelerate healing, build mental and physical strength, and find hope."

Dr. Andy Smith (President and CEO of Sunnybrook Health Sciences Centre)

"Dr. Dwight Chapin has a gift for translating complex concepts into everyday language. *Take Good Care* will help you craft a formula guided by leading research and an inspiring call to action."

Dr. Greg Wells (Performance Physiologist, CEO of Wells Performance, Author)

"There is nothing better than expert advice, based in science, yet tested through years of hands-on application where it matters most: In people's daily lives. *Take Good Care* contains a career's worth of hard-earned knowledge in readable, actionable, and relatable steps. Make yourself healthier, smarter, and happier: get this book."
Michael Grange (Professional Basketball Analyst for Sportsnet)

"Dr. Chapin has a unique understanding of the lifestyle practices required to unlock the body's healing potential. He also understands the pitfalls that make it difficult to do so. In *Take Good Care*, he skillfully shares his knowledge and the leading evidence in an inspiring call to action that will add quality years to your life."
Randy Lennox (Former President of Universal Music Canada and Bell Media)

"In addition to being a skilled medical practitioner with the writing of *Take Good Care*, Dr. Dwight Chapin has demonstrated a gift of storytelling and translating complex concepts into a very readable and actionable script. I only wish that I had been able to access all of his insights many years ago!"
Lynn Langrock (VP of People for Bimbo QSR)

"Through this captivating book, readers will discover how small changes in their daily habits can make a big difference to overall health, performance, and even longevity. Dr. Chapin reveals an empowering path of performance tweaks that anyone can take to improve well-being, gain strength both mentally and physically - all while rediscovering hope! It's essential reading for those seeking maximum potential from self-healing strategies."
Alison Dantas (Senior Executive & Executive Coach, Potential Actualized)

"*Take Good Care* offers candid insights and tools for prioritizing your health from a practitioner's vantage point who knows what it takes to be well. It is refreshing to read and learn from diverse perspectives that approach health in their own unique ways yet share the common goal of being well to be of service to others."
Dr. Robyne Hanley-Dafoe (Author, Psychology and Education Instructor, Stress Resiliency Expert)

"In *Take Good Care*, Dr. Chapin reveals how even small changes to our daily routine can have a profound effect on health and wellbeing - allowing us to become stronger in body and mind, ward off illness more effectively, and experience an overall sense of hope. An inspiring guide for anyone looking to unlock their healing potential, this is essential reading!"
Michael Richardson (CEO and Co-Founder of Eclipsys)

"Everyone has a vision of what they want a healthy life to look like. But a vision is more than the end result, it is the daily plan, the "process" to get there. In his book, Dr. Dwight Chapin lays it out for you in seven easy yet disciplined steps to get a healthy, more fulfilling life journey and why those steps matter."
Marc Trestman (Head Coach in NFL, Three-Time Grey Cup Champion Head Coach in CFL, and University of Miami Lecturer, Adjunct Faculty and Advisory Board Member, Entertainment, Arts and Sports Law LL.M)

Take Good Care

DR. DWIGHT CHAPIN

B.SC. (H), D.C.

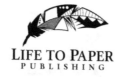

LIFE TO PAPER
PUBLISHING

To request permissions, contact the publisher at info@lifetopaper.com.

Paperback: 978-1-990700-23-1
Ebook: 978-1-990700-24-8

First paperback edition May 2023.
Edited by Katrina DeLiberato, Jennifer Goulden & Don Loney
Cover Design by Tabitha Rose & Monty Langford
Photography by Monty Langford
Layout by Jennifer Goulden

Printed in the USA.
1 2 3 4 5 6 7 8 9 10

Life to Paper Publishing Inc.
Toronto | Miami

www.lifetopaper.com

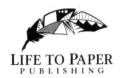

LIFE TO PAPER
PUBLISHING

To my patients,
Thank you for your trust.
It was the inspiration behind this book.

CONTENTS

FOREWORD

Dear Reader,

If you're like me, you've picked this book up and have turned it over in your hands a few times. You may be intrigued — may even believe there's something within these pages for you — but you hesitate. Believe me, I get it. There are so many volumes of texts out there. How's anyone to know which are actually helpful?

In *Take Good Care*, Dr. Dwight Chapin aims to share a series of practices that may be of help to you. It's not a compendium of advice from people who have it all figured out. (If it were, I'd be patently underqualified to write this foreword). Rather, this book is a compendium of learnings from people who have found some success — in sport, medicine, leadership, commerce, or education — and who've also struggled to find balance. This is a book about humans, like us, who sometimes falter in our bodies. This is a book for humans who sometimes lack the enthusiasm we need to attack the day. This book is about the tools we can develop to live lives full of strength and hope. I can't be certain, but I'm pretty sure this book's gonna help you. And me too.

Full disclosure: I've been a patient of Dr. Chapin's for the past few years. I'm a professional writer who suffers through chronic pain from both injury and repetitive stress. My life partner is a gridiron quarterback who has his own share of corporeal strain. Dr. Chapin's care is prismatic enough that he's able to see us both, to treat our individual ailments holistically, and to do so with great specificity. He takes really, really good care of us — engaging our minds and hearts — as we move toward a shared vision of health.

In the time I've seen him, Dr. Chapin has honored my own experience and has never been didactic or preachy. Every single time I leave him, I do so feeling more like myself. I don't get to visit nearly as often as I'd like. Selfishly, I'm elated to *finally* be able to extend the work we do on site. I'm thrilled to take a piece of Dr. Chapin's care home with me.

I'm confident that any book he's penned will be an extension of his thoughtful practice. Truthfully, I'm excited for anyone who chooses to read.

If you're still hesitant, don't be. There's no theory in this book that Dr. Chapin hasn't inspected, stress-tested, and put through the proverbial ringer. You shouldn't listen to him because of any letters before or after his name. Don't listen because he's celebrated as one of the most respected healthcare providers in the country. I'd encourage you to read through, earnestly and hungrily, as the Dwight Chapin I know has pored over the interviews and lessons doggedly, with your best health in mind. I'm confident he's culled only what may be of use to you. I know he'd only write this book as an offering — with a wish that after reading, digesting, and enacting you, dear reader, begin to *feel better*. That's it. That's the whole ball game. You might feel more determined, more energetic, more focused, or even just better rested after using this book.

Wouldn't that be worth it?

In strength and hope,

Chinaka Hodge
Californian Poet, Educator, Playwright, and Screenwriter

INTRODUCTION

WHERE THIS BOOK BEGAN

*A*s a chiropractor and co-owner of a large multi-disciplinary health clinic, Team Chiropractor for the Toronto Argonauts, lead clinician of the onsite repetitive strain injury prevention clinic for Globe and Mail employees, and corporate wellness innovator, I have made it my life's mission to care for, educate, and inspire others in their journey toward optimal health.

> *There is nothing like a full-stop health crisis to bring the collateral damage of a dysfunctional lifestyle into focus.*

I lived at the outer margins of my clinical skills, physical endurance, and mental fitness in the early days of the COVID-19 pandemic. At the two-month mark, I was already leaning hard into my twenty-four years of experience as a frontline primary care clinician. Novel virus infections, fractures, heart attacks, cancer detection, unmanaged diabetes, and mental health crises all belong upstream from a chiropractor's treatment table.

My days in the clinic are usually spent managing back pain, sports injuries, and supporting the health and performance of high-level executives and athletes. But in the chaos of the first wave, my patients needed my help differently. Fearful of entering a hospital or unable to see their family doctors, patients knew I was a voice they could trust, and that my door was still open to those in need of urgent care. As word spread, patients started coming in with everything. Each day presented new challenges and tested my capacity. I helped those I could within my scope of practice and did everything in my power to ensure everyone else landed in capable hands. In the months to come, I would be recognized by the City of Mississauga as a COVID Hero for staying in the fight. Most days, I felt like that wasn't enough.

As we entered 2021 and people began to confront the extent of their grief, loss, and sacrifice, there was a noticeable shift in the attitude of patients seeking care. Fear and anxiety were beginning to give way to frustration and a determination to emerge from COVID-19 stronger and healthier. The coping strategies many developed to endure the early isolation and restrictions were never intended to support such a long haul and had left many raw, vulnerable, and in poor health. *Physical health reveals a truth there is no hiding from.*

As a musculoskeletal expert, I have a unique vantage point from which to observe the health impact of daily routines. An individual's approach to life, their process, and the priority they place on their health have always fascinated me. I am blessed with the ability to put people back together, but patients today want and need more than a return to normal. The disruption caused by the pandemic has brought many to a tipping point by exposing the distractions and poor choices that cut our lives short and rob us of our potential. As the pace of work and life continues to increase, competition intensifies, and peak performance has become the expected norm. This pace is not sustainable; consequently, how we work and the choices we make must change.

My patients are telling me they have zero interest in returning to their frantic pre-pandemic pace and are proactively seeking guidance and support to gain a performance edge and elevate their health. They want to feel better, move better, think better — *be* better. The trend emerging is a strong desire to push the limits of our biological potential and chronological age by leveraging the advances in lifestyle medicine.

Having supported the health of individuals at the top of their game for many years, I know the science and the behavior required to activate the body's healing potential. I'm also familiar with the common pitfalls and health challenges holding many people back from doing so. Excited by my patients' heightened level of curiosity and engagement, I sensed an opportunity to use my influence to help drive transformational change in the health and well-being of a much larger audience.

By early 2021, I had gained clarity around this book's purpose and began my research. I knew that the world did not need another introductory wellness guide. Patients wanted confirmation that "better" was possible. And so I took up the challenge of writing a wellness performance playbook to show them how to get there. It is based on the leading scientific research, my twenty-four years of clinical experience, and the health journeys of twenty-one remarkable Canadians.

In football, a playbook is a carefully curated, ready-to-go collection of a team's strategies and plays; essentially their formulas for success on the field. Divided into offensive, defensive, and special teams plays, it is based on hundreds of past games and countless hours of top level experience. *Take Good Care* is your playbook for better health, strength, and hope. It's divided into wellness rituals, strategies, and formulas for success in life. It is based on countless scientific studies, my twenty-four years as a leader in healthcare, and first hand accounts by twenty-one of Canada's most remarkable people.

In my practice, I see patients in pain every day whose struggles are rooted in unhealthy day-to-day lifestyle choices. Our bodies are remarkably resilient, but only to a point. Left unchecked, unhealthy lifestyles can lead to premature aging, metabolic and cardiovascular disease, hypertension, joint and skeletal disorders, obesity, cancer, mental illness, and premature death. Unfortunately, this outcome awaits far too many traveling in today's fast lane. The good news is that evidence-based science explains how we can push the boundaries of human health, performance, and longevity beyond what we have come to accept as the societal norm. In short, our daily routines hold tremendous influence, but people lack the knowledge to tap into this power in a meaningful way. Adopting advances in lifestyle medicine makes it possible to elevate performance on demand and significantly reduce the risk of future disease.

Having worked closely with professionals who have successfully converted their casual awareness of healthy habits into hard-wired, strategic Wellness Rituals, I know what the human body is capable of when healthy choices are stacked together. I needed to share these stories and show people the power of their healing potential. Waiting for the weekend or a future holiday to nurture your mind and body is not a winning game plan. To inspire action, this book would have to do more than just present current evidence and leading practices. I needed to set it apart and ensure it made a significant impact by bringing real-life examples of well-known and respected individuals to the table. I had to assemble a group of mentors whose lives and experiences would illustrate to the reader that "better" was not just possible but within their reach.

The selection of this group became my passion. I did not want to showcase masters of clean living or set some unrealistic standard with their profiles. I wanted to share motivating stories of individuals recognized for their influence and talent who walked the walk — people who intentionally prioritized their health and were willing to share the details of their formula for success and the struggles they had overcome in its development. I called on the group of twenty-one mentors featured in this book and invited them to participate in this project because of their resiliency, discipline, passion, consistency, and influence. Every one of them has learned how to take good care of themselves so they can perform at their best in all facets of life.

In an honest and vulnerable exchange, they opened their lives to me, inspired by my purpose and genuinely altruistic in their intention to help others. Poring over the fine details of their daily routine, I was determined to understand their approach to adversity, discipline with self-care, and strategies for extending and recovering from peak performance. As they walked me through their lives, I was surprised to discover even more. Embedded within each of their formulas were 7 specific Wellness Rituals practiced by all twenty-one. There was common ground in their excellence.

Take Good Care is my moonshot, evidence-based call-to-action. My hope is that the practice of the 7 Wellness Rituals presented in this book will provide readers with a springboard to emerge from the pandemic in full command of their healing potential.

In addition to the lifestyle practices and experiences shared by the twenty-one mentors, the content is based on my professional experience from twenty-four years of practice as a musculoskeletal (MSK) expert and leader in Corporate Wellness and from the leading evidence-based research and science.

I also relied on an advisory team of clinicians that helped review the evidence behind the Wellness Rituals and graciously shared their clinical wisdom with me. This book is undoubtedly better thanks to their input and support. A special thank you to Dr. Patrick Welsh, Dr. Noah Litvak, Nazima Qureshi, Dr. Ian Dawe, and Dr. Michael Odlozinski.

HOW THIS BOOK IS ORGANIZED

Similar to the way a football playbook is divided by types of plays (offensive, defensive, and special teams), *Take Good Care* is divided into seven sections — 7 Wellness Rituals. These rituals have been shown to promote healing, improve physical and mental strength, and encourage hope. While the health-boosting effect of each is significant, the evidence shows us that when all seven rituals are practiced together, the benefits are even further amplified. To illustrate this effect, mentor profiles are woven between the sections explaining the science to provide a practical, behind-the-scenes look at the mentors' unique formula for health and success. While the mentors practice all 7 Wellness Rituals, they give them different weights and have learned how and when to lean into each one. Within the mentor profiles, I have embedded self-care exercises and reflections to encourage you to examine your understanding and consider how you may incorporate the rituals into your daily routine. I have also included a section dedicated to activating each ritual to help you in your journey toward optimal health.

WELLNESS RITUAL #1: PRIORITIZE SLEEP, REST, & RECOVERY

Sleep is a complex, dynamic process that affects every organ, tissue, and system in our body. In sleep we tap into our healing potential. Failing to prioritize this daily reset puts you on a fast track toward burnout and chronic disease. Wellness Ritual #1 is fundamental to good health.

WELLNESS RITUAL #2: CONSUME HEALTHY FUEL

Hidden within our DNA is the genetic blueprint for healing. Our dietary habits will either help our body unlock this code and promote good health or suppress it and put our body on the defensive. Wellness Ritual #2 is all about developing an appreciation for how our diet influences health and performance. It looks at what, why, and when we eat. Consuming a variety of nutrient-dense foods and eating in response to hunger in a time-restricted window allows your body to mobilize calories efficiently and minimize chronic inflammation.

WELLNESS RITUAL #3: FIGHT FOR YOUR WAISTLINE

Wellness Ritual #3 always gets a lot of attention. We want to feel good, but we also want to look good. One of the reasons that maintaining a healthy weight is difficult is that evolution favored those with the reserves to weather unexpected adversity; in other words, a little extra fat stored when times were good might mean you had a better chance to survive a difficult season when resources were scarce. In our sedentary lives, where calories are abundant, we are still genetically programmed to make and store fat in preparation for potentially tough times ahead. Learning to eat less, consume a variety of nutrient-dense foods, limit processed foods, get active, and practice mindful eating puts you back in this fight.

WELLNESS RITUAL #4: MOVE TO STAY YOUNG

When we challenge our range of motion, balance, coordination, and strength by moving often, we improve the quality of our movement and slow the aging process. To enjoy the ability to move well, we must practice moving. Stiffness and poor movement are not inevitable consequences of aging.

Wellness Ritual #4 is about bringing a variety of movements to every day, challenging our physical capacity, and limiting time spent in sedentary postures.

WELLNESS RITUAL #5: PROTECT YOUR STRENGTH

Resistance training is essential to healthy aging. By the time you reach the age of 40, your muscular strength is already a decade into decline if you are not actively protecting it. The practice of Wellness Ritual #5 will keep you strong, but it will also help improve sleep, energy levels, insulin sensitivity, and weight management. With a surprisingly small investment in time, this ritual will also reduce visceral fat and boost cardiovascular, bone, and brain health - regardless of age.

WELLNESS RITUAL #6: NURTURE MENTAL FITNESS

The wave of mental illness accompanying the pandemic is alarming. Prolonged exposure to stress decreases activity in areas of the brain that handle high-order tasks and stimulates more primitive parts focused on our emotional response and survival. If you are stuck in a fight or flight stress response all day, you are training your mind to constantly look for threats.

Choosing to operate from this position will cut your life short. Wellness Ritual #6 is about breaking free from that pattern, learning how to harness the power of our thoughts and improve our resiliency to find a state of mental, emotional, social, and spiritual well-being.

WELLNESS RITUAL #7: PLAY WITH PURPOSE

Play is an integral part of developing and maintaining a healthy lifestyle. Studies have shown a direct link between play and improved creativity, imagination, energy levels, problem-solving ability, stress resiliency, cognitive function, mindfulness, and enhanced relationships. Play is invigorating; it eases our burden and renews our optimism and hope. Wellness Ritual #7 is about bringing more happiness, joy, excitement, and wonder into your life. Playful people are happier, and happiness boosts health.

A NOTE TO THE READER

If you are reading this in paperback or hardcover, I encourage you to use this book actively. Take a pen and highlighter to it. Dog-ear the corners and make notes in the margins! And if you're on an e-reader, bookmark what resonates most to you. Much like football teams watch game tapes to spot winning moves and flag areas for improvement, take time to reflect on the self-care exercises as you make your way through the book. Record your thoughts as you go. You will find a complementary journal available for download at **7WellnessRituals.com**.

It is my hope that you will be inspired and encouraged by the mentors' stories, celebrate what we are capable of when we set our minds to it, learn from their experiences, and be moved by their honesty and straight talk.

I ask you, too, to be honest and consider how your daily decisions affect your health. Become aware of your lifestyle habits — healthy or not. The strategies presented in this book will not elevate your health or performance if their practice is regarded as a simple add-on list of recommended healthy habits. On the surface, that may appear to be the case. It is not. Habits are defined as a settled or regular tendency or practice. Tendencies are not strong enough to command the attention of our biology. The strategies within your formula must be hard-wired with a much greater intention and purpose. For that reason, these strategies must become rituals, not merely habits. This distinction is essential.

Defining the 7 Wellness Rituals as "rituals" links their consistent practice to your everyday thoughts, activities, and behaviors. Bring this level of commitment to your journey, and you will enjoy greater health, happiness, and performance.

Humans do not have a "best-before date." Your body has tremendous potential to heal. Unlock this potential by learning how to take good care of your body, mind, and spirit.

I look forward to supporting you in your journey toward optimal health.

Let's get to work.

Dr. Dwight Chapin

Having worked closely with professionals who have successfully converted their casual awareness of healthy habits into **hard-wired, strategic Wellness Rituals**, I know what the human body is capable of when healthy choices are stacked together. I needed to share these stories and **show people the power of their healing potential.**

MENTOR PROFILES

JIM TRELIVING
CLAUDETTE MCGOWAN
JIM LEECH

This was **the first shot across the bow**. Jim was in his early forties and realized **his formula for success would kill him** if he did not make some serious changes. "At the time, I was pushing the limits really, really hard...Going hard is what I did. It was easy for me." **Hitting the wall surprised him.** "I was having so much fun and just got caught up in it..."

JIM TRELIVING

Boston Pizza Co-owner and Dragons' Den Investor

As far as Canadian entrepreneurs go, Jim Treliving is a legend. His story is one of hard work, integrity, sacrifice, and profound, well-earned respect for the importance he ascribes to a healthy lifestyle. In his presence, you feel protected. His eyes and smile are kind. His wisdom and insight have the heft of a seasoned professional. He is a master storyteller who is generous with his time and advice. I witnessed his unique talent firsthand as I joined him virtually at his vacation home in Hawaii a few months before his eightieth birthday.

As chairman and owner of Boston Pizza International (BPI), he has been the man behind the successful restaurant brand for over fifty years. Under his exceptional leadership, his company has been recognized as a member of Canada's 50 Best Managed Companies Platinum Club and Canada's 10 Most Admired Corporate Cultures. It has also won the Henry Singer Award from the Canadian Institute of Retailing and Services and the Canadian Franchise Association's Lifetime Achievement Award. Despite this success, his role as a TV personality on CBC's *Dragons' Den* is likely what he is most widely recognized for. The reality television show features budding entrepreneurs pitching their business ideas to a panel of venture capitalists. Jim is one of the investor "dragons" and true to form, is known as the "nice dragon."

The "nice dragon" is highly regarded for his moral compass. Growing up in the small town of Virden, Manitoba, Jim's parents ran a tight ship. His father was the provider. His mother ruled the roost. Jim's world as a young boy had little gray area. There was right, and there was wrong. He vividly remembers a day at age fifteen when his behavior fell short of what was expected in the presence of his mother. His father marched him to the basement where he made it clear that he was to honor his mother above all else, without exception. Jim shares, "My dad looked me in the eye and said, 'I don't care if it is the middle of July. If your mother says it is snowing, you better not second guess with a peek out the window. You better go grab a shovel. Do I make myself clear?'" Jim apologized to his mother and the day was forever etched in his memory.

A STOP FOR LUNCH REVEALS A PASSION

Jim left home at eighteen to begin his career as a Royal Canadian Mounted Police (RCMP) Officer. During the punishing eleven-month training regimen, he made friends for life with his troop mates and went on to proudly serve on the force for eight years. Then one day much like any other, a first bite of pizza at Boston Pizza and Spaghetti House in Edmonton, Alberta, opened his eyes to opportunity.

Walking away from his established and well-respected career as an RCMP officer, he jumped into the pizza business. He bought a franchise for Penticton, BC, in 1968. Fifteen years later, he and his business partner, George Melville, purchased the entire chain of forty-four restaurants from founder Gus Agioritis. There are now over 400 Boston Pizza locations across Canada, the US, and Mexico. Jim's reach has extended well beyond pizza, with operations in hospitality, food and beverage, manufacturing, and real estate, with annual system-wide sales exceeding $1 billion.

I found it inspiring to listen to Jim speak of the priority he places on health and explain his understanding of the intimate link between health and performance. One of the first questions he asks new executives on his team or business leaders he mentors is who their family doctor is. The practice of prevention has become a topic of particular interest to him, sparking his curiosity in this book.

WINNING AT ALL COSTS HAS A FATAL FLAW

Prioritizing his health did not come easily to Jim. He admits this journey has taken him the better part of fifty years, and he is still learning. It was not until Jim had pushed himself to complete exhaustion and his body quit on him that the power of lifestyle choices came into clear focus.

Jim shared, "I went into RCMP police training at 200 pounds and graduated weighing 185, as solid as concrete." At six-foot-four, he was a physical specimen, which earned him the nickname "Big." His strength was impressive, and Jim's confidence in his health and constitution fueled his pace long after he had left the police force. He never gave the long hours he worked or the neglect of his diet much thought.

Of course, it is a different time now. In the 1980s, leaders were not encouraged to pursue personal growth and development in the ways they are today. The very idea of strategically developing a personal formula to support health, performance, and happiness when he started in business would have been as far-fetched as a business proposal featuring a young Canadian police officer with zero experience in the restaurant industry partnering with a Greek friend to sell Italian food in a small town in Western Canada. For all the *Dragons' Den* fans, you should know that when Jim approached his father with this very idea and asked for some financial assistance, his father told him that he didn't need a loan — he needed a psychiatrist.

Given the opportunity to travel back to 1976 and ask a thirty-five-year-old Jim about his rituals and approach to business and life success, I am guessing the conversation would have been very short. If you were even lucky enough to get Jim to agree to sit down to have this conversation in the first place, he likely would have told you two things: work hard and love your work. The restaurant business rewards those willing to work long hours at a frantic pace. It has zero patience or compassion for those who do not. Jim, not one to shy away from hard work, took to these rules of engagement. They suited him, and he quickly realized that success was granted to those who could and would outwork the business down the street. He saw sleep as a waste of time or a luxury that he could get by with very little of as a young man.

SELF-CARE REFLECTION #1

The restaurant business has one set of rules of engagement. How do the rules of engagement for your work align with the priorities you have set for your health and well-being? Please record your response to this question in the downloadable journal available at **7WellnessRituals.com** that accompanies this book. The journal has been designed to help you record and track your responses to the self-care exercises presented throughout the book.

Jim pressed hard for seven days a week. After a full week at his restaurant in Penticton, he would jump in his car and drive nine hours north to Prince George to work weekends at another restaurant. On Friday and Saturday nights, he would close the restaurant at 2 a.m. or later. On Sunday nights, he'd drive back to Penticton to rinse and repeat.

A formula that honored hard work above all else was cast. This idea was not new to Jim.

Hard work was the model his father presented as the way a man provided for his family. His father, the town barber, worked twelve-hour days six days a week and never showed a crack in his armor. It was also the model drilled into him during his RCMP training and eight years policing the streets. When applied against the satisfaction of an honest day's work, the formula further motivated Jim, and his days got even longer. At one point, one of Jim's former police buddies asked him, "Hey Big, what are you trying to do, be the richest guy in the graveyard? Come on out and play some golf with us and have some fun."

Eventually, Jim's body could no longer keep pace. His formula was built to support a sprint, not a marathon. The belief that he could set and sustain a pace that others could not compete with was initially rewarded with opportunity, growth, and success.

This set a trap that many entrepreneurs fall into. Hidden from the unaware, hardworking, and driven entrepreneur lies a fatal flaw in the *work-hard-at-all-costs* formula for success.

SELF-CARE REFLECTION #2

Think back to the last time you worked yourself to exhaustion. Besides fatigue, did you notice how your performance started to fall off? Learning to recognize how your physiology changes as your body responds to stress is an essential skill. Stress is a necessary ingredient for peak performance. However, prolonged exposure will lead to a decline in health and performance. In your journal, describe the following:

- ▸ How do you feel when you have pushed past the point of exhaustion? List your symptoms.
- ▸ How is your sleep quality and sleep duration impacted?
- ▸ How is your mental state and experience of physical pain affected when you are tired?
- ▸ Begin to recognize how your body feels, thinks and moves when you are in the zone and at your peak compared to when you are spent. Record your reflections in your journal.

INDIFFERENCE IS A RECIPE FOR POOR HEALTH

Turning a blind eye to his lifestyle choices, Jim had allowed his chiseled frame to become soft. "I never gave my weight much thought. I just kept buying bigger clothes." Any feelings of fatigue or drag on his endurance lead Jim to push harder.

> ❝ **I was go, go, go — until I just couldn't go anymore."**

Many business leaders caught in a sprint discover the flaw in their formula just as their first summit comes into view. This was Jim's experience. His restaurants were thriving, new locations were opening, and his hard work was paying off. He admits, "I was go, go, go — until I just couldn't go anymore."

He woke up one day and did not have the strength to get out of bed. He struggled to get to the shower, hoping to find his typical morning energy there. With a long list of essential tasks to attend to, he was already running behind. Getting out of the shower, he toweled off and labored to get dressed. Within five minutes, he was once again soaking wet, having completely sweat through his clothes. At his wife's insistence, he returned to bed, and she called his doctor, who immediately came over to the house. Jim was diagnosed with double pneumonia, told to stay in bed for the next five days and informed that he should not expect to return to work for about a month. The doctor told him, "I'm going to give you a medication cocktail that will put you on a trip like you have never been on before." Four days later, Jim woke up, and his fever had broken.

This was the first shot across the bow. Jim was in his early forties and realized his formula for success would kill him if he did not make some serious changes. "At the time, I was pushing the limits really, really hard. I had this confidence that I was this big, strong guy. It had carried over from my RCMP days. Going hard is what I did. It was easy for me." He acknowledged that he was working long hours, but compared to the demands of police work, the restaurant business was fun. Hitting the wall surprised him. "I honestly didn't realize that I was going too fast. I was having so much fun and just got caught up in it. Sure there were days I was tired, but I kept pushing the time to catch up down the road."

The very idea that he might be vulnerable did not sit well with him. But his body had hijacked his attention, giving him no option but to rest. It would be a few weeks before he felt strong enough to attempt a full reentry.

While this experience forced Jim to slow down, it would still be a few years before his formula would evolve beyond the "work hard" and "love your work" framework to what it is today. With his weight up to 275 pounds, he found himself back in his doctor's office with severe back and hip pain. After some clinical uncertainty, the suspicion of a young intern that he may be suffering from gout was confirmed by blood work. Jim had developed the habit of taking a couple of swigs of concentrated pop syrup without any carbonated water multiple times a day. The shot gave him an edge in exchange for uric acid levels that were off the charts. The habit was also contributing to his weight gain. Cutting pop from his diet resulted in a complete resolution of his joint pain, and in short order, he dropped close to thirty pounds. At the recommendation of a good friend, he joined Weight Watchers® and got his weight back down to 225 pounds, where it has been since.

JIM'S FORMULA FOR HEALTH, STRENGTH & HOPE

PLAY A NEW GAME

Jim's energy began returning. He developed a respect for sleep and recovery, had tweaked his diet and gotten his weight back down, and was exercising daily. Jim channeled this energy into his work. What he was missing was finding time for play. He finally clued in when a friend and police officer pleaded with him to come out for a round of golf and kick back with some friends. Jim grew up playing football and hockey, so the idea of chasing a little white ball around a field did not hold much appeal — at least not initially. By the third hole of his first round, the game had a firm grip on him.

Golf has since become a treasured pastime for Jim. He loves the challenge the game presents, the time spent walking the course outdoors, and the camaraderie found on the tee box and in the clubhouse. Learning to golf at age forty-seven was not easy, but Jim was not about to let a simple thing like age slow him down. With work and practice, his handicap has dropped from thirty-two to eight. He has golfed at many of the top courses the world has to offer and plays in a couple of Pro-AM tournaments every year. Golf brings him joy and has helped him prioritize fun. He attends the Masters tournament every year and has Augusta committed to memory. It is his favorite course. Playing it, which he has done three times, is the ultimate reward for hard work.

"SHOW TIME"

His restaurant chain's success requires more than attentive service, good food, and well-run kitchens. Jim shares, "You have to create an atmosphere, a sense of community." He calls it "show time": "You are putting on a show. I want franchisees to provide for their guests as they would if they were serving them in their own home."

This business truth parallels Jim's journey with his own health, performance, and happiness. The attention he pays to every detail of a customer's dining experience is equivalent to the attention he now applies to his health and success. It's his personal "show time." It took Jim a while to figure it out, but he got there. Working harder and longer would have only capped his impact or cut his life short.

> **I've had to adapt my approach over the years, respect sleep, add in more time for social fun, and watch my daily choices."**

Jim exemplifies the practice of the 7 Wellness Rituals in this book. With the intentional discipline he developed as a youth, he has established accountability with his family's love and support and under the watchful eye of his doctor. He lives and enjoys a full and active life in great health in his eighties.

"You have to love change or learn to love it, to be successful in both business and in health. I've learned that life can get too serious sometimes. I've had to adapt my approach over the years, respect sleep, add in more time for social fun, and watch my daily choices. I hope I can help others get there sooner than I did. I feel great, but once you are in your eighties, every day is a great day."

CLAUDETTE McGOWAN

CEO of Protexxa and Former Global Executive Officer for Cyber Security at TD Bank

*C*laudette McGowan has lived and continues to live an extraordinary life. She is a mother, wife, author, technologist, global cybersecurity executive officer, corporate board member, podcast host, and robot maker. Capable of bending time to her advantage, she has learned how to stretch the potential of a day with energy to spare.

Among her honors is her recognition by the Women's Executive Network as one of the 100 Most Powerful Women in Canada. She is a member of Canada's Task Force on Women in the Economy, and as chair of the Coalition of Innovation Leaders Against Racism (CILAR), she leads a diverse group of senior leaders committed to a) creating new pathways for Black people, Indigenous peoples, and people of color, and b) ending systemic racism within the innovation economy. The United Nations recently invited her to lead a discussion on her passion — digital literacy. She leads with confidence and humility, and the world is drawn to her insight.

When Michelle Obama arrived in Toronto in the fall of 2019 to promote her book *Becoming*, Claudette was at center stage with the former First Lady, guiding a candid conversation about their life experiences and the importance of being a change-maker in today's world.

Claudette's authenticity, kind heart, and sharp intellect matched Michelle's. Reviewers called it one of the best interviews of the tour and marveled at the chemistry shared by the two leading women. To those in Claudette's inner circle, this was no surprise; Claudette was just being Claudette. To everyone else in attendance, this was their introduction to a superb role model.

NEW IDEAS AND WELL-LOVED ROUTINES

Claudette knows her lane, and any deviations from it are strategic and intentional. Her confidence is forged by discipline and preparation. She thinks, moves, and influences with unwavering positivity. Her curiosity is rewarded by a voracious consumption of information. As a young girl, her father would tell her, "Reading is the key to knowledge." Early in her career, she would consume a book a day on her commute to work by train. She enjoys the daily practice of challenging her thinking by reading and listening to podcasts on a wide variety of subjects. She told me, "At any one time, I'm probably surrounded by over seventy books."

With over eighteen years of success leading digital transformations and optimizing infrastructure, Claudette is currently the CEO of Protexxa and former Global Executive Officer for Cyber Security at TD Bank. "I've been in operations basically my whole career. Running a 24/7 shop, supporting critical operations, like banking systems behind ATMs, to my cybersecurity focus with TD Bank." If things went sideways digitally, Claudette was the one to lead the bank's response. Helping the world elevate its cybersecurity is one of her top priorities.

To live and deliver at the high standard Claudette has set for her life, she has forged a formula that leaves nothing to chance. She understands the influence her decisions carry and gives every one careful consideration. Open to new ideas, she is also a creature of habit — habits that have proven their worth have become rituals and are now locked down on autopilot, at least until a worthy upgrade is discovered. As we unpacked her day-to-day routine, her level of self-awareness immediately stood out as unique. She knows what makes her happy and keeps these sources close. She has developed a sixth sense for the finely-honed inner workings of home and work without losing sight of her needs. The question on the minds of those who have seen her in action is, how does she do it? How does she find the time to skillfully juggle the significant demands of her corporate jobs with the busy athletic and academic schedules of her two children and still have time to chair boards, write children's books, tackle racism, and join Canada's deputy prime minister and minister of finance's economic advisory committee?

Her secret lies in how she has turned time into an ally.

SELF-CARE REFLECTION #3

Please reflect on these questions and make notes in your journal:
- ▸ Is time an ally or are you constantly chasing the clock?
- ▸ How did you practice self-care this week?
- ▸ Where does self-care fit into your schedule?

FINDING A SUSTAINABLE PACE

Claudette does not chase the clock. With the assistance of her EA, her calendar operates like a finely tuned instrument. In tandem, they adapt quickly if a crisis demands her immediate attention. "The day changes shape quickly. At the bank, I would move from an all-hands team meeting with more than 700 employees on the call, to a regulatory meeting, and then to a smaller, high-level cybersecurity discussion or talent management discussion in a day. I have to be able to pivot on the fly." To stay sharp, she no longer pretends she can get by on only three to four hours of rest a night. She said she learned this lesson the hard way. "Early in my career, I was one of those people that went super hard all the time."

> ❝ **With the helpful encouragement from close friends and some of my own research, I realized my pace was not sustainable and have since developed a respect for rest."**

Claudette's mother was a gifted and giving nurse. Like her mom, Claudette immediately built a reputation as someone who would show up and get the job done. But she came to a realization, "With the helpful encouragement from close friends and some of my own research, I realized my pace was not sustainable and have since developed a respect for rest."

She now locks in six to seven hours of sleep a night, in bed by 11 to 11:30 p.m. and up by 6 a.m. A sleep story on the Calm App gently completes her end-of-day wind down as her head hits the pillow. She rarely hears the end of a story. There is no alarm clock on her bedside table. She wakes on cue, ready to go.

The remaining seventeen to eighteen hours in her day bend to her formula. She creates pockets of time to sufficiently support her priorities, allowing for adequate preparation and a meaningful investment in self-care.

For starters at TD, Claudette experimented with a four-day work week. Barring a critical system outage, Mondays were hers. "If there was an outage or my boss needed me, he would call; otherwise, he was super respectful of this time and was happy I took Mondays and wanted me to enjoy it. It's in the DNA of TD Bank to make sure people have balance and wellness in their life. A three-day weekend every week was very empowering. It energized me and allowed me to be intentional about how I spent my time." Her Mondays may include writing, reading, preparing for the week ahead, or just being ever-present for her kids. What is important is that the time was hers to use as she saw fit.

Tuesday to Friday mornings generally allow for an hour of quiet time before she launches into her calendar. Once the day kicks into gear, it plays out at an intense pace. At the end of each workday, she deliberately pushes pause and completes a daily retrospective review with her executive assistant. They discuss how the day went, what tomorrow looks like, and any final preparations required for upcoming events. This relationship and exchange is essential to Claudette's success and time management. "I spend a fair bit of my time speaking with regulators, and these conversations require a thoughtful approach." Whether she is working from home or in her downtown office, she strives to turn her attention to her family by 7 p.m. This creates another four-hour window each day to connect with her family, exercise, and uncoil daily stressors. In addition, the importance of protecting her schedule and honoring the time she sets aside for herself has grown as her influence has expanded. She has learned to say no.

The McGowan family life also moves at a quick pace. Claudette is passionate about her work but is a mother first. The health and well-being of her children are her north star. Having healthy meals prepared for the family buys her additional quality time with her family, which she treasures.

CLAUDETTE'S FORMULA FOR HEALTH, STRENGTH & HOPE

When it comes to food, Claudette likes what she likes and sticks with it. Her mom, as a dedicated healthcare worker, advocated for healthy eating. For breakfast, she rocks a protein shake. She is not a coffee drinker. Lunch is often avocado toast or a grilled chicken or salmon salad, and dinner consists of lean protein accompanied by fresh vegetables. Given a choice, she would choose crispy, savory snacks over sweets. Despite her family's love for ice cream, she does not have a sweet tooth and is just as happy without dessert.

For exercise, Claudette hops on her recumbent bike for twenty-minute power cycles. Having a bike in the home and not traveling to the gym creates additional time in her day. On days she feels her energy flagging, she will opt for a session of yoga or meditation instead of a ride or resistance training.

She says, "Physical activity was a huge part of my life growing up. Before having kids, I'd be at the gym training hard several times a week." Parenthood challenged this ritual. Falling out of her fitness routine as a new mom was difficult. She craved exercise, felt depleted without it, and struggled with weight management. As her kids got a little older, she reclaimed the time needed to return to regular physical activity. She drew inspiration from her father, a professional boxer. Her brother is a tennis coach. Her husband played varsity basketball, coached competitively, and now plays ultimate frisbee for fun. Both of her children play rep-level sports. She likes the way exercise makes her feel; she likes to sweat and is motivated by the satisfaction of completing a physical challenge. Keen to keep her workouts interesting, challenging, and age-appropriate, her focus has turned to dynamic movement, strength training, and flexibility. While not an outdoors person, Claudette was convinced by some close friends to join them on hikes during the pandemic, she went begrudgingly but now admits to enjoying the experience.

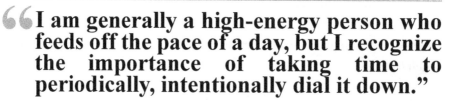

I am generally a high-energy person who feeds off the pace of a day, but I recognize the importance of taking time to periodically, intentionally dial it down."

If the hours or intensity of a day leave her feeling spread thin, her self-awareness sharpens. In contrast, many leaders lose energy and focus to stress, especially when stress becomes chronic. The investment Claudette made in her post-stress recovery has given her the ability to navigate chaos and prevent physiological decline. "I get quiet when things get noisy." In the eye of a storm, Claudette begins pruning all non-essential demands pulling at her attention. Asking her inner circle for feedback and assistance helps her complete this task. She has a small group of close friends, trusted colleagues, and a large family to turn to for perspective, love, and support and is never shy of asking for help.

Claudette explains, "I am generally a high-energy person who feeds off the pace of a day, but I recognize the importance of taking time to periodically, intentionally dial it down. I'll take time on weekends but also schedule time to slow down mid-week with a ninety-minute massage every Wednesday."

Much like her cycling workouts and four-day work weeks, the treatment provides another powerful boost to her ability to deliver. "The massage gives me a mid-week reset."

SELF-CARE REFLECTION #4

Claudette places tremendous value on her time and works hard to structure her week around self-care. Proactive scheduling is one of her tricks. Most of us, even those with the best intentions, approach self-care in the opposite direction and look for holes to squeeze it into. This habit marks self-care as a second-tier priority. It is tempting to look at Claudette's formula and say, "Well, if I could work a four-day week, afford help on the home front, and get a weekly massage, I'd have time for self-care too." But Claudette didn't build a big life and then decide to prioritize self-care. Her commitment to this discipline came first. How can you develop practices to take better care? This book will help you do so, and ensuring adequate time for sleep is an excellent place to start.

AGEISM, RACISM, AND DIVERSITY AS STRENGTH

I was curious about how Claudette remains so steady and self-possessed in a male-dominated industry where she started her career as the youngest in the room, the only female in the room, and the only person of color in the room. One of the reasons she provided is that she enters every room prepared, confident, and positive. She believes in being kind to herself and to others.

She is no stranger to adversity. A scar on her lip reminds her daily of the schoolyard bully who pushed her to the ground because of the color of her skin. Multiple failed pregnancies remind her of the value of life and keep her present in parenthood. "As a young girl, the realization that someone who didn't even know me would want to hurt me because he didn't like Black people was difficult to accept."

At points throughout her career, people have made comments about the color of her skin. "I am not naïve to this perspective, but it is still surprising when and where it reveals itself. Because of the way we are in Canada, racism is not always overt. Truthfully, ageism, more so than racism, has been a hurdle I've had to clear in my career. I believe that sharing stories, humanizing experiences, and being honest about questions and concerns all help bring the world one step closer to where we want to be."

She has shared the story of the schoolyard bully with her daughter. She wants her kids to work hard and experience joy but does not want them to feel as though they are less-than, especially in today's world that rewards creativity and initiative. "I grew up hearing that I was going to have to work twice as hard to have half as much as everyone else. I would never say this to my kids; in fact, I don't believe it to be true. I think if you keep telling yourself something, the more likely it is to become your reality." Her children are learning to see their diversity as their strength.

PLAY, PURPOSE, AND THE CREATIVE FORCE

When it comes to play, Claudette finds enjoyment in helping to make cyber digital security digestible to the world. In this sandbox, she plays alone. On occasion, she indulges in a guilty-pleasure podcast or some frivolous fiction but never strays too far from her calling to help elevate cyber literacy. "I know how compromised people are, and the world is oblivious to it, and it frustrates me. Helping people become more aware and change online behaviors is very rewarding." Her podcast titled *C Suite*, which launched in early 2021, is dedicated to this passion. She tackles topics like demystifying the Dark Web, cyberbullying, online security, ransomware, robocalls, and email hacks. The podcast's sizable following is evidence of the content value she offers. In 2023, she will launch a new podcast branded *Conexus* with a focus on cyber challenges with the fourteen billion Internet of Things (IoT) devices currently connected to the Internet.

Switching gears, writing also gives her creativity an outlet. Her most recent publication titled *Triple Threat* is a children's book about the power of perseverance. She currently has seven books at different stages of completion in the works, with some ready for print and others still in the outline stage. Yes, Claudette McGowan, the children's author, is also Claudette McGowan, the cybersecurity expert.

Once awarded with success and a high level of recognition for her efforts, she is quick to move on. The challenge around the next corner holds greater appeal than any celebration for a job well done ever could. Her neurons are wired to solve complex problems on multiple fronts. In pursuit of additional summits, she keeps her formula in full view. Recently, Claudette completed a leadership course designed to help leaders define their unique purpose. "After three months of training and surveys, my purpose was revealed. I was to help people. It made me laugh because I started my career in technology on the help desk." Ever efficient, it was no surprise to learn that Claudette was on the correct path from the very beginning.

JIM LEECH

Chancellor Emeritus, Queen's University and Former President of the Ontario Teachers' Pension Plan

*I*n the spring of 2014, Jim Leech was a member of Canada's largest expedition to ski to the magnetic North Pole. The purpose of the expedition was to raise awareness and money for Canadian veterans suffering from post-traumatic stress disorder (PTSD).

With fifty-three members on the team, the trip still stands as the largest expedition ever mounted north of the Arctic Circle. Jim recounts, "There were twelve ill and injured soldiers, all with PTSD at various stages. The goalie and the captain of the Canadian women's Olympic gold-medal-winning hockey team from Sochi — Carolyn Ouellette and Geneviève Lacasse — were there, as well as a journalist and eight guides. The rest were crazy businesspeople."

The flight from Resolute Bay to King Christian Island was 250 km. From there, the group skied 100 km to reach the magnetic North Pole. The expedition raised $2.1 million, which helped fund five critical programs supporting servicemen and women, veterans, and their families. At the finish line was a mountain of snow constructed by Canadian Rangers who planted a Canadian flag as a symbol of hope and renewal for everyone on the team. All on the expedition had formed meaningful relationships and completed the final stretch in tears, singing the Canadian national anthem in English and French in a continuous loop.

Reaching the flag was one of the greatest moments of Jim's life.

The ground surrounding the Canadian flag at the finish line became sacred as the soldiers placed mementos from tours of duty that they had brought with them on the expedition at the base of it. In celebration of his physical accomplishment, the accomplishment of his crew members, and the answers he found along the way, Jim opened his pack and pulled out a Santa costume. He put the costume on and took pictures to show his grandkids that he met Santa Claus at the North Pole.

To tackle something like this at 68 when your day job has you behind a desk is bold. Jim enjoys adventure travel, but this trip was a notch or two above hiking the Skyline Trail in Nova Scotia or the West Coast Trail in British Columbia. I asked Jim to help me understand his motivation. "It was a transition period in my life, as I was preparing to leave Ontario Teachers'. The expedition gave me time to get clear on what I wanted to do next. I also wanted to prove to myself that I could still do something physical like this."

At the time, there was considerable pressure on Jim to join several boards as he walked away from Ontario Teachers'. By agreeing to join the expedition, he felt the freedom to tell all of his suitors, "Come see me in five months. Right now, I'm focusing on trying to stay alive on this trip."

A LIFE OF SERVICE

Jim retired in 2014 as president and CEO of the Ontario Teachers' Pension Plan (Ontario Teachers'). The plan is one of the largest and most innovative pension funds in the world. Protecting the retirement security of over 331,000 working and retired teachers, the fund's net assets were over $220 billion at the end of 2020. During Jim's tenure as CEO, Ontario Teachers' eliminated its funding deficit and was ranked first in the world amongst peer plans for absolute returns over five and ten years, value-added returns over five and ten years, and service to members.[1]

Before he was appointed CEO, Jim led Ontario Teachers' Private Capital, the pension plan's private investment division, where he oversaw the growth in private equity, venture capital, and infrastructure investments from $2 billion in 2001 to over $20 billion by 2007.[2] Upon his retirement, he was invested as a Member of the Order of Canada for his contributions as an innovator and author in pension management and for his community involvement.

In 2013, he co-authored *The Third Rail: Confronting Our Pension Failures*, a best-selling book that received the 2013–2014 Best Canadian Business Book Award. Shortly thereafter, he was awarded the Queen's Diamond Jubilee Medal in recognition of his work with True Patriot Love Foundation, an organization dedicated to inspiring every Canadian to contribute to the resilience and well-being of the Canadian military, veterans, and their families.

He is currently a Board Member (previous Board Chair) of the MasterCard Foundation, a foundation committed to advancing learning and promoting financial inclusion for people living in poverty. He also serves as an honorary colonel in the Canadian Armed Forces, and was the Chancellor of Queen's University from 2014 to 2021.

In short, his long list of accomplishments reads like the life story of a fictional hero. In person, he is every bit as impressive and lives up to his reputation. A proud husband, father of three, and grandfather of seven, he is a disciplined man of action and principle who places family above all else. His A-game is played at the next level. Time with Jim leaves you with a greater appreciation for the present moment, a desire to give back, and a craving to squeeze a little more out of each day.

SLEEP DISCIPLINE AND PERFORMANCE

Jim has always maintained an acute awareness of the link between sleep and performance. Even during stretches where he was sprinting toward a deadline and may have been averaging only five hours a night, he never lost track of why he prioritized sleep.

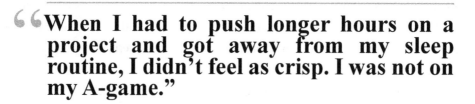

66**When I had to push longer hours on a project and got away from my sleep routine, I didn't feel as crisp. I was not on my A-game."**

Fatigue's drag on his performance did not go unnoticed. Any longer than two weeks away from his sleep ritual would come at a cost that Jim recognized and would not tolerate. "When I had to push longer hours on a project and got away from my sleep routine, I didn't feel as crisp. I was not on my A-game."

Throughout Jim's career, he frequently used the expression "come to play your A-game" with his staff. He held himself to the same standard and made a conscious effort to bring the best version of himself to work every day.

Jim's father, George Leech, was a brigadier-general in the Canadian Armed Forces. His uncle, Lieutenant-General Don Laubman, was also a career officer. Given his military upbringing, I was not surprised to discover Jim's comfort with routine. As a young boy, there was a structure to his day that started with a good night's sleep. "I have always been a good sleeper and have really benefited from not having any trouble sleeping in my life. I consistently have got eight to eight and a half hours my entire career."

In retirement, his day now starts to wind down sometime after 10 p.m. Typically in bed by 10:45 p.m., he will read until 11:30 p.m. and then quickly fall asleep. He is up and at it by 7:30 a.m., rarely needing the assistance of an alarm clock. At the peak of his career, his day would usually start closer to 6 a.m. to allow for a morning workout between 7 and 8 a.m. before heading off to work. On weekends, he may steal an extra thirty to forty-five minutes in bed, but otherwise, his sleep and exercise rituals are locked in. The priority he places on sleep and his physical health appear to be rooted in lessons learned at a young age that continue to serve him well.

"There were stretches in my life where this sleep schedule was not always possible given work demands or travel, but I can only think of a couple of times in my career when I had any trouble with sleep." He shared that there was a two-month stretch in the middle of his career when a business challenge started disrupting his sleep ritual in a new and profound way. For the first time, sleep was hard to come by for Jim, and he could feel the impact. He would lay down ready to sleep, his body fatigued, but his mind would fight the transition and could not be silenced. Turning to a mentor for help, they offered, "You have a dog, don't you? Go and walk the dog from 10:30 to 11 p.m. every night, and then go straight to bed." Jim gave it a try, and it worked like a charm. The walk presented him with a physical cleanse and a mental distraction. It was a simple solution that provided the necessary reset of his sleep cycle.

SELF-CARE REFLECTION #5

Please reflect on these questions and record your answers in your journal:

- ▸ Do you have a formal sleep routine?
- ▸ How do you unwind at the end of the day?

SELF-DISCIPLINE — THE KEY TO RESILIENCE AND LONGEVITY

Holding a position of authority at work from a young age provided Jim with a degree of freedom to set his schedule. He shared that he would actually get up from meetings at 5 p.m. and say, "Sorry, I've got to be on the ice in forty-five minutes," and leave to go coach his son's hockey team."

Jim never missed a game. He would take work home if necessary, but he avoided going into the office on weekends. "Even though I had the responsibility of CEO, I lived a very disciplined life with respect to my family."

Jim's father modeled this discipline. Despite his dad's high-ranking military position, he never missed one of Jim's childhood hockey games either. Jim recalls, "I was organizing a big social community event at our high school in Edmonton, and my dad showed up in his uniform, having left a formal work function to be there." His father's presence that day had a direct impact on the man Jim wanted to become. George held a strong belief in the importance of self-discipline that his son now models. "Growing up in a military family, you would think my home was horribly strict, but actually, my parents were quite liberal in that sense. They threw responsibility on us at an early age."

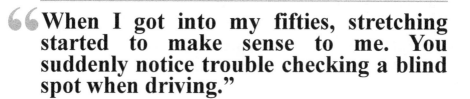

When I got into my fifties, stretching started to make sense to me. You suddenly notice trouble checking a blind spot when driving."

In studying Jim's life, it is clear that he believes in putting in the work. The man does not cut corners. "I was always at my best if I exercised first thing in the morning." Leaving the office, changing, working up a sweat, and then trying to cool down after a midday workout held zero appeal. Jim enjoyed the practice of investing in his health with a morning workout as his first meaningful action of the day. He would meet with a personal trainer and keep his mind on the workout before turning his attention to his professional responsibilities. Jim's trainer helped him stay one step ahead of the influence of aging by bringing a greater focus to the importance of maintaining functional range of motion and flexibility.

As a former rugby player in his days at the Royal Military College of Canada, Jim never developed much love for stretching. "When I got into my fifties, stretching started to make sense to me. You suddenly notice trouble checking a blind spot when driving."

On his fiftieth birthday, he had an appointment to see his family doctor and take his car in for maintenance. The reality of aging hit him square in the chest when he realized that the list of things wrong with his body was longer than the list of things wrong with his car. "It was then that I realized I needed to make a few changes and committed to working on my flexibility."

Rehabbing three significant surgeries and recovering from a skiing injury, all within the last decade, drove home Jim's appreciation for his mobility even further. With operations on his ankle and lower back, hip replacement surgery, and rehabilitation to restore the range of motion in his shoulder following a significant clavicular fracture, he developed tremendous respect for the body's healing potential. He also formed a strong bond with his physiotherapist and surgical team.

Two months prior to their departure to the North Pole, the crew members completed a full health examination to assess their physical ability to meet the trip's demands. Jim cleared this hurdle. However, as one of the older members on the crew, the trip was not without risk. With the guidance of his trainer, time to prepare, and an appetite for adventure, Jim agreed to go. His training program was designed to maximize his flexibility and balance. "With sixty pounds on your back and pulling another ninety pounds behind you while on skis all day, if you fall over, you need to have the strength to get up." The guides familiar with the route made sure Jim understood that the falls toward the end of the day, as fatigue settles in, can be dangerous. To mitigate the risk, the primary focus of Jim's training was fall prevention. "One of the best exercises they gave us is to stand with my feet lined up heel to toe — one foot directly in front of the other. I still practice this today when standing at cocktail parties." NOTE: You will find a video demonstrating this exercise at **7WellnessRituals.com**.

JIM'S FORMULA FOR HEALTH, STRENGTH & HOPE

Jim's mother prepared the family meals. Everything was homemade, simple, and healthy. After leaving home, Jim kept to those habits. He recalls attending a corporate dinner in his twenties where he found himself seated next to the CEO of a major global bank. The executive was German, all business, and had the physical presence of Michelangelo's *David*. Jim remembers asking him about his eating habits on the road as an executive. He shared with Jim that his secret was to eat only half of what was served. He would cut every meal in half and set the untouched food aside. The importance of portion control stuck with Jim. Whenever eating on the go, he is mindful and appreciative of this exchange. Ten years ago, Jim turned to a vegan diet to regulate his cholesterol levels. At sixty-five, his family doctor wanted to see his total cholesterol under 2.0 mmol/L. Under the direction of his daughter, a naturopathic doctor, he set out to drop his levels by 10% before agreeing to commit to a statin medication. His daughter informed him that a drop of this magnitude was within reach if he was willing to make changes to his food choices, including letting go of his love for BBQ steaks. Within weeks, his cholesterol dropped to 1.8 mmol/L.

Given the success of this lifestyle modification, he stuck with it and has grown to enjoy eating vegan. On occasion, he will still have white fish or a chicken breast when a vegetarian option is not available. He reports that there has been no appreciable decrease in his strength or energy levels and that his weight initially dropped from 200 to 192 pounds, where it has since stabilized. In support of his general health, he also takes the following: vitamin D, omega-3 fish oil, magnesium, resveratrol, coenzyme Q10, and garlic. After his seventieth birthday, he started a low dose of statin for added protection. Jim told me that his favorite time of day was the subway ride into work. The ride was twenty-five minutes on the nose. For twenty-five minutes, he could melt into the crowd of commuters. He found the anonymity therapeutic and comforting. He arrived at work ready to play the A-game.

As our discussion came to an end, he offered, "The only real risk is not knowing you are taking a risk. Do your homework, understand the risk, evaluate the cost of the decision, and then make a move." Jim Leech is an extraordinary Canadian. If countries had an all-star team of nonpartisan advisors made up of their most impactful citizens, the best of the best, and this team was charged with providing their nation with innovative leadership, sage guidance, and a moral compass, Jim would make an excellent team captain for Canada.

SELF-CARE REFLECTION #6

Skiing to the magnetic North Pole may seem like an unattainable achievement for you, but consider setting a stretch goal for yourself to complete within the next twelve months. Record your response in your journal.

PRIORITIZE SLEEP, REST, & RECOVERY

7 WELLNESS RITUALS
FOR HEALTH, STRENGTH & HOPE

WELLNESS RITUAL #1: THE SCIENCE

Pre-pandemic, many lived in a frantic state of "busy-ness" with their monster list of "to-dos" ruling the roost. But it is easy to mistake being busy for being productive. Sacrificing sleep, rest, and recovery in an effort to get more out of a day is a dangerous habit. So is accepting poor sleep quality and moving through the day exhausted. When you consistently deprive yourself of sleep, you jeopardize the health of your entire body and the quality of your performance in all areas of life.

*H*umans are brilliantly complex organisms made up of trillions of cells, each with a unique design and purpose. To define this complexity, scientists continue to debate the exact cell count. Current estimates predict it to be somewhere north of thirty-seven trillion.[1] The lifespan of a cell varies significantly, some lasting days, others months, while neurons in our brain can last a lifetime. Each cell contains a biological power in the form of a genetic blueprint that directs a remarkable, altruistic balance with neighboring cells. The efficient execution of this power is a requirement for our survival. It calls on cell-to-cell coordination of data exchange, defense, memory, reproduction, adaptation, and repair that defines what it is to be human and determines our state of health and the quality of our performance. It is a masterful symphony whose execution cannot be left to chance or, even worse, bad habits.

And yet, so many do, starting with the low priority placed on the need for sleep and recovery. Who hasn't consciously cut their pillow time short to prop up longer work hours or force a ruthless to-do list into retreat? We often make the trade — sacrifice sleep to meet that next deadline or prepare for an early morning call. We do this even if we are aware that it's a bad trade with diminishing returns.

As we have evolved, we have developed an ability to dig a little deeper and push in fifth gear a little longer. At our best, we call this "hitting our stride" or "finding our flow" (more on this in Wellness Rituals #6 and #7). However, when we chase peak performance all the time and try to convince ourselves that we can be productive for eighteen or twenty hours out of every twenty-four, our fifth gear will fail. Eventually, our third and fourth gears will fail as well. Let me burst the fantasy bubble that extended days are available to those who train their bodies to operate on less sleep. You cannot get water from a stone. And if you find yourself looking for a shortcut, it doesn't exist. Unhealthy lifestyle choices made to mask fatigue and declining performance only compound the ripple effect of the behavioral causes of sleep deprivation.[2,3]

Escalating levels of stress, unrealistic targets, and unforgiving deadlines are defining our workplace, and the consequences are impacting our work and our family lives. Simply put, sleep is not getting the respect it deserves. To continue to push through life ignoring the irrevocable biological requirement for rest and recovery is akin to expecting Beethoven's Third Symphony — *The Eroica* — to sound equally brilliant with every seventh note removed.

Welcome to Wellness Ritual #1: Prioritize Sleep, Rest & Recovery. To truly examine the impact of poor rest and recovery habits in the light of day, we must turn to the science of sleep for a quick "Sleep 101" crash course. Understanding sleep will help motivate a change in both behavior and mindset surrounding this daily requirement. The twenty-one mentors profiled in this book regard sleep as a precious secret weapon. They do not resent the need to unplug and recharge — they embrace it.

KEY FACTS, TRENDS, AND STATISTICS YOU NEED TO KNOW

Let's start with the elephant in the room. Sleep is an essential biological process. It is as fundamental a need as oxygen, food, and water.

Insufficient sleep is now considered a public health epidemic. A 2013 study published by the Centers for Disease Control and Prevention (CDC) raised a red flag by making this declaration, drawing attention to poor sleep habits and the significant adverse health effects of insufficient sleep.[3] In fact, depriving yourself of adequate rest is now a classified, distinct clinical disorder. It is called Insufficient Sleep Syndrome (ISS) and can be found listed in the third edition of the International Classification of Sleep Disorders (ICSD-3) along with other sleep disorders, including sleep apnea and restless leg syndrome.[4,5]

SLEEP DISORDER DEFINITIONS

Insufficient Sleep Syndrome: This condition occurs when you regularly fail to get enough sleep at night. When you are deprived of sleep, you cannot be mentally alert. You will feel aggravated and irritable because of constant fatigue. You will make choices that prevent you from getting the sleep your body needs. Insufficient sleep syndrome is the most common cause of daytime fatigue.[6]

Sleep Apnea: If you suffer from this disorder, your breathing becomes shallow or may stop altogether for a few seconds or much longer during sleep. There are several types of sleep apnea, but the most common is *obstructive sleep apnea*, which is increasing in prevalence given the rise in obesity.[6] Disrupted breathing is caused by the relaxation of the muscles in the back of the throat, causing the airway to narrow or close. Interestingly, people with sleep apnea may not be aware that their breathing is interrupted. The list of serious complications from this disorder is long and includes severe daytime drowsiness, difficulty concentrating, poor memory, cardiovascular stress, and an irritable, sleep-deprived partner.

Restless Legs Syndrome (RLS): This disorder is characterized by a strong urge to move your legs often because you notice strange or unpleasant sensations: creeping, crawling, pulling, itching, tingling, burning, aching, and even electric shocks. When you move your legs, it relieves the strange sensations. The unpleasant feelings are strongest when you are resting or inactive, and they can make it difficult to fall or stay asleep.[6] Often there is no known cause.

When we are up against a deadline, we seem to have little choice but to cut back on our sleep. But it's a nasty tradeoff. In a thorough review of the scientific studies on insufficient sleep by the National Center for Biotechnology Information (NCBI), a division of the United States National Library of Medicine, an accumulating body of evidence has identified insufficient sleep as the first cause of impairments in physiological functioning, mental and cognitive deficits, and mood or emotional effects.[7] In other words, lack of sleep can cause weight gain, elevated blood pressure, diabetes, and poor mental health.[8] Figure 1.1 provides an overview of the clinical ripple effect of insufficient sleep.

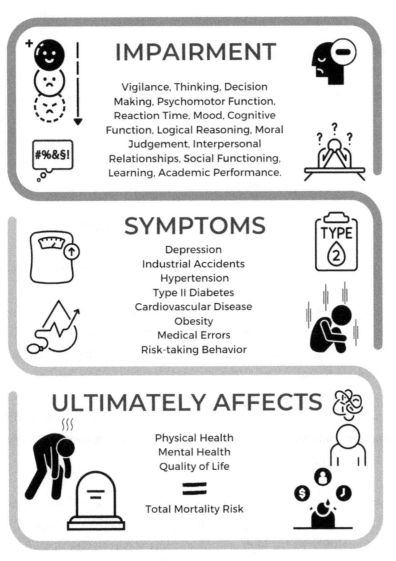

Figure 1.1: Adapted from the National Centre for Biotechnology Information[7]

While this graphic drives the point home, several additional epidemiological studies have revealed that shorter durations of sleep are associated with increased mortality and altered gene expression.[9-12] Translation: depriving yourself of enough sleep can alter how your DNA blueprint plays out or even cut your life short. It is dangerous. If knowing this does not make you want to adjust your bedtime ritual, then I suggest you put this book down, have a nap, and then re-read that last page and a half.

CURRENT TRENDS

Misery loves company. According to a 2017 Statistics Canada health report on the duration and quality of sleep among Canadians aged eighteen to seventy-nine, about one-third sleep fewer hours per night than recommended for optimal physical and mental health.[13] This group also experiences poor sleep quality more frequently than do those who sleep for the recommended number of hours.

Here are some additional important statistics from this report:

- Women's average sleep duration is significantly longer than that of men (7.24 versus 7 hours per night).
- 43% of men and 55% of women aged eighteen to sixty-four report finding it difficult to go to sleep or stay asleep "sometimes/most of the time/all of the time."
- Similarly, among seniors aged sixty-five to seventy-nine, women are 19% more likely than men to report difficulty going to sleep or staying asleep "sometimes/most of the time/all of the time."
- Around a third (33%) of people aged eighteen to sixty-four and 30% of seniors report difficulty staying awake during normal waking hours "sometimes/most of the time/all of the time."

The story in the United States is perhaps even slightly worse. Population-based studies indicate that nearly 30% of American adults report sleeping an average of six or fewer hours per night, while 69% of high school students report having less than eight hours of sleep on an average school night.[14-17] The National Sleep Foundation's 2020 Sleep in

America® poll found that Americans feel sleepy on an average of three days a week, with many saying it impacts their daily activities, mood, mental acuity, productivity, and more.[18]

HOW MUCH SLEEP DO WE REALLY NEED?

Genes may play a significant role in how much sleep we each need. Scientists have identified several genes involved with sleep and sleep disorders, including genes that control the excitability of neurons and "clock" genes that influence our circadian rhythms and the timing of sleep.[19] Additional research is still required to better understand inherited sleep patterns and the risks of sleep disorders.

As a general rule, the National Sleep Foundation (NSF) recommends that school-age children should receive at least ten hours of sleep daily, while the minimum requirement for adults aged eighteen to sixty-four is seven to nine hours, and seven to eight hours for adults aged sixty-five and over.[20-23] If this is not your reality, you may have forgotten that the characteristics of a good night's sleep include waking up feeling refreshed, alert, and able to be fully productive throughout your waking hours.

REGULATION AND STAGES OF SLEEP

There are two main biological mechanisms at play in healthy sleep, both of which are influenced by lifestyle practices. Their coordination regulates our sleep-wake daily cycle. They are our circadian rhythm and sleep-wake homeostasis, and their command centers are found in the middle of our brains, in our hypothalamus.

Circadian rhythms direct a wide variety of functions, from daily fluctuations in wakefulness to body temperature, metabolism, and the release of hormones.[19] This mechanism will cause you to feel sleepy at night and is responsible for your tendency to wake in the morning without an alarm at a consistent time. It is based on the body's twenty-four-hour biological clock and is synchronized with environmental cues like light and temperature.

Sleep-wake homeostasis keeps track of your need for sleep. This homeostatic sleep drive reminds the body to sleep after a certain time and regulates sleep intensity. Think of it as a built-in autopilot feature hard-wired to your mainframe. Your sleep drive gets stronger every hour you are awake and after a long day, will cause you to sleep longer and more deeply.[19]

External factors can have a dramatic influence on both of these mechanisms and the interplay between them, influencing your body's recovery, sleep needs, and quality of rest. These factors include a host of different medical conditions, medications, stress, sleep environment, and what you eat and drink. Interestingly, one of the most significant influences on sleep is exposure to light. Specialized cells in the eye's retina process light and tell the brain whether it is day or night. They can advance or delay our sleep-wake cycle. Exposure to light can make it difficult to fall asleep and return to sleep when awakened.

STAGES OF SLEEP

There are two basic types of sleep, rapid eye movement (REM) sleep and non-REM sleep, which play out over four different stages. Each stage is linked to specific brain waves and neuronal activity, with memory consolidation most likely requiring both non-REM and REM sleep.[19]

We cycle through all non-REM and REM sleep stages several times during a typical night, with increasingly longer and deeper REM periods occurring toward morning.[19,23-24] This pattern also occurs for those on shift work who must sleep in the daytime or evening hours.

Stage 1: Non-REM sleep: During this stage, we fall asleep, and as we do, our heartbeat, breathing, and eye movements slow. Our muscles also start to relax, with occasional twitches. Brain waves begin to slow from their daytime wakefulness patterns.[19]

Stage 2: Non-REM sleep: This stage is a period of light sleep before entering deeper sleep: heartbeat and breathing slow, and our muscles continue to relax. Body temperature drops, and eye movements stop. Brain wave activity slows, but there are brief bursts of electrical activity. We spend more of our repeated sleep cycles in Stage 2 sleep than in other sleep stages.[19]

Stage 3: Non-REM sleep: This stage is a period of deep sleep necessary for us to feel rejuvenated in the morning. It occurs in longer periods during the first half of the night. In this stage, our heartbeat and breathing slow to their lowest levels. Our muscles become totally relaxed, and it may be difficult to be awakened, as our brain waves become even slower.[19]

Stage 4: REM sleep: REM sleep occurs during the first ninety minutes after falling asleep, during which time, our eyes move rapidly from side to side behind closed eyelids. Brain wave activity becomes closer to that seen in wakefulness. Our breathing becomes faster and irregular, and our heart rate and blood pressure can increase to near waking levels.[19,23] REM sleep is where we do most of our dreaming. Our arm and leg muscles actually become temporarily paralyzed at this point, which prevents any acting out of our dreams. On average, we move through three to five REM cycles each night, with each episode lasting a little longer. If your sleep ritual permits seven to eight hours of sleep, roughly ninety minutes will be in REM. As we age, our REM sleep time gradually decreases. [19, 23]

HOW THE BODY RESETS AND REPAIRS DURING SLEEP

Research shows that sleep is among the most critical factors for peak performance, memory, productivity, immune function, and mood regulation.[7] What actually happens when our head is on the pillow is biologically spectacular.

Here is a quick review of some of the critical functions of sleep necessary for the masterful cell-to-cell coordination mentioned at the beginning of this chapter:

SLEEP DECLUTTERS THE MIND. Your brain is quite busy when you are asleep. It sorts and stores information it has taken in from the day. This process is critical to maintaining the pathways in your brain that let you learn and create new memories, concentrate, and think.[19] Sleep is vital to several brain functions, including how nerve cells (neurons) communicate and how the brain manages waste. Studies show that sleep plays a critical housekeeping role by removing toxins in your brain, including beta-amyloid and tau proteins, which are associated with Alzheimer's disease. Researchers have discovered that the coupling of slow brain wave activity and the flow of cerebrospinal fluid (CSF) during sleep flushes these toxic, memory-impairing proteins from the brain.[25]

SLEEP ACTIVATES NEUROTRANSMITTERS AND HORMONAL SWITCHES. These chemical messengers play an essential role in sleep regulation. According to the National Institute of Neurological Disorders and Stroke, clusters of sleep-promoting neurons in many parts of the brain become more active as we prepare for bed and "switch off" or dampen cellular activity that signals arousal assisting with sleep.[26] For example, the neurotransmitter GABA is associated with sleep, muscle relaxation, and sedation. Other neurotransmitters that shape sleep and wakefulness include acetylcholine, histamine, adrenaline, cortisol, and serotonin.[23]

Hormones also have a role to play in priming the body for rest and repair. Melatonin, which is released by a small gland in the middle of your brain called the pineal gland helps control the sleep-wake regulation described above. Its release is triggered by darkness; hence the name "hormone of darkness."[27] The pituitary gland also gets in on the action by releasing growth hormone once we are asleep, which helps stimulate essential growth and repair neural pathways.

SLEEP HELPS OUR NERVOUS SYSTEM DE-STRESS. When we sleep, our sympathetic nervous system, which controls our fight or flight stress response, is allowed to drop its guard. Studies have shown that depriving healthy subjects of sleep acutely increases blood pressure and sympathetic nervous system activity.[24] Prolonged short sleep durations could lead to hypertension through extended exposure to increased blood pressure, heart rate, elevated sympathetic nervous system activity, and increased salt retention. Such forces place the cardiovascular system under operational stress.[24]

SLEEP REGULATES CORTISOL. Cortisol levels have tremendous authority over your biology. It is known as the "stress hormone" and has an intricate relationship with the hormone insulin, which controls your blood sugar. Among other things, its chronic elevation is linked to weight gain and obesity (more on this in Wellness Ritual #3). Your cortisol levels fall off during the first few hours of sleep and then rise to a peak soon after we wake up.[27] Consistency in sleep routine helps to regulate this hormone, which after a good night's sleep, will help you feel alert in the morning and switch on your appetite.

SLEEP GIVES US AN IMMUNE BOOST. While you sleep, your inflammation-fighting, immune-system-priming proteins called cytokines are released.[18] They help drive your repair and recovery process and signal the immune system to do its job. If cytokine release is compromised by sleep deprivation, it leaves the immune system short-handed and under-resourced.

CHAPIN CLINICAL CORNER

Our best intentions to catch up on a sleep debt can lead to inconsistent patterns of sleep. This is a slippery slope. Unfortunately, an hour less tonight does not equal an extra hour tomorrow. The belief that people can adapt to chronic sleep loss without a negative influence on brain function is no longer supported. Loading up on caffeine and other stimulants only further disrupts the sleep-wake cycle.

In addition to nutritional and consumption habits that amplify sleep deprivation, many people wake up feeling tired thanks to insomnia or more subtle sleep disturbances caused by problems like nighttime acid reflux and sleep apnea.

Not all sleep is equal. Recovery or catch-up sleep is characterized by abnormal brain waves as the brain attempts to resynchronize with the body's circadian rhythm and declutter your mind. Even a mild sleep reduction or change in sleep routine can produce detrimental effects on cognitive performance for many days afterward.

Our twenty-one mentors structure their lifestyle formula around the framework of their sleep-wake requirements. As mentioned above, they prioritize sleep without compromise to ensure their body's ability to repair and recover is optimal. As Jim Leech shared, "If your body and mind are not rested, everything you attempt will be below your ability and standard."

Maintaining a consistent sleep schedule and feeling well-rested are related; those with the most regular and consistent weekday sleep schedules are about 1.5 times more likely to report feeling well-rested than those without consistency to their sleep patterns. Fifty-two percent to 56% of Americans reporting the most regular sleep schedules wake up feeling well-rested on weekdays. In comparison, only 34% to 38% of those with the most varied sleep times report the same.[14-15]

There is great individual variance in sleep cycles. Some can fall asleep as soon as they are horizontal; others may take an hour. Both are considered within the normal range. A sleep ritual that leads to normal, quality nighttime sleep and full daytime alertness, referred to as sleep hygiene, is best supported by consistency seven days a week.

If you are having trouble falling asleep, staying asleep, not feeling rested when you wake up or feeling tired during the day, talk to your doctor or primary healthcare practitioner. Do not continue to suffer in silence or tolerate sub-par performance because of fatigue. If sleep hygiene is not an area of expertise among the team of clinicians helping to manage your health, request a referral to a sleep specialist or sleep clinic. They can be very helpful in providing a clinical pathway forward through the challenges of restless leg syndrome, sleep apnea, or chronic pain, which may be preventing quality sleep.

In my practice, I also frequently emphasize the importance of sleep posture with my patients. Unfortunately, sleep quality for many individuals is limited because of back, neck, shoulder, or hip pain. Please visit the book's website **7WellnessRituals.com** for sleep posture tips that will help you improve the quality of your sleep.

RITUAL ACTIVATION

In sleep, you unlock a powerful therapeutic force that protects the mind and body. Think of it as a daily reboot. The goal is not perfection. Mentor Dr. Robyne Hanley-Dafoe adjusts her sleep patterns to a three-day average to reduce sleep anxiety if a night doesn't go as planned. There will be days or nights when sleep is fleeting. Shift workers; new parents; and patients with sleep disorders, pain, or mental health challenges can struggle to find consistency in their patterns of sleep despite their best efforts. I encourage this group to find rest when they can. A short ten- to twenty-minute power nap can be rejuvenating. Give yourself permission to rest. It will charge your performance. If sleep continues to be difficult, bring your desire to improve the quality of sleep to your next appointment with your primary healthcare practitioner. There is help available.

Getting your sleep-wake cycle regulated is essential to living up to your potential. Set your bedtime like an important business meeting. Show up to this meeting on time and prepared — lights out, TV off, and phone out of reach. If logging seven to nine hours a night is a challenge, start by going to bed twenty to thirty minutes earlier each night for a few weeks until you meet the recommendations.

RITUAL TARGET:

Go to bed and wake up at the same time every day. Schedule seven to nine hours of sleep every night if you are between the ages of eighteen and sixty-four, and seven to eight hours if you are aged sixty-five and over. This is the most important meeting of your day. Take these steps to show up for this meeting prepared:

- **Avoid stimulants such as caffeine late in the day.** My rule is no caffeine after lunch. Caffeine hits the body quickly, and its impact can linger with a half-life (the time it takes your body to eliminate half of the substance) of roughly three to five hours. Consuming caffeine late in the day can cause lighter and more disturbed sleep that night. In a 2013 study, researchers found that consuming 400 mg of caffeine (a large Tim Hortons coffee has approximately 140 mg of caffeine) six hours before bed cut total sleeping time by more than one hour.[28]

- **Avoid alcohol consumption too close to bedtime.** Alcohol may speed the onset of sleep, but it disrupts your sleep quality in later stages as the body begins to metabolize the alcohol. This process causes arousal. Alcohol will also reduce the amount of time that you spend in deeper sleep stages, which has an adverse effect on memory, concentration, and physical coordination.[28]

- **Exercise can promote good sleep.** Keep your vigorous exercise to the morning or late afternoon. A relaxing exercise, such as a gentle yoga class or a casual neighborhood stroll with your dog is fine and can be done before bed to help initiate a restful night's sleep.

- **Do not consume large meals close to bedtime.** Eating can be disruptive right before sleep. Pre-bed snacks will also sabotage your efforts with Wellness Ritual #3 - Fight for Your Waistline.

- **Ensure adequate exposure to natural light.** This is particularly important for people who may not venture outside as frequently. Light exposure within the first thirty to sixty minutes of your day will help you maintain a healthy sleep-wake cycle. If you are up before the sun, turn on artificial lights and get outdoors for a few minutes once the sun rises.[29]

- **Establish a regular relaxing bedtime routine.** Prior to your committed bedtime, take twenty to thirty minutes to begin to unwind. This practice cues your mind and prepares you for sleep. Try to avoid emotionally charged conversations and activities right before bed. A hot bath or shower, reading, or listening to a meditation app may be helpful. (I recommend the Calm App. As a side note, listen to LeBron James' seven-minute podcast on "The Power of Sleep" featured on this app for extra sleep motivation). Do your best to maintain a consistent sleep schedule seven days a week.

- **Associate your bed with sleep.** If falling asleep is a challenge, avoid watching TV, surfing the web, or reading in bed. Keep your bedroom dark and at a comfortable temperature. If you are still tossing and turning after thirty minutes, get up. Listen to some relaxing music or read a book until you feel sleepy, then return to bed. Research has shown that this helps to train your mind to associate your bed with sleep instead of struggle.[30]

- **Track sleep patterns.** Tracking the trend line of your efforts to practice this Wellness Ritual helps link the quality of your daytime performance with the quality of your sleep. Download a smartphone app or purchase a wearable smart bracelet or watch. Smart technology can record sounds and movements during sleep, journal hours slept, and monitor heart rate and breathing patterns.

- **Ask for feedback.** Discuss your sleep patterns with your partner. If you snore loudly, gasp, or seem to choke during sleep, you may have sleep apnea. There are treatments available, including weight-loss strategies and pressurized masks to facilitate better breathing, which can dramatically improve sleep quality.

IN SUMMARY

Sleep has a profound impact on every part of the human body and drastically influences our mental and physical health. Research shows that a chronic lack of sleep or frequent poor-quality sleep increases the risk of disorders, including high blood pressure, cardiovascular disease, diabetes, depression, and obesity.

In Jim Leech's words, "The only real risk is not knowing you are taking a risk." Thus, now that you know the science behind, and the danger of, insufficient sleep, it is easy to place very real importance on making sleep, rest, and recovery part of your daily Wellness Rituals moving forward — just as Claudette McGowan and Jim Treliving have.

Those who are committed to their well-being and achieving their potential do not sacrifice sleep. Averaging seven to nine hours a night with disciplined intention builds the foundation for proper self-care and a higher quality of life.

"I can take an athlete that doesn't eat breakfast—never has, and never will—and discuss a healthy approach to **intermittent fasting** that will set them up for success. But then their teammate, who may also be **underutilizing breakfast** for different reasons—but is open to the idea—may see **a huge jump in their performance** by introducing an early morning protein source. **Both strategies can work; it just depends on the individual.**" - Jenn Sygo

MENTOR PROFILES

—————

JENNIFER SYGO

KHAMICA BINGHAM

JEFFREY LATIMER

JENNIFER SYGO

Dietitian for Toronto Raptors, Athletics Canada, and Gymnastics Canada

*T*aking a peek inside the fridge of one of Canada's leading nutrition experts feels a little like being invited to an exclusive party. The very idea piques my curiosity. If anyone holds the secret to healthy eating, it is Registered Dietitian Jen Sygo. As team dietitian for the NBA World-Champion Toronto Raptors, Athletics Canada, and Gymnastics Canada, Jen has helped many of our country's very best athletes reach the summit of their sport and compete on the world stage. As a busy professional, married with two active kids, she also walks the walk. Talking about lifestyle rituals with Jen reveals an accessible on-ramp to healthy living for those looking for a place to start.

Jen is determined to bring the healing power of food to the forefront and to empower her patients and athletes to take accountability for their diet and general health. The clinical reward of helping a patient improve their relationship with food, speed their recovery, maximize their training, or elevate their performance is what drives her. She shares, "There is an old saying that what you eat before you play won't win you the game, but it could make you lose it."

SELF-CARE REFLECTION #7

Please reflect on these questions and record your thoughts in your journal:

▸ Do you have the energy you need when you need it?
▸ How would you rate your relationship with food on a 10-point scale, from 0 (very poor, my diet is not supporting my health and performance goals) to 10 (excellent, my diet allows me to bring my best effort forward when needed and recover quickly)?

In addition to seeing private clients at Cleveland Clinic Canada, Jen is hired by teams to help their athletes make simple dietary changes to improve their health and performance and reduce the risk of injury. Somehow, in the middle of all this activity, she has carved time out to pursue a part-time Ph.D. at Manchester Metropolitan University with a Canadian grant from *Own the Podium's Innovation 4 Gold* program. In conjunction with the Canadian Women's Gymnastics Team, Jen is studying the impact of chronic under-fueling (under-eating) on performance outcomes. She hopes her research will lead to a greater understanding among athletes, coaches, parents, and administrators of the effects of pressuring athletes to eat or not to eat in harmful ways.

"I found myself at the midway point of my career with a choice of which direction to head next. One option was to continue along the same path doing the work I'm doing with my client base. This is work that I am good at and comfortable with. The other option was to take a chance, advance my career, and create an opportunity to learn and push my skill set."

Her clinical curiosity made the second option an easy choice. Completing her Ph.D. will provide Jen with a platform to shine a bright light on issues paramount to athletes' emotional and physical well-being. The pressures emerging from social media for young athletes to look a certain way while delivering flawlessly on cue is destructive, and Jen intends to do something about it.

SELF-CARE REFLECTION #8

Connecting with your internal motivation to live a healthier life is essential to making the 7 Wellness Rituals stick. Common motivators include physical appearance, performance, medical history, and age. Where does your motivation to improve your health come from?

A DISCIPLINED SLEEP RITUAL

Clinicians hard-wired to lift others up sometimes require a little coaxing to turn the focus back to themselves. Before I asked Jen about her own nutritional practices, I started with an easy question about her bedtime. As a general rule, she is in bed by 11 p.m., although she often does so with some reluctance.

Jen lives in the fast lane and acknowledges that she has developed a nagging sense of FOMO — Fear Of Missing Out — which makes the process of closing out her day a challenge. To quiet her FOMO, Jen's pre-bed ritual includes dimming the lights, avoiding email or scrolling on her phone, and stepping away from her to-do list at least thirty minutes before bed.

Exercise too late in the day will also disrupt her sleep quality, so she avoids it. An 11 p.m. to 7 a.m. sleep routine provides Jen with eight hours a night. The rain hitting a bedroom window or her husband jumping into an early-morning shower does not go unnoticed by her as a light sleeper. Once up, sleep can be a challenge for her to re-enter.

A sleep-in on the odd lazy family weekend can be a nice reward, but given the choice to hit the snooze button or jump in the shower, Jen will grab a towel and start her day.

THE IMPORTANCE OF MICRO-BREAKS IN A BUSY DAY

During the Raptors' season, the medical and performance teams convene for a standing meeting at 9 a.m. before breaking out to support the players. "In pro sports, you have to grab the players when you can. In my work, I have a lot of one- to two-minute conversations with players. You might catch them in a break or coming off the treatment table. Sometimes I'll set up formal one-on-one meetings if a player is looking for more support, but most of the work of checking-in happens on the fly. When I am onsite and have a presence, I can be a voice in their ear and help guide decisions."

When Jen has pushed through a long day, she closes her laptop and looks to retreat to her family and get active. As a dietitian, patient consultations stacked back-to-back can result in prolonged periods of sitting. As postural fatigue creeps in, she knows she has been still for too long. Low back pain draws her attention to this misstep and triggers her to move.

Jen admits to falling into a pattern of ignoring her needs to stay present for her patients above all else and is actively taking steps to change this behavior. By scheduling more frequent micro-breaks for a bathroom visit, a sip of water, or a quick stretch between clients, she can provide the standard of care she aspires to deliver without sacrificing her health in the process.

Jen is also working on setting boundaries in the evening and now limits the after-hours charting and administrative work that results from her busy practice. Learning to protect her downtime and proactively schedule time to tie off loose ends has become a critical feature of her formula. "I will now make the intentional decision to take my kid to hockey instead of extending my day and block a thirty-minute window the next morning to complete my paperwork or respond to emails." She keeps her work emails to working hours, protecting her weekends, and has learned to respond to the late Friday-afternoon email on Monday morning without guilt.

Jen credits the lockdown during the COVID-19 pandemic with helping her to slow down and develop a greater appreciation for rest and recovery. She now prioritizes unscripted play with her kids, spontaneous family pub nights, a stroll through the park, a tennis match with a friend, or just quiet time for reflective meditation in a whole new way. "I routinely talk to clients who have sixty-plus hour work weeks about the cost of their pace and the huge uptick in creativity, energy, and the quality of execution when they make rest a priority." Turning inward, Jen has found a comforting peace in the practice of meditation. She likes the version of herself that has emerged as a result of putting her own advice to work.

"I have gobs of energy and can typically push through a fair bit before I feel fatigued. What I have learned is that meditation really helps me manage my energy. It is a steadying force that grounds me. I have passed that point in my career where the goal was to accomplish as many things as possible. My focus now is to cherish and experience everything as much as I can in the richest way possible — my family, my athletes, and my clients. Prioritizing rest and recovery and learning to meditate has helped me lock in on these goals."

❝I want a body that doesn't lose its ability to function as it ages."

When it comes to exercise, Jen prefers to work out in the morning. Running is her default, but she also enjoys free weights, yoga, and pilates. Once a week, she also plays in a women's ball hockey league. Jen's eye is on her immediate and future well-being when it comes to exercise. "I want a body that doesn't lose its ability to function as it ages. I grew up playing a little bit of everything — basketball, volleyball, track, swimming, and Ultimate Frisbee. I try to continue to bring variety to my workouts and practice different movement patterns to ensure that I will be able to move freely as I get older. My approach to fitness is an intentional hodgepodge of activity."

JEN'S FORMULA FOR HEALTH, STRENGTH & HOPE

As our conversation turned to nutritional practices, Jen quickly emphasized the importance of developing an individual approach when it comes to food. As an example, she prefers to exercise on an empty stomach in the morning. She says, "I literally have allergic reactions if I eat in advance of my morning workout. This approach is not for everyone, but it works for me." Jen shared her approach to eating for this book with the caveat that no one should follow her script without first speaking to their healthcare team. She suffers from food sensitivities and allergies that influence what, when, and how she eats.

Breakfast usually consists of oatmeal with various hemp seeds, pumpkin seeds, or walnuts with a little cow's milk or non-dairy milk. Too much dairy appears to aggravate her skin. If she needs an extra boost while at the Raptors' training facility in the morning she will grab a pressed juice or extend her breakfast to include some fruit, an egg, or if she skipped her oatmeal at home, cold cereal with nuts on top. She drinks tea, not coffee.

For lunch, she will commonly pack an avocado and egg salad or grab the lunch prepared by the Raptors' team chef. "I have a food allergy to chicken and fish, so my meat protein comes from lean cuts of beef, pork, or lamb. If this isn't an option, I'll turn to beans, eggs, cheese, or nuts." Accompanying her protein selection is always a healthy serving of fresh vegetables and a carbohydrate.

Jennifer feels her body performs at its best in workouts if she includes a starchy carbohydrate at every meal. Potatoes, whole-grain bread, rice, and whole-wheat pasta do the trick. When it comes to fueling after a workout, she recommends including a protein and carbohydrate within thirty minutes of exercise to help fast-track muscle repair and replenish muscle energy stores. Whey protein is particularly effective for recovery. A protein smoothie on the go can help sustain performance and avoid a mid-afternoon crash.

Afternoon snack options include yogurt and fruit; veggies with hummus; or a handful of cashews, walnuts, almonds, and dried fruit. Jennifer recommends keeping a small bag of nuts in your car or briefcase. She says it can be a real lifesaver for executives or athletes on the move. Nuts offer a good energy source and are nutritionally diverse. A can of tuna or salmon, Greek yogurt, or cottage cheese provides an excellent, quick protein source to sustain energy as well.

In anticipation of her kids coming home from school hungry, Jen will often put out a tray of options for them to graze on, to tide them over until dinner. The tray may include grapes, apple slices, cheese, veggie sticks, and salami. Another family favorite in the Sygo household is protein pancakes. She will make up a big batch using whey protein and keep them cold in the fridge for a family snack. She admits that healthy eating requires extra planning, but hungry people make poor choices when good options are not readily available.

Jen and her husband share dinner responsibilities and enjoy family mealtime with the kids. Meal plans are kept varied, and their kids are expected to have at least one bite of everything. No food is labeled bad or off limits. She says, "We try to enter the week with a family meal strategy to ensure we have all the ingredients and know which one of us is preparing which meal." On the night of our first interview, the scheduled dinner was skirt steak sandwiches with garlic aioli and homemade coleslaw on the side. They tend not to order in often but enjoy the spontaneity of heading down the street to a local family restaurant.

> Visit the book's website **7WellnessRituals.com** for a list of micro-breaks and easy desk stretches to bring movement to your day.

When pressed for a framework for healthy eating, Jen reminds her clients that "there is no one diet that fits all, no master plan for us to follow. Developing an approach to eating that elevates your individual performance takes time, patience, and experimentation." To develop this plan, Jen listens to her clients to understand how their day works and studies the preferences and tendencies that influence their choices. She seeks to understand the complexity of their home and work life and any external pressures from schedules, travel, or health concerns.

Dispelling food myths for clients is also a part of her professional role. Jen states, "The idea a certain berry will help you lose weight or a particular vegetable will prevent cancer in isolation is unrealistic." And the six to eight glasses of water we are told to drink? Two liters of fluids (not exclusively water) ensure proper hydration, which is essential for good health. She cautions that sports drinks, which tend to have a high sugar content, are not required after a walk around the block. They are best served to athletes in extreme heat or following prolonged, aggressive physical exertion greater than ninety minutes, not to weekend warriors.

For executives who challenge their cognitive limits to meet the demands of their day, she emphasizes consuming calories from food sources that will help stabilize energy early in the morning. Replacing a croissant and coffee breakfast with a meal that provides a healthy protein and fat source can dramatically reduce the feeling of brain fog or sluggishness in the morning. Jen encourages working with a professional who can introduce you to different foods to ensure you have a broad palette for delicious and nutritious fuel. She asks her clients to take risks in the kitchen by trying new recipes and having some fun with friends and family in food preparation.

In the end, the contents of Jen's fridge did not offer a surprising reveal. In fact, her inventory is likely not that much different than yours, with milk, yogurt, cheese, eggs, a few condiments, the odd container of leftovers, and a variety of fresh fruits and vegetables on the list. Health is not found in a strict diet or delivered through a particular grocery list. There is no one secret to healthy eating. Good health is dynamic and must be nurtured. Jen's rituals stand as a reminder of our body's favorable adaptation to studying our habits — healthy and unhealthy — and responding with a formula rooted in evidence, self-care, and a passion for helping others.

SELF-CARE REFLECTION #9

Turn to your journal and complete the One Week Diet Diary. Let's see what you discover about what, why, and when you consume fuel for your body.

KHAMICA BINGHAM

Olympic Track and Field Athlete for Team Canada, Motivational speaker

*I*n 2016, at twenty-two years of age, Khamica Bingham ran a personal best of 11.13 seconds in the 100 m sprint and qualified as the fastest woman in Canada. She averaged almost nine meters per second, her top speed that year. In July 2016, she was added to Canada's Olympic team. Now a celebrated two-time World Championship finalist, Pan Am bronze medalist, and Olympian, she has consistently represented Canada with tremendous poise and grace.

As a nationally ranked gymnast, her original Olympic dreams lay in a different sport. However, pursuing a gymnastics dream was expensive, and her speed, discipline, and competitive drive made sprinting a more natural fit. In her first year of competition, she won gold in the 2010 Ontario High School Track and Field Championships in the 100 m and 200 m sprints. From this moment forward, she dedicated her life to pushing the limits of her athletic talent.

In 2015, Khamica anchored the Canadian Women's 4x100 m relay at the World Relay Championships, missing third place by 1/100th of a second. This performance earned the Canadian women an opportunity to compete in the 2016 Rio Olympic Games. By capturing the Canadian National 100 m title shortly thereafter, Khamica qualified for the Olympic 100 m and 200 m races as well. With each race, she gained more confidence and speed, and the relay team won bronze at the 2015 Pan Am Games hosted in Toronto. This victory on home turf was particularly sweet and remains one of her proudest accomplishments to date. In Rio, her Olympic debut, Canada's women's 4x100 m relay team, anchored by Khamica, finished sixth, earning Canada its first Olympic final in the event since the 1984 Games in Los Angeles.

Athletes that specialize in the 100 m sprint must train for hours every day for most of the year in order to possess the ability to explode on demand at their peak for a ten- to eleven-second burst of speed. There is no room for doubt or hesitation in their preparation or execution. Success can swing on a hundredth of a second, so each step is given consideration, and biomechanics must be perfected.

Before diving into Khamica's formula, I asked her to describe what it felt like to sprint at world-class speed in perfect kinetic motion. Did she feel fast? She sat quietly for a moment, pondering my question, appearing to temporarily lose herself in the vision of a perfect race, sampling the thrill and exhilaration of peak speed privately in her mind. She smiled and then shared, "It feels smooth — really, really smooth."

Khamica's story illustrates the powerful connection between mindset and performance and not only strength of body, but strength of will.

KHAMICA OVERCOMES EARLY INJURIES

From 2016 to 2019, Khamica struggled as injuries started to pile up and threatened to derail her promising career. Four months before the 2016 Olympic trials, shortly after being crowned the fastest woman in Canada, she suffered a cartilage tear in her knee. In 2017, she experienced a partial tear of her left Achilles tendon. In 2018, she tore her right Achilles. Athletes in running sports suffer higher incidences of Achilles tendon injuries, which can be particularly tricky to overcome, especially for speed athletes. The Achilles is the large tendon that attaches your calf muscles to the back of your heel and acts as a powerful elastic band allowing you to push off while walking, running, and jumping. Rehab for any of these injuries demands considerable rest and time away from sport, which comes at a high cost to an athlete's confidence.

Khamica told me, "My Achilles is my worst enemy. Honestly, after three consecutive seasons dealing with injuries, I thought too much time had passed and my sprinting days were done. I just wasn't hitting the times I once could, and my body was no longer responding to training like it always had. Completing an entire competition season is really important to my rhythm and confidence. Injuries kept me out, and I lost my race fitness. There is a fundamental difference between training fitness and race fitness."

Suddenly, running was no longer easy. It was hard and painful. "I remember thinking in 2019, 'I don't know if I've got it anymore.' I was so used to competing at an elite level, and I found myself trying to come back from injury, struggling to beat times I was running back in high school. I knew my recovery would be slow, but I wasn't seeing the expected progression in my recovery. It was a really challenging time for me. The field of women at the top was only getting faster, and I was working super hard just to catch up to where I was."

Where she was would no longer be good enough, and Khamica knew it. She wanted more, and her sport demanded it. Uncertain of whether or not a successful comeback was even possible, she set what felt like a huge goal — qualifying for the Tokyo 2020 Olympic Games as a two-time Canadian Olympian and running a personal best on that stage.

Standing in Khamica's way, complicating her return to peak form, were two additional factors — a diagnosis of iron deficiency anemia and the devastating disruption of the COVID-19 pandemic. The discovery of her anemic condition came as a surprise; however, it offered some answers as to why her body was suddenly breaking down with one soft-tissue injury after another. The body's wound-healing process relies heavily on oxygenation. Low oxygen levels caused by her anemia were likely responsible for her slow healing and susceptibility to injury. By identifying and addressing this issue with her medical team and undergoing PRP-Plasma Rich Protein injections to facilitate tendon healing, Khamica overcame her Achilles trouble, and her stamina and resiliency started to return. There was still considerable rest and rehab required before her frame would tolerate a full training schedule, but she could feel momentum on her side once again. As for the COVID-19 pandemic, she took the opportunity to slow down, get quiet, and develop the mental fitness she would need to have a shot at achieving her dream.

SELF-CARE REFLECTION #10

Think about Khamica's words, "I don't know if I've got it anymore." For an athlete pursuing an Olympic dream to run for their country, this admission is devastating. But we all have those moments when we feel we just don't have any more to give. In your journal, describe such a moment and the steps you took to heal and overcome. What aspects of your being helped you through your challenge — physical, spiritual, mental? Did you have the benefit of a mentor or support network?

HEALING FROM PERSONAL LOSS

As Khamica started posting competitive times once again, her mental fitness and conviction were further tested by the unexpected news of her mother's passing. On her Instagram account, Khamica wrote, "I lost my mom. Training for the Olympics while grieving has been mentally, physically and spiritually draining." Her mom would have wanted her to continue striving toward her goal. To do so, she had to embrace the adversity of injury and grief, release the outcome, and trust her formula.

"I had got to a dark place where coming to the track to train was no longer fun. I doubted my body's ability to compete. Coming off three years where the more I pushed, the more injury trouble I had, I had to take a hard look at my approach. Training and competing injury-free are completely different from mounting a comeback from injury. To bounce back, I needed to tear down and rebuild my process. I had to relearn my body. When you try to force speed, when you try to feel fast, your body and processes break down. The time that opened up with COVID-19 gave me the respite I needed to rebuild, mentally and physically."

Blocking out all external noise and creating space for her body to heal and her mind to find a positive direction, Khamica got to work on rebuilding her formula from the ground up. Leaning into her faith helped her manage her grief and the mounting anxiety surrounding the uncertainty of her future. "I learned to trust my mindset, the hard work I was putting in, and my process, and let everything else go. I could only control what I could control, and that is where I put my energy. Walking by faith and not by sight allowed me to accept all of the surprise bumps along the way and continue to work on my dream without distraction. My faith kept me moving forward; without it, the journey would have ended a while ago."

Logic suggested her dream was over. The gap between where she was and where she needed to be was still too great, and time was running out. However, there is no quit in Khamica. She credits her mom and Athletes-in-Action chaplain Herbie Kuhn (another mentor profiled in this book) for modeling a way forward and helping her rediscover her purpose and love for sprinting.

"Track athletes are goal-oriented. We like having a plan and executing that plan. The uncertainty in the months leading up to the Olympics was extremely difficult."

With only a handful of meets to qualify remaining on the calendar, the restrictions surrounding her ability to travel and compete at these meets — or maintain access to coaches, teammates, and training facilities — left big question marks. Nevertheless, her demanding training had to continue if she were to have a shot. The stress was extraordinary.

With COVID-19 pushing the Tokyo Games into 2021, Khamica had a little more time. She decided to train at Louisiana State University. To make the Canadian team, she had to run the Olympic standard time of 11.15 seconds. If she fell short in the remaining meets in the US, she would need to return to Canada, quarantine for two weeks, and then compete in the 2021 Canadian Olympic and Paralympic Track and Field Trials in Montreal in late June. This is exactly what happened, and on July 3, 2021, Athletics Canada revealed which athletes would compete in Tokyo. Khamica was on the list. She was going to compete in her second Olympic Games. The bet on herself had paid off. Turning to Instagram, she posted, "If you ever felt like you've been down too long and cannot come back, I am telling you that with God it is possible."

Khamica's formula to make this dream come true is outlined below.

KHAMICA'S FORMULA FOR HEALTH, STRENGTH & HOPE

PREPARATION FOR RACE DAY

Khamica's sleep routine is non-negotiable. She gets eight to nine hours of quality sleep every night and naps daily for up to an hour. Within two weeks of a big event, she adjusts her sleep regimen according to the time zone she will be competing in. Before getting into bed, her wind-down process includes a dark, cool room and limited screen time. She falls asleep quickly and wakes rejuvenated, typically without the aid of an alarm clock. Her circadian rhythm is locked in and valued as an essential performance tool.

She visualizes race day often to leave nothing to chance. "I dial into what race day will feel like. The time I wake up, the breakfast I'll have, the time I'll arrive at the track, my warm-up, my pre-race ritual, the music I listen to; it is all scripted to simulate race day."

Drake kicks off her pre-race music playlist. Every effort is made to make the actual race day feel familiar. Travel, time zones, elevation changes, climate differences are all given consideration. In the minutes before a race, her earbuds come out so she can hear the sound of her spikes hitting the track in warm up. The sound is comforting and connects her to the rhythm and cadence of her event. By the time the gun goes off, Khamica has already run the race hundreds of times in her mind.

Guided meditation, deep breathing exercises, journaling, and visualization of how she wants her body to move and which thoughts she wants to dominate her mind all help to prepare her for excellence. "Sprinting requires a state of relaxed tension. If you are too tense, too hyped, you slow yourself down. However, races where I haven't felt some level of stress and excitement in the blocks are never my best."

> 66 **In the end, it is really all about mindset, hard work, and trusting the process. I learned that as soon as I release all expectations, my performance will improve."**

This balanced state is delicate and comes with experience. "When I was younger, I would show up at a meet over-stressed and anxious, and by the time of the race, I'd be exhausted." To break this cycle, she has learned how to preserve and protect her energy by studying past races. "More experienced Olympic athletes taught me the value of journaling and studying the small details of my preparation." Her journal now acts as an additional coach that offers great insight as her formula evolves. She enjoys working on her process and rises to the challenge of improvement.

Khamica's practice of meditation and visualization, combined with prayer, form her intentional mindset. She surrounds herself with positive people who support her singular focus and prevent her from getting distracted by her competitors.

She trusts in her body's ability to respond favorably to the work she inputs. "In the end, it is really all about mindset, hard work, and trusting the process. I learned that as soon as I release all expectations, my performance will improve."

When it comes to nutrition, Khamica is all business. With the guidance of her team dietitian and sports nutritionist, she is serious about the fuel she puts in her body. Her breakfast is usually split into two parts by her morning workout. Part one is typically a slice of whole-wheat toast with peanut butter and sliced bananas, sprinkled with chia seeds. After training, she grabs a vanilla-flavored whey protein shake (she likes the brand Core Power) and then heads home for breakfast part two, which is more substantial. "This is where I will enjoy scrambled eggs, toast, yogurt, fruit, or maybe some potatoes on the side."

Following her morning workout, cool-down, and second breakfast, she turns her attention to a well-scripted recovery process. Because rest and recovery played a huge role in her comeback, she takes a power nap that can last up to an hour. Some days, she will actually sleep; on others, the quiet time is spent in reflection. After the nap, she begins a routine of foam rolling, dynamic stretching, leg compression and pulse therapy (using a Normatec unit), Epsom salt baths, and manual therapy, all designed to speed recovery and reset her mind and body for the next workout.

This pushes her lunch to late afternoon, usually sometime between 3 and 4 p.m. This meal is light, like a small tossed salad with grilled chicken. Time remaining in the afternoon is spent coaching young athletes, reading, journaling, catching up with friends, or working on an initiative she co-founded called Meet My Melanin (see below). Dinner is pushed to 7 or 8 p.m. and includes a plate of lean protein surrounded by fresh veggies. As for snacking, chips are her weakness. "I'll devour the whole bag if I'm not careful, so I need to pre-portion a handful of chips in a bowl, and when it's done, I'm done."

Khamica plans her meals according to her training regimen. The night before a big race, she might enjoy a plate of penne pasta with Bolognese sauce. Salmon with mashed potatoes is another favorite. Desserts and sweets are restricted.

As an elite athlete, her body composition, body fat, lean muscle mass, and bone density are measured every three months or so with a DEXA scan, and her formula is tweaked accordingly. Her target performance body fat is 15%. As someone who competes with the fastest humans in the world, this number is particularly important for her to maintain.

THERE IS BEAUTY ON THE OTHER SIDE

Returning to the Olympic Games for another opportunity to race for Canada is a dream come true for Khamica. In her life, a winning formula could shave a hundredth of a second off her time. Performance judged by such a razor's edge is unforgiving — and also exhilarating. The willpower to create this opportunity required a level of resiliency and maturity far beyond her years. Khamica reminds us that when big dreams are supported by hard work, you can reject negativity and noise from the cheap seats and focus on mastering the ability to drive to the goal you have set.

As the Tokyo Games came to a close, she discovered a reward hidden in her journey: "To my God, angels, supporters, therapists, coaches, friends, family, and sponsors, thank you for carrying me through to the finish line as a semi-finalist. It didn't go the way I wanted, but if I learned anything in this season of losses, it is that there is beauty on the other side of the lesson. There were many curveballs and many, many times where I felt completely lost and broken and had no clue how I was going to make it. Grieving the loss of my mom while training for the Olympic Games forced me to make room for painful growth, more love and appreciation for the little things, never to stop fighting, and most importantly, to take one day at a time."

Today, in addition to competing as a world-class sprinter, Khamica is a motivational speaker, fitness model, and an advocate for women empowerment, racial equality, and youth mentorship. She is the co-founder of Meet My Melanin (*meetmymelanin.com*), a movement created to celebrate and honor the experiences of people of color on a platform that is both healing and revealing. Khamica and her team offer motivational workshops and virtual events on racial inclusion and equality for Black, Indigenous, and People of Color (BIPOC). Her passion for helping minority communities to be heard, seen, and known, represents a lifelong race she is committed to running well beyond her track and field career.

Khamica is a beautiful person with infectious energy, an electric smile, and a kind heart set on helping others to the finish line.

SELF-CARE REFLECTION #11

Khamica has a ritual of studying past performances and journaling about them. She says, "More experienced Olympic athletes taught me the value of journaling and studying the small details of my preparation." Do you take the time to reflect on your own "past performances," be it at work, with family, or even in self-care rituals? Is there potential for you, like Khamica, to use your journal as a kind of coach?

JEFFREY LATIMER

CEO of Canada's Walk of Fame, Owner of JL Entertainment

For a man only in his late fifties, Jeffrey Latimer has already lived ten full lives. As CEO of Canada's Walk of Fame and Owner/CEO of JL Entertainment, a globally renowned artist management and event production agency, he is a veteran producer of live theater, musical entertainment, special events, film, and TV. Known for his creativity, his passion is getting the deal done, whether that be securing funding for a big production or assembling a team of creative artists to deliver on a new project.

> **I am not looking forward or backward to some other time or day. I'm right where I want to be, doing what I want to do, living my best life. I feel very blessed."**

Jeffrey's charity work is also extensive. He is currently on the Sarah McLachlan Foundation Board, and was on the boards of the Jays Care Foundation, the David Foster Foundation, and others.

Together with his husband, Larry, and their beautiful daughter, Maddie, he appears to have settled into a formula and stage of life that has allowed him to truly tap into his full potential. He is currently healthier and happier than he has ever been and as a result, is executing professionally at the highest level of his career. "I am not looking forward or backward to some other time or day. I'm right where I want to be, doing what I want to do, living my best life. I feel very blessed."

This was not always the way.

CRASHING IN THE FAST LANE

At the age of thirty, after living in LA for five years, Jeffrey was back in Toronto where the shows he produced were bringing in a million dollars a week. He lived the lifestyle that a lot of money could buy. Industry parties for the industry players and professional networking engagements for high-flying influencers were bridged by alcohol and cocaine. It was a wild time and Jeffrey got caught up in it.

"Those at the top have this stupid insecurity, and it drives us to do more and more."

Jeffrey's sexuality added a layer of complexity to this competitive landscape. Fueling his insecurity, at age twenty-two, he made the courageous decision to come out as a gay man while still trying to find his footing professionally. "For me, it was like being gay was this terrible thing. I felt I should at least be super rich or super successful in hopes that people would not judge me by my sexuality but would judge me instead by my success."

When the money started to roll in, he began spending it, playing the role of the successful entertainment executive and playing it well. Those in the Jeffrey Latimer camp were envied by those on the outside looking in.

But the fast lane came to an abrupt end. When confronted with business failure and personal unhappiness, Jeffrey was forced to take stock of the choices he was making. Bankruptcy is brutal and unforgiving.

But true to form, he was back on his feet quickly. A front-page newspaper article detailing his failure still hangs in a frame in his home office. I am guessing it reminds him of how far he has come.

SELF-CARE REFLECTION #12

As you read the rest of Jeffrey's story, you will see how he overcame the challenges he faced by drawing inspiration from love. Practicing the 7 Wellness Rituals, particularly when life feels like a struggle, is easier when you are clear on your priorities and what motivates you. Think of this clarity as your True North. Defining it, repeating it, and sharing it helps to suppress outside noise and avoid distraction. In your journal, define your True North.

LIFE BEGINS AT FIFTY

> ❝ **It is a fascinating thing…what not putting any substances into your body does to bring out greatness.** ❞

It has been fifteen years since Jeffrey has had a drink. Sobriety gave him his acute focus back. He shared, "The difference in my mind, the way I think, how I feel in the morning, and how I use my time is extraordinary. It is a fascinating thing…what not putting any substances into your body does to bring out greatness."

Clear-headed, he became more strategic with where he put his energy. As a result, he says his "batting average went way up."

Jeffrey sees the world differently now. "What I have learned is that the greatest success in your life starts after the age of fifty because you need all your failures to position you to succeed." If his life were a Broadway play, the intermission between Jeffrey Latimer Act One and Act Two would now be over. The curtains have risen, everyone is back in their seats, and Jeffrey is standing in the spotlight, ready to charge into the second half of his story. Leaning on the depth of his experience, he is now much more productive, closing a higher percentage of business deals and making more money. And he is having a lot more fun.

LOVE OF FAMILY AND FRIENDS MAKES LIFE COMPLETE

As exciting and fulfilling as his success has been, the love he shares with Larry and Maddie is what adds texture and meaning to his life. The unconditional love provided by his family allows Jeffrey to play with purpose (Wellness Ritual #7). He comes alive when describing Larry. After twenty-five years together, they have become quite the dynamic team. Their love is resolute and appears to have had a calming influence on Jeffrey's competitive drive, helping him even out his pace.

While Jeffrey acknowledges that he moves and thinks quickly, he appreciates the balance Larry brings to their relationship with his methodical and thorough approach. "Larry has helped me slow down and become a better listener. I am a really good salesman, but learning to listen to the nuance of what people are really asking for has been very helpful for me." Jeffrey is free to be himself, vulnerable with all of his faults exposed, with Larry. He credits Larry for helping him more completely understand his weaknesses and strengths. To be loved for both is profound.

Becoming parents together has been the greatest gift of Jeffrey's life. Maddie's grade school would be fortunate to have Larry and Jeffrey co-chair the PTA.

Jeffrey also draws on the emotional support provided by a small group of close friends he has known since he was a teenager. They, too, make frequent appearances in Jeffrey's life and love him for who he is, not the access he offers. He now allows only a select handful into the Jeffrey Latimer camp.

JEFFREY'S FORMULA FOR HEALTH, STRENGTH & HOPE

Jeffrey's success is built on structure. The closer he stays to the script, the better his performance. Here is a description of a sample day in the life of Jeffrey Latimer:

He wakes between 5 and 5:30 a.m. every day. Setting his sleep ritual to a consistent schedule five or six days a week gives him the performance kick he needs to maintain a busy lifestyle. He values the first 120 minutes a day offers above all else. "What I get from the morning between 5:30 and 7:30 is a complete sense of peace. It is the most powerful time of the day." The morning is his playground. It is a time when "anything is possible." He cherishes the daily opportunity to reset, reflect, and calmly ease into the demands of the day. It grounds him and is vital to his performance. "You are not expected to be available between five and eight in the morning." By the time the rest of the world is waking up, Jeffrey is primed and ready to embrace whatever is coming his way, on his terms.

He will write, think, and respond to emails over a coffee and a bowl of fruit with some yogurt for breakfast while the house remains silent.

Monday through Friday, he turns to exercise: a morning routine following breakfast at least three days a week, and tries to get another day or two in whenever possible. His workouts vary. Today, he exercises at home and at a private club. For the last few years, running has been his main focus. Three to four kilometer runs give him an endorphin kick, allow big ideas to come to him, and clear his mind of certain distractions.

This offline time sparks Jeffrey's creativity. When the weather is less inviting, he will bang out thirty to forty-five minutes on the treadmill while watching *Modern Family*. He also enjoys playing tennis and skiing. Resistance and flexibility training are newer focuses for him. He understands the role of exercise and massage in maintaining a full range of motion.

By 7:30 a.m., Maddie is usually up and comes down to say good morning. Jeffrey turns his attention to the back-to-back Zoom calls stacked for the remainder of his morning only after enjoying getting her ready for school.

For a mid-morning snack, he fires up his Bluicer — a high-performance juicer — and enjoys a protein-rich, antioxidant power shake consisting of blueberries, strawberries, blackberries, bananas, pineapple, melon, apples, oranges, tomatoes, kale, spinach, beets, carrots, celery, hemp, flaxseed, and a scoop of protein powder. The shake helps him carry a high energy level through the day.

By 11 a.m., the incoming email traffic starts to build for Jeffrey, and this has a weight to it. He compares managing his inbox to being a master juggler. At any point in the day, he may have a dozen different plates in the air. The odd one gets away from him, but not often. "I have ADHD, and distraction is hard for me." The complexity of the deals in Jeffrey's world have sharpened his management skills, allowing him to effectively nurture a very dynamic daily to-do list. Follow-ups with multiple players on each file is the norm. A derailing distraction lurks around every corner. To ease this burden, Jeffrey relies on systems and structure to his process, right down to the particular placement of what goes where on his desk. Finding order in the chaos assists in his execution and lessens his anxiety linked to ADHD. Jeffrey recognizes the drop in his performance when he attempts to multi-task too many complex demands at the same time and will actively manage his daily to-do list to narrow his focus and stay on track.

Lunch consists of a salad. He will dress-up a salad pack from his local grocery store with some additional vegetables and sliced chicken and slowly graze on it into the early afternoon while on Zoom calls with his video disabled.

By 3 p.m., fatigue appears. "By mid-afternoon, I've been working on several opportunities. I'll have five big wins, three losses, and feel drained." There is no caffeine consumed after mid-afternoon. This is one of Jeffrey's hard-and-fast rules, and it required him to give up Diet Coke, which was not a small thing. "A lot of high-functioning alcoholics drink Diet Coke because it gives us our caffeine, and it's got a great buzz, but it's just so bad for your belly."

Between 3 and 5 p.m., he prioritizes his outstanding to-do list and continues with conference calls. Finding time in the afternoon for recalibration helps him stay focused on which plates he still has in the air and which ones he can set down.

At 7 p.m., the day is done, and he turns his full attention to the family. "We put on our Sonos system throughout the house and play piano music, light candles, and sit down together and have a beautiful dinner." Phones are off and computers are powered down. A skilled chef, Larry is in charge of planning and making dinners. They eat with their health top of mind. Most meals feature fish or chicken garnished with a rainbow of colorful, fresh vegetables. Maddie, at age five, loves it all. Dessert is limited to a small piece of sea salt dark chocolate. Despite this treat being one of Jeffrey's favorites, he takes pride in making a single chocolate bar last three to four days.

Dinner is followed by family time and bedtime stories with Maddie. This routine has become very special. It is also a bookend to Jeffrey's morning ritual and helps him take the edge off any anxiety lingering from the day. Setting boundaries — some of them virtual, some of them in his day-to-day rituals surrounding mealtime, workout schedules, conference calls, or time to decompress — protects Jeffrey from the pressure created by incoming demands. This is the key to Jeffrey's formula, and without it he feels scattered.

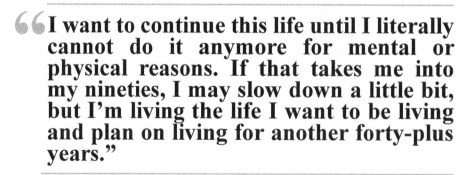

"I want to continue this life until I literally cannot do it anymore for mental or physical reasons. If that takes me into my nineties, I may slow down a little bit, but I'm living the life I want to be living and plan on living for another forty-plus years."

He is predictably in bed by 10:30 p.m. — and strives for seven hours of sleep a night. For years, he failed to see the worth of sleep, rest, and recovery and as a younger man, was determined "not to waste thirty years of my life sleeping." When sleep is evasive, he can usually put together five hours and get by. Recognizing that this is not enough, Jeffrey is prioritizing sleep as one area of his life that he needs to improve. There is no device use in the bedroom. His pre-bed ritual is designed to calm his mind and prepare him for rest. If he struggles, he literally counts sheep.

SELF-CARE REFLECTION #13

The pandemic presented many people with more time for family and self-care. Did you establish any healthy rituals during this time that you intend to bring forward? Did you develop any bad habits that need to be dropped? Make a list of both in your journal.

ADVERSITY AND PURPOSE

Jeffrey has found his happy place. His work is his passion and his play. His family is his love.

He credits his struggles for the love and success he has cultivated in his life. Dealing with adversity allowed him to develop the confidence he lacked in the early days of his career, tighten up his inner circle, and get sober.

Jeffrey would never push his formula or approach to life, business, or success on anyone else. He knows better than most the blood, sweat, and tears that must be invested if you are to discover your purpose. Gratitude is his guiding force now. Every morning, he greets his formula with the greatest respect and appreciation. Here is a man who has lived large at the top of his industry and yet appears to be only just now catching his stride. His talent and influence are legendary, but it seems that Jeffrey's best work still awaits him.

The **common thread** to their eating habits lies in their deliberate use of diet to achieve a desired energy and performance outcome. Each one eats with this intention, but it is important to highlight that they all enjoy food and drink. **Not one expressed feelings of deprivation linked to their diet.**

CONSUME HEALTHY FUEL

7 WELLNESS RITUALS
FOR HEALTH, STRENGTH & HOPE

WELLNESS RITUAL #2: THE SCIENCE

> The science is clear — our well-being and overall quality of life depend on making good food choices and understanding how, when, and why we eat alters our energy and performance. Choosing to consume healthy, nutrient-dense foods and learning to eat in response to hunger within a restricted window of time allows the body to mobilize calories with remarkable efficiency and minimal inflammation. This Wellness Ritual translates into improved energy, reduced risk of disease, and perhaps even greater longevity.

*Y*ou will not find a one-size-fits-all super diet in the pages that follow. I wish it were that simple. It is not. We would do well to stop searching for a single solution. Our individual needs are far too unique. I would suggest approaching anyone who states otherwise with caution. Food offers many powerful medicinal properties, but promises of cure-all elixirs and magical diets are as plentiful as snake oil.

The influence of our diet choices, the local resources that may or may not be available to us, our different cultural preferences and experiences, our emotional state, our varied medical histories and nuanced metabolic differences, the biodiversity and health of the microorganisms that live in our gut, and the responsive expression of our genetic code all add to our variability and the complexity of healthy eating. Nevertheless, fueling our bodies well is an essential life skill. So much so that you'd think we'd have had a better grip on it before space tourism became available. Sadly, this is not the case. The *2017 Global Burden of Disease* (GBD) study revealed that poor diet causes more deaths than all other risk factors — more than smoking, high blood pressure, or alcohol consumption.[1] We are sowing what we reap — prioritizing convenience over healthy meals prepared at home and completely disregarding our individual needs.

Registered Dietitian and *Mentor* Jen Sygo explains, "You have to put in the work to discover what diet works best for you. There is no one script. There is no shortcut."

Welcome to Wellness Ritual #2: Consume Healthy Fuel. What we are going to do first is explore your nutritional habits and from there, build a framework to support healthy eating.

EATING WELL IS A LIFELONG JOURNEY

The first step is to recognize patterns in the choices you are making, expand on what is working, and begin pivoting away from what isn't. Be thoughtful and patient with this process. Our bodies tend to respond best to incremental changes. The twenty-one mentors remind us that learning to eat well is a lifelong journey that requires daily attention. As we age and the needs and responses of our bodies change, so must our fueling strategy. This Wellness Ritual must remain dynamic. Craft your formula to the principles highlighted in this chapter, and you will advance your biological potential.

Our mentors all come to the dinner table with a different approach to fueling. Some eat a whole-foods, plant-based diet while others eat steak regularly. Some consume the bulk of their calories early in the day by kick-starting their mornings with a hearty breakfast, and others go light on breakfast and lean on the boosts offered by healthy snacks to energize the back half of their day. There are coffee drinkers, tea drinkers, water lovers, smoothie makers, and fine-wine experts in the group. There are supplement users, sweet-tooth chasers, and sugar-avoiders. Some employ intermittent fasting or restrict their calorie intake windows; others eat five to six smaller meals a day. Their choices are diverse and seldom overlap.

The common thread to their eating habits lies in their deliberate use of diet to achieve a desired energy and performance outcome. Each one eats with this intention, but it is important to highlight that they all enjoy food and drink. Not one expressed feelings of deprivation linked to their diet.

BUILDING A SENIOR EXECUTIVE TEAM OF HEALTH PROFESSIONALS TO SUPPORT YOUR FORMULA

When selecting a clinician to join your team, do your homework first. Think of these professionals as the senior VPs of your company. One of them should have expertise in clinical nutrition. As CEO, start with a short list of referrals from trusted sources. Review the clinician's experience prior to interviewing them for the job. Look for clinicians who are gifted listeners who practice through the lens of an evidence-based, patient-centered model of care. Working with the right team of clinicians who are open to collaboration will advance your health further and help you avoid false starts and unnecessary frustration. There will be times when you need an extra kick of motivation. Empower your senior VPs to hold you accountable. Once you establish your health targets, facilitate your team's communication to develop a customized treatment strategy.

THE CHOICES WE MAKE

What you eat, when you eat, and why you eat are all critical choices that profoundly impact your state of health and well-being. Unfortunately, far too many relinquish this power and bounce from one fad diet to another, destroying their relationship with the healing power of food along the way. Our emotional response will hijack the best intentions if a healthy eating strategy isn't structured with support, discipline, and authority. Turning a blind eye to the cumulative consequences of poor nutritional choices is dangerous. The commanding biological force you are looking to control has a dark side too.

Statistics Canada reports that two out of three adults in Canada are overweight or obese.[2,3] This group is at higher risk of heart disease, high blood pressure, type 2 diabetes, stroke, gallbladder disease, osteoarthritis, sleep apnea, cancer, and mental health problems.[3] Many organizations, including the Canadian Medical Association and the World Health Organization, now consider obesity a chronic disease. It is estimated that one in ten premature deaths among Canadian adults aged twenty to sixty-four is directly related to obesity.[4] Take a good look at the people walking next to you in the mall or grocery store. As shocking as these statistics seem, you will see that they are accurate. We are no longer alarmed by excess weight and have become complacent to it. The good news is that a different reality is available to you.

There may have been a season in your life when you could rock a mid-week, late business dinner that included a couple of pre-dinner cocktails, half a dozen tasty appetizers, a starter Caesar salad, a twelve-ounce peppercorn New York Striploin steak with a loaded baked potato, a glass or two of wine, and crème brûlée for dessert and still feel like you could perform well the next day. There may have been a season when the fast-food drive-thru was the only thing keeping you and your family alive, as night after night, you hurried home from work to grab your kids and get them to the ball diamond or hockey arena with minutes to spare. Full disclosure, I've done both. During my boys' baseball seasons, we were on a first-name basis with the local Subway restaurant staff. There are times that life rolls this way or our pace appears to present limited nutritious options. The goal of healthy eating is not one of perfection. This pursuit results in feelings of failure, shame, and misery. However, extended seasons of poor choices will shorten your life.

The desired outcome of healthy fueling is a consumption strategy that provides you with the energy to be the best version of yourself. In other words, how can you use food and drink as a therapeutic tool to intentionally elevate your health and performance and bring an end to self-sabotaging behavior? The number on your bathroom scale or photo of you in a bathing suit may have some influence, but for most, this influence is fleeting. In my experience, patients inspired by the healing potential of the body, who are armed with the current evidence and an understanding of how the body works, are the ones most likely to make meaningful, lasting changes.

Humans tend to make poor choices when "hangry" (bad-tempered or irritable due to hunger) or simply when they are ill-prepared and haven't given much thought to what, when, and why they need to eat. To avoid this pitfall, I would ask you to accept the following three principles of Consuming Healthy Fuel. If these principles do not sit well with you, I suggest you voice your opposition to the senior VPs on your healthcare team and clear up any misinformation or old baggage you may still be carrying from days past. The Consume Healthy Fuel Wellness Ritual requires a discipline that leaves zero room for doubt.

THREE PRINCIPLES OF CONSUMING HEALTHY FUEL

1. A healthy diet will add quality years to your life. An unhealthy diet will shorten it.
2. Healthy fuel today will give you more energy to bring to tomorrow.
3. You are what you eat, when you eat, and why you eat.

Healthy Fuel Principle #1:

A healthy diet will add quality years to your life. An unhealthy diet will shorten it.

The foods we eat get broken down into many active substances that interact with receptors found in our body. This chemical exchange defines our performance. Nutritional habits, healthy or not, drive a trend line at these receptors, which will lead to one of two possible outcomes: balance and homeostasis or instability and chronic inflammation. While more research is needed to fully understand the impact of diet on our inflammatory response and the onset of disease, it is clear that a dangerous inflammatory firestorm results when a North American, calorie-rich diet is combined with overconsumption and a sedentary lifestyle. Chronic inflammation appears to be the body's defensive response to this assault. In contrast, a healthy diet provides the essential ingredients required to alter your internal chemistry and extinguish the flame of chronic inflammation.

To be clear, inflammation is essential to our survival. It plays a vital role in our immune system's response to infection and injury.[5] When exposed to a virus, bacterial pathogen, or a chemical toxin or when we suffer from a physical injury, inflammation signals the immune system to attack invaders and launch into its well-rehearsed tissue repair and healing processes. With the threat neutralized, the attack is called off and things return to normal. In the short term, this process is life-saving.

However, sometimes our inflammatory activation lingers, persisting long past an acute response, which triggers chronic inflammation. In this state, our immune system can begin to target healthy cells for destruction. This is bad news biologically and signals the start of illness for many. Research shows that chronic inflammation can damage healthy cells and prevent our vital organs from working as well as they should, making us more susceptible to cancer, heart disease, diabetes, arthritis, depression, and Alzheimer's as a result.[6,7] It is also known to cause muscle and joint pain.

Think of your inflammatory and immune response like a campfire. The fire brings light, warmth, comfort, and the ability to cook dinner, but left unattended or smoldering after you've left the campsite, it holds the power to burn the forest to the ground.

Dr. David Sinclair, a leading world authority on genetics and longevity, Harvard professor, and author of *The New York Times* bestseller titled *Lifespan: Why We Age*

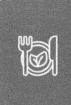

— and Why We Don't Have To declares aging a treatable disease. Research coming out of Sinclair's lab explores the key hallmarks of aging and the diseases that come with it, including altered intercellular communication and the production of inflammatory molecules perpetuated through poor lifestyle choices. Sinclair states that "inflammation is a driving force in the development of age-related diseases." In *Lifespan,* he presents an argument that "no matter who you are, where you live, how old you are, and how much you earn, you can engage your longevity genes, starting right now."[8] For those who do, Sinclair sees a future where individuals will routinely live — and live well — well past their one hundredth birthday.

Studies indicate that a well-balanced diet helps to keep our immune system and inflammatory response attentive and finely tuned, meaning that it turns on and off at appropriate times, while an unhealthy diet stokes a low-grade inflammatory response.[9,10]

A review published by Harvard Medical School titled *Can Diet Heal Chronic Pain?* presents evidence that the immune system reacts to an unhealthy diet in much the same way it would respond to a bacterial infection.[11] The specific mechanisms behind this triggered response remain unknown; however, some evidence suggests that deficiencies in various micronutrients — such as zinc, selenium, iron, folic acid, and vitamins A, B6, C, and E — may alter immune function. The review further highlights the strong scientific evidence that foods rich in antioxidants known as polyphenols, which are protective micronutrients found in plants, can have a powerful anti-inflammatory effect that helps reduce chronic pain.[10,11]

Nutrient-dense polyphenol compounds, considered "lifespan essentials," have the power to prevent or reverse damage to cells caused by aging, the environment, and lifestyle.[8,11,12] Research shows that polyphenols promote healthy bacteria growth in our gut, which supports digestion and is essential to our immune system function.[13] People with diets rich in polyphenols (more than 650 milligrams per day) enjoy longer lives, improved heart health, reduced chronic inflammation, improved immunity, and lowered risk of diabetes and cancer.[8,12,13]

These health boosting micronutrients are easily added to your diet from foods like fruits, vegetables, teas, and spices. There are over 8,000 different types of polyphenols. These eight foods have the highest polyphenol content per serving:[13] *See figure 2.1.*

Dr. Rangan Chatterjee, popular television host of the BBC One series *Doctor in the House* and author of *Feel Great, Lose Weight: Simple Habits for Lasting and Sustainable Weight Loss*,[26] offers a simple, creative way to ensure you are consuming a diet rich in polyphenols. He recommends we "eat the rainbow" by literally using a rainbow chart and aiming to eat at least one fruit or vegetable for each color of the rainbow every day.

Dr. Dean Ornish, renowned American physician, researcher, and champion of lifestyle medicine, has demonstrated the powerful impact diet and lifestyle practices can have on reversing chronic disease. His scientifically proven lifestyle program centers around a diet that features low-fat, plant-based foods and limits animal products, refined carbohydrates, high-fat foods, and processed ingredients.

Here are some of the milestone results of Ornish's work:

- A randomized, controlled trial showed, for the first time, that even severe heart disease could be reversed by the Ornish Program, as demonstrated by reductions (reversal) in coronary artery blockages after one year.
- A randomized controlled trial showed, for the first time, that the progression of early stage prostate cancer may be stopped or even reversed by the Ornish Program after one year.
- After only three months on the Ornish Program, over 500 genes were changed among participants. Genes that enhance health were turned on; genes that promote heart disease, prostate cancer, breast cancer, and colon cancer were turned off.
- The Ornish Program increased the length of telomeres, the ends of chromosomes that control aging and how long we live. As telomeres get longer, our lives get longer. This is the first study showing that any intervention may lengthen telomeres.

Visit *ornish.com* for more information.

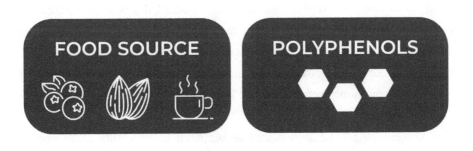

Berries	Polyphenols delivered per half-cup serving: Elderberries 870 mg; blueberries 535 mg; blackcurrant 485 mg; blackberries, raspberries, and strawberries 160 mg
Herbs and Spices	Polyphenols per ounce: Cloves 542 mg; peppermint 427 mg; star anise 195 mg; oregano, celery seed, sage, rosemary, and thyme ~30 mg
Cocoa	Polyphenols per tablespoon: Cocoa powder 516 mg; dark chocolate 249 mg
Nuts	Most nuts contain polyphenols. The highest content is found in chestnuts. Polyphenols per ounce: Chestnuts 347 mg; hazelnuts and pecans 140 mg; almonds 53 mg
Flaxseed	229 mg per tablespoon
Vegetables	Most vegetables contain polyphenols. The highest content is found in artichokes. Polyphenols per cup: Artichoke 260 mg; red onion 168 mg; spinach 40 mg
Olives	Polyphenols per 20 grams (roughly 5 olives): Black olives 113 mg; green olives 70 mg
Coffee; black, green, or ginger tea	~35 mg per cup

Figure 2.1. Source: webmd.com/diet/foods-high-in-polyphenols

Research like this turns Sinclair and other longevity experts toward populations applying these findings. Writer Dan Buettner sparked the world's interest in five regions where humans live much longer than the average and enjoy greater health. These so-called Blue Zones include Okinawa, Japan; Sardinia, Italy; Nicoya, Costa Rica; Ikaria, Greece; and Loma Linda, California. The diets from centenarians living in these areas, commonly referred to as "longevity diets," have naturally become a key point of interest.

The centenarians have shown us that we need to be eating more vegetables, legumes, and whole grains while consuming less meat, dairy products, and sugar. They eat local and seasonally available produce, avoid processed foods, and share their meal times with loved ones in social settings. Their guidance may appear simple, but it is difficult to argue with the results.

The Mediterranean diet has also been widely studied and recognized for its positive influence on health, including weight loss, heart and brain health, cancer prevention, and diabetes prevention and control.[12] It is based on the consumption of high quantities of vegetables, fruits, cereals, legumes, nuts, fish, and olive oil as the central culinary fat.[11,12]

Several trials have shown that a Mediterranean dietary pattern is associated with reduced metabolic and cardiovascular risk and lower levels of blood serum markers of inflammation.[12] The therapeutic antioxidant and anti-inflammatory properties of the diet's featured foods prevent and counteract DNA damage, slowing down the development of cancer.[12]

In my practice, I've worked with patients who have found relief from migraines and muscle and joint pain and have lost weight following a variety of different diets, including longevity and Mediterranean diets as well as a host of low-carb, high-protein, low-fat diets. Some benefit from the structure of counting calories; others find this practice sparks feelings of deprivation and guilt. For every weight-loss success story, there is a story of struggle and defeat — same diet, opposite outcome. This low level of success leads to diet confusion, a lack of meaningful action, and a return to the old habits responsible for poor health in the first place. There is comfort in a familiar menu. However, within this confusion and the copious amounts of nutritional research, there are guideposts to healthy eating that consistently produce favorable results.

Your Fuel Strategy

A number of mentors profiled in this book share their struggles in developing a healthy relationship with food. They highlight the need for patience and the importance of trial and error when setting this ritual. Life experience, clinical assistance, and the determination to live and play at or near peak levels helps them find success. Their rituals invite variety and prioritize the enjoyment of eating within a structure that keeps them at their best. Here are the guideposts they follow.

Anti-inflammatory Foods to Consume

To fight inflammation, choose whole, unprocessed foods with no added sugar at every opportunity. By making this choice, you will be ingesting a higher concentration of natural antioxidants and polyphenols. This list included fruits, vegetables, whole grains, legumes (beans, lentils), fish, poultry, nuts, seeds, a little bit of low-fat dairy, and olive oil. Nazima Qureshi, a gifted registered dietitian I collaborate with, promotes diets rich in antioxidants found in brightly colored fruits and vegetables, like blueberries, cooked tomatoes, carrots, squash, and broccoli. Qureshi states, "They act to neutralize the negative effects of unstable molecules called free radicals, which damage cells and promote disease." Spices like turmeric, cinnamon, ginger, garlic, cayenne, and black pepper have also been shown to have anti-inflammatory properties.[6]

Consuming more of the following foods will also help to fight inflammation:

- **Fiber:** Food sources include fruits and vegetables, especially legumes and whole grains, such as barley, oats, and bran.
- **Omega-3 Fatty Acids:** Food sources include fish (salmon, mackerel, sardines, tuna); vegetable oils (flaxseed and canola); walnuts; flaxseeds; and leafy green vegetables (spinach and kale). Omega-3 fats have also been shown to improve mood, memory, and cognitive function.
- **Polyphenols (Plant Chemicals):** Food sources include berries, dark chocolate, tea, apples, citrus, onions, soybeans, coffee, and red wine (see Polyphenol chart above).

- **Unsaturated Fats:** Food sources include almonds, pecans, walnuts, flaxseeds, pumpkin and sesame seeds, and plant oils (olive, peanut, canola). Nuts are a good source of fiber, protein, and essential fatty acids but do deliver a higher calorie punch, so moderate portions.

Foods to Avoid

When possible, take a pass on pre-packaged foods. It will help dial back inflammation. Pre-packaged, heavily processed foods are convenient, taste good, and are aggressively marketed to attract our attention, but they are also largely unhealthy and pro-inflammatory. Loaded with sugar, sodium, and unhealthy fats, highly processed foods come at too high a cost.

Qureshi advises her patients to start in the kitchen and transform their pantry, freezer, and fridge so that the foods there are going to provide more nutritional value. Replace over-processed foods with those high in nutrients. Remove the temptation. Microwaveable dinners, hot dogs, chicken nuggets, dehydrated soups, packaged baked goods, sugary cereals, processed meats, biscuits, and sauces will not support your health.[6] Stock your shelves with foods that haven't been modified. Mac'n'cheese out of the box is considered heavily processed. The powdered cheese is chemically altered with flavors and additives. Making healthier choices at each meal gets easier when you start thinking about your fuel in terms of inflammation. Will this meal provide me with the energy I need today, or will it dial-up my inflammatory response?

A study commissioned by the Heart & Stroke Foundation of Canada reveals that nearly half of our daily calories come from ultra-processed foods.[10] According to Dr. Jean-Claude Moubarac, assistant professor at the University of Montreal and author of the report, Canadians are consuming far too much packaged sweets, cookies, salty snacks, margarine, sauces, reconstituted meat, burgers, pizza, and sugary beverages.[10] These foods are nutritionally poor choices, high in salt, sugar, and unhealthy fat and low in protein, fiber, minerals, and vitamins.

Here are some additional anti-inflammatory guideposts:

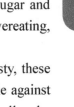

- **Avoid refined carbohydrates.** This group includes white bread, white pasta, and white rice as well as pastries and many sugary breakfast cereals. These foods are stripped of almost all their goodness, so with little fiber, vitamins, and minerals to offer, they are considered empty calories. They also tend to have a high glycemic index that will result in a rapid spike in your blood sugar and insulin response after consumption. Refined carbs are also linked to overeating, risk of obesity, and a laundry list of diseases you want no part of.[11,12]

- **Avoid fried foods.** Just about anything can be deep fried. While tasty, these foods are high in calories and trans fats, which tip the cholesterol scale against you and are hard on your heart. A few years back, a deep-fried butter ball and a bacon-wrapped deep-fried Mars bar were feature menu options at the Canadian National Exhibit (CNE) in Toronto. Comical, but also deadly.

- **Avoid high-sugar beverages.** Soda, pop, most fruit juices, lemonade, sweetened powdered drinks, as well as sports and energy drinks should be eliminated from your regular diet or significantly limited. Drink water instead. There are close to forty grams of sugar in a twelve-ounce can of soda. This is roughly equivalent to ten teaspoons or eighteen packets of sugar. That is as outrageous as it sounds. As for sports beverages, they are designed to provide pro-athletes with carbohydrates, electrolytes, and fluid during high-intensity workouts lasting longer than an hour. For the rest of us, they provide unnecessary calories and sugar. Remember the intention behind your choices. Centenarians limit sugar intake and drink water instead.

- **Avoid processed meats.** Bacon, hot dogs, sausages, lunch meat — meat that has been processed in some way to preserve or flavor it — is bad for your health, according to experts.[14] Frank Hu, a Fredrick J. Stare Professor of Nutrition and Epidemiology and Chair of the Department of Nutrition at Harvard T.H. Chan School of Public Health, suggests that eating a small amount of processed meat occasionally, such as once or twice a month, is unlikely to significantly harm health. However, he also warns that "the current evidence suggests the higher your intake of processed meat, the higher the risk of chronic diseases and mortality."[14]

- **Reduce Unhealthy Fats.** Not all fat is created equal. Saturated and trans fats are the ones to try to limit. Most of the foods that contain these types of fats are solid at room temperature, like butter, margarine, shortening, and beef or pork fat. These food sources can contribute to elevated LDL (bad) cholesterol levels, suppress HDL (good) cholesterol, and increase risk of inflammation in the body.

HEALTHY FUEL PRINCIPLE #2:

Healthy fuel today will give you more energy to bring to tomorrow

Energy is something we all want more of. To have it is to feel youthful, confident, resilient, and healthy. Possessing it can give you an edge and at times, the feeling of momentum that tips life to your advantage. On the flip side, struggling to maintain or find it can be frustrating and lead to poor choices.

In an article titled "Energy, and How to Get It" published in the November 8, 2021 issue of *The New Yorker*, journalist Nick Paumgarten describes energy as a "misnomer, or at least an elision."[15] He refers to what we commonly call our energy as our "metabolic mood," which reflects our perception of our metabolism and the efficiency with which we convert energy to work. "Energy is biochemical and psychophysical, vaguely delineated, widely misunderstood, elusive as grace. You know it when you got it, and even more when you don't."[15] The quality of your fuel will profoundly impact which group you find yourself in — the haves or the have nots.

The nutrient-dense choices listed in the previous section will not only prolong your life by reducing chronic inflammation but will also boost energy, adding quality to your years. Healthy fuel provides your cells with the nutrients to maintain optimal cellular energy and a healthy metabolism. This translates into more energy.

As you will discover as you read this book, our mentors employ the following energy boosting nutritional strategies:

- **Break away from eating only two or three meals a day.** If boosting energy is one of your top priorities, try eating five to six small meals a day. Our brains need a steady fuel source, and some people are more sensitive to blood-sugar drops than others. By introducing strategic mid-morning and mid-afternoon snacks and consuming smaller meals at lunch and dinner, you will experience an energy boost and avoid late-afternoon energy dips. Have real-food snack options readily accessible. Real food is the best source of real energy. Good snack options include a combination of complex carbohydrates with protein and fat. Fiber, protein, and fat will slow down the release of sugar into your blood, which helps to maintain energy levels. Try mixing nuts and dried fruit, or a small serving of Greek yogurt with natural granola, or sliced veggies dipped in hummus. A small Ziploc bag of walnuts and blueberries is my favorite go-to. Note: This technique takes self-control. To keep your body weight from increasing, you will need to reduce your lunch and dinner portions.

- **Avoid weight-loss crash diets.** Poor nutrition or severe calorie restricted diets without medical supervision can cause fatigue and a sluggish metabolism.[16] In Wellness Ritual #3, we will take a closer look at weight management, but a diet that results in weight loss any faster than one to two pounds a week will be difficult to maintain.

- **Keep alcohol consumption within recommended limits.** The risk of alcohol-induced ailments increases with the number of drinks you consume per week. In January 2023, the Canadian Centre on Substance Use and Addiction published updated alcohol consumption guidelines. The guidelines suggest that drinking any amount of alcohol increases your risk of adverse health effects, including an increased risk of several types of cancer. One to two drinks per week represents a low risk, three to six, a moderate risk, and seven or more per week, a high risk. Note: Alcohol consumed before bed will interrupt your REM sleep.

- **Stay well hydrated.** This is one of the easiest ways to maintain energy levels. The body needs plenty of water to function optimally. Fatigue is one of the early signs of dehydration. Water is the main component of our blood. Nutrients and waste products are carried to and from our cells through our blood stream. Keep a reusable water bottle close and take a sip every hour.

- **Avoid artificial energy boosters.** Super-caffeinated energy drinks will give you a short burst, but they are also linked to obesity, high blood pressure, and cardiovascular issues. Large amounts of caffeine may cause serious heart and blood vessel problems and have also been linked with anxiety, sleep disturbances, digestive problems, and dehydration.[17] Caffeine ingested via a morning cup of coffee or tea or through a piece of dark chocolate has health benefits, but keep your consumption reasonable (less than 400 milligrams of caffeine a day) and enjoy it in the front half of your day.

- **Drink herbal tea.** The antioxidants and vitamins found in herbal teas can protect against oxidative stress, boost immune function, and lower the risk of chronic disease.[18] Talk to your healthcare team about the medicinal properties of chamomile, ginger, black, and green teas.

- **Eat breakfast.** Priming your body with healthy calories in the morning will help keep you alert and satisfied until your next meal. When you wake up, the blood sugar your body needs to move, think, and act is low. This first meal of the day replenishes your fuel stores, which helps fuel your metabolism as you start your day. Simple-carbohydrate-rich breakfasts are of no value. Eat a breakfast that is balanced in terms of protein, complex carbohydrates, and fat.

HEALTHY FUEL PRINCIPLE #3:

You are what you eat, when you eat, and why you eat.

The intimate relationship between health and diet is not a new concept. The first mention of the phrase "you are what you eat" came from the 1826 work of French author Anthelme Brillat-Savarin. He wrote: "Tell me what you eat, and I will tell you what you are."

What You Eat

The first two healthy fuel principles provide the ritual framework to establish what we need to be eating more — and less — of. Talk with your healthcare VPs about what healthy and energy-boosting foods to look for, and clear your fridge and kitchen of processed foods that will steal your health.

The foods we choose matter to the active and rather wonderful communities that live in our gut. Our gut's microbiome is made up of trillions of bacteria, fungi, parasites, and viruses. Collectively, they are considered a vital supportive organ that plays an essential role in our well-being.[19]

In a state of good health, the inhabitants of our microbiome coexist peacefully. We each possess a uniquely diverse collection of microorganisms that begins to take shape as an infant, during delivery in the birth canal, and through the mother's breast milk.[19] The first exposure depends solely on the species found in the mother. Later on, environmental exposures and diet can change our microbiome to be either beneficial to our health or place us at greater risk for disease.[19]

Increasing the fiber in your diet by consuming a wide variety of colorful vegetables, fruits, whole grains, and legumes keeps your microbiome happy and well fed and offers many downstream health perks. We lack the ability to digest dietary fiber and must rely on these microorganisms to complete the job for us. In doing so, they release Short Chain Fatty Acids (SCFA), which have a wide range of benefits, including the stimulation of immune cell activity, stabilization of blood sugar and cholesterol levels, and reduction of inflammation.[19] SCFA also help to lower the pH in the colon, which influences the type of microorganisms that can thrive in your gut, creating a welcoming environment for the "good" bugs to work their altruistic magic. The microbiome also aids with the production of vitamins and other essential nutrients. While more research is needed, we know that if the microbiome isn't healthy, then neither are you, so eat your fiber.

Dedicate an appropriate block of time with a qualified health professional to define your fuel needs — your "what" of healthy eating — with the microbiome in mind. Without high-quality calories, no matter how hard you practice the other six Wellness Rituals, you won't reach your best.

Why You Eat

Many patients struggle with a deep dive into why we eat, but it is a conversation that cannot be avoided. Our emotional connection with food represents a strong bond. We celebrate with food in good times and bad. Birthdays, anniversaries, graduations, promotions, or times of stress, fatigue, boredom, and heartache commonly feature food. Left unchecked, our emotional state yields a dominant influence over why and when we choose to eat. And this rarely occurs in response to hunger and the need for fuel.

In exploring why you eat, it is important to acknowledge that emotional eating is normal and enjoyable. The goal is not to set a rigid expectation of shutting this down and stripping away the enjoyment of eating. Research shows that punitive, restrictive diets lead only to feelings of deprivation, guilt, and more intense cravings.[20] Our mentors know how to celebrate and do so regularly with food and drink. The key is to develop a level of awareness and control over when you choose to eat for reasons other than hunger and when you choose to ignore your satiety signals. In these moments, you can extract important insights that will help you appreciate what is behind your cravings and the desire to eat when not queued by the need for fuel. Emotional triggers are only temporarily satisfied by eating and are more appropriately dealt with through the stress resiliency practices discussed in Wellness Ritual #6.

Identifying and understanding the source of the emotional states that bring you to the kitchen on the hunt for food will help you break away from behaviors that compromise your health. It is here that your team of health professionals can provide guidance because with practice, it is possible to read and measure the sensation of hunger. Set a hunger scale where only a 6 or higher out of 10 will require food intake. Have only healthful foods on hand. Desires to eat not connected to a need to re-fuel, whether in response to a stressful day or a desperate craving, can be addressed through a mindfulness exercise like yoga, meditation, a warm bath, or a short walk. In some cases, a glass of water or conversation with a good friend may be enough to help the craving pass.

When You Eat

The final variable to consider when building this ritual is when you eat. The window of time between your first and last meal of the day is known as your *daily eating duration*. Research suggests there are significant health benefits to keeping this window consistent and possibly restricted.

Most nutrition experts recommend starting the day with breakfast. Jumping into the day with an empty tank will lead to a sluggish start and set you up for bad choices later in the day when your hunger commands your attention. Aim to have breakfast within an hour of waking. If breakfast is not your thing, it is likely because you have ignored the morning hunger signals for too long, and your body knows not to expect morning fuel, so the signal has gone dormant. The choice to skip breakfast entirely will harm your performance. Your car will not run on an empty tank or drained battery, and neither will your body. We need fuel to start our day. By reintroducing a daily breakfast, your morning hunger cues will gradually return. Include a protein at this meal to give your morning energy a boost. Coffee shop donuts, croissants, muffins, and other baked goods do not make for a good breakfast and will only slow you down. If pressed for time in the morning, a protein smoothie to go is an option.

A small, healthy, mid-morning snack that includes protein and a carb will carry your energy into lunch, which ideally would follow four to five hours after breakfast. A mid-afternoon snack (similar to the morning snack) will carry you to dinner if you find your energy falling off in the afternoon. A well-timed afternoon snack provides another opportunity to bring calories forward in the day and reduce dinner portions even further, preventing overeating in the evening. Front loading calories and cutting back at dinner time has been shown to be an effective weight management strategy[21] and is a trend practiced by a number of our twenty-one mentors. Many keep a stash of healthy snacks with them in their car, briefcase, or small fridge in their office and snack to maintain their energy throughout the day.

A healthy schedule may look like this: breakfast at 7 a.m., mid-morning snack at 10 a.m., lunch between noon and 1 p.m., mid-afternoon snack around 3 p.m., and dinner before 7 p.m. Consistent predictability of your next meal influences your metabolism and how your body stores energy in a positive way — more on this in Wellness Ritual #3. Our circadian rhythm is signaled in part by our calorie consumption. Our bodies are best at digesting food when we are up and active and light is present. Wild swings in when you eat can throw this biological clock out of sync, negatively impacting numerous biological systems.[22]

Time-restricted eating, or limiting your food intake to a set number of hours each day by taking the schedule above and compressing it into a narrow window, is gaining popularity. Preliminary studies show this pattern of eating has a positive influence on health and longevity and may improve metabolism and cardiovascular health by optimizing our circadian rhythm.[21] In mice, time-restricted eating prevents and reverses obesity and diabetes, supports healing bacteria in the gut, and reduces inflammation.[22,23] Small studies in humans have tested daily eating durations of four to eleven hours a day and found that this strategy decreases blood pressure, improves blood sugar, and can help with weight management, energy levels, sleep, and appetite.[20,22,23] While the mechanism and effectiveness of this diet require more research, it appears fasting allows the body to focus on repair, improving the overall health of many organs, including the brain.[22-25]

In an effort to test the boundary of human longevity, Dr. Sinclair fasts for close to twenty hours a day, restricting his calorie consumption to a four-hour window. He skips breakfast and lunch and chooses to load the bulk of his calories at dinner. In his *Lifespan* podcast, he reviews how intermittent fasting with adequate nutrients has trained his liver to produce glucose at a consistent level, regulating his blood sugar and helping him avoid big swings in energy. He also reports an improved cognitive ability and a return of his twenty-year-old body thanks to this diet. His research is showing that fasting places the body in a state of adversity that alters the expression of our genes in favor of a longer life. While a twenty-hour daily fast will not be a realistic diet for most, Sinclair's research highlights the favorable biological response to time-restricted eating.

Dr. Rangan Chatterjee promotes the practice of keeping the consumption of all daily calories to a twelve-hour window to protect against the metabolic effects of diet-induced obesity. Meaning, if you have breakfast at 7 a.m., then you will want to have finished dinner by 7 p.m., providing your body with a full twelve-hour fast before your next meal.

There still isn't enough information to know which eating window is best. However, a consistent daily eating duration of twelve hours or fewer, the consumption of the bulk of calories in the earlier part of the day, and the avoidance of bedtime snacks appear to be good guideposts to adopt.

CHAPIN CLINICAL CORNER

The cellular damage caused by poor food choices is often hidden from view until the day it is not. And on that day, illness and disease can be well underway. You are less likely to be caught by this unwelcome surprise if you become an active observer of your body and its function. Smartphone apps make it easy to maintain a performance dashboard that tracks key health metrics. Body weight, body mass index, blood pressure, resting heart rate, fasting insulin levels, cholesterol profile, steps per day, and any noticeable changes in bowel or bladder function provide valuable insight over time and can be easily monitored without much effort, expense, or inconvenience.

It is worth emphasizing that what many patients consider to be a decline in health related to aging commonly has more to do with poor choices than with the advance of

INTERMITTENT FASTING:

INVOLVES REDUCING OR REFRAINING FROM CALORIE INTAKE FOR VARIOUS PERIODS OF TIME. THERE ARE NUMEROUS APPROACHES INCLUDING:

ALTERNATE-DAY FASTING:

COMPLETE FASTING (WATER ONLY) EVERY OTHER DAY.

ALTERNATE-DAY MODIFIED FASTING:

CONSUMING A CALORIE RESTRICTED DIET (25%) EVERY OTHER DAY.

PERIODIC FASTING:

COMPLETE FASTING (WATER ONLY) ONE DAY PER WEEK OR A FEW DAYS PER MONTH.

WHILE A FEW MENTORS SHARED THAT THEY HAD EXPERIMENTED WITH TIME-RESTRICTING EATING, NONE OF THEM REPORTED ADOPTING AN INTERMITTENT FASTING STRATEGY INTO THEIR FORMULA.

the clock. Watching the trend lines on your dashboard can help trigger an early warning bell, allowing more time to course-correct. Surviving the scare of a heart attack, stroke, or cancer diagnosis will spark urgency to change lifestyle practices, but there is no need to wait for that day.

Dr. Noah Litvak, a trusted naturopathic doctor in my inner circle who shares my passion for the medicinal properties of food, states that "the Standard American Diet (SAD) is typically considered inflammatory. Any dietary practice that reduces ultra-processed foods, added sugars, and saturated fats will have health benefits. Individuals have the power to reduce inflammation by focusing on eating more anti-inflammatory foods and less inflammatory foods, an approach that helps to promote microbiome health and support blood sugar regulation."

Nutrition experts will often ask their patients to complete a diet diary to reveal eating patterns and help patients identify emotional triggers and unhealthy behaviors. As a simple exercise, make a note of everything you eat and drink over the next two weeks. Record the "what, when, and why" before your first bite with complete honesty and zero judgment. A typical entry may read, "It is 12:15 p.m., and I am hungry (6.5 out of 10) and ready for lunch. I enjoyed a chicken salad, an apple, and a glass of water." Other entries may surprise you: "It is 11:15 p.m., and I am not hungry (2 out of 10) but am REALLY craving a scoop of ice cream. Enjoyed it at the time, then immediately felt guilty. Not worth it."

The message is to be a mindful eater and place a high value on the food choices you make in addition to *why* and *when* you eat. When tempted, make a healthy choice.

If you have been eating without a strategy designed to support your performance and longevity, you likely have picked up a few bad habits along the way. You may have also misplaced, forgotten, or never fully developed an appreciation for the influence of meal-time choices. Consumption that features fast food, refined sugars, unhealthy fats, and processed foods comes at a high cost. Dietary indifference is like playing Russian roulette with all but one chamber loaded. Find the urgency to set this ritual right. Remember, the goal is not perfection; there is no such thing. Connect with the three principles of healthy fueling, and your body will do the rest.

RITUAL ACTIVATION

As you look for opportunities to clean up your diet, be kind to yourself. Hold firm expectations, but keep eating fun. Bring variety to your choices. Deprivation will not work, so introduce changes slowly. When missteps happen, and they will, enjoy them in the moment and then move on. Carrying guilt forward is a waste of energy, and you are trying to win the long game. Reset at the next meal and then the next. By stacking good decisions and giving your body time and space to respond, your ritual will begin to take shape. As it does, you will be amazed by what happens next.

RITUAL TARGET:

Eat to fuel for the long game by exercising the discipline to make healthy food choices most of the time. Take these steps:

- **Keep a consumption diary.** For two weeks, track what, why, and when you eat.

- **Make an appointment with a nutrition expert.** Seek professional guidance to help you develop your ritual, incorporating all three principles of healthy fueling and a thorough review of your consumption diary.

- **Connect with your hunger scale before your first bite.** Begin to introduce dietary changes slowly.

- **Consume less sugar, and eat more foods from the ground and fewer sold in packages.**

- **Aim for variety.** The more color and variety in a meal, the better.

- **Remind yourself every day of the profound impact dietary choices have on your long-term health.**

IN SUMMARY

Fueling for success requires attention to what, when, and why you eat. The nutritional value of the foods in our diet runs on a spectrum. Try not to think of your diet as simply good or bad. Begin to actively choose to consume healthy, nutrient-dense foods and eat in response to hunger within a restricted window of time. This practice will allow your body to mobilize calories and minimize inflammation efficiently, which translates into improved energy, reduced disease risk, and perhaps greater longevity.

By stacking **good decisions** and giving your body time and space to respond, your ritual will begin to take shape. As it does, **you will be amazed by what happens next.**

MENTOR PROFILES

HERBIE KUHN
FRANCOIS OLIVIER
PATTIE LOVETT-REID

HERBIE KUHN

Public Address Announcer for the Toronto Raptors, Chaplain to the Toronto Argonauts, Toronto Raptors, and Athletics Canada

*T*chaikovsky's *1812 Overture* would be an appropriate soundtrack for Herbie Kuhn's life. A personal favorite of his, the piece opens gracefully and builds to a crescendo of cannon fire and brass fanfare. For Herbie, the musical masterpiece accurately mimics the emotional ebb and flow of life and captures the true excitement of living. Having served as the "voice" of the Toronto Raptors' home games since the team's inception in 1995, he knows a thing or two about excitement. However, not as well-known as his iconic voice is his role as team chaplain for the Raptors and the Toronto Argonauts. This lens provides Herbie with a unique perspective on what it takes to deliver peak performance with professional consistency.

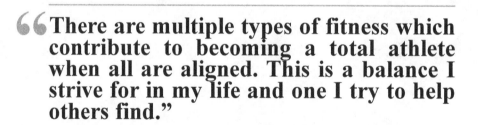

There are multiple types of fitness which contribute to becoming a total athlete when all are aligned. This is a balance I strive for in my life and one I try to help others find."

Herbie's ministry work through Athletes-in-Action (AIA) encourages athletes to adopt a holistic approach to health and become a "total athlete." Becoming a "total athlete" requires physical, emotional, mental, social and spiritual fitness. To only focus on physical fitness will undercut performance.

As host of AIA's podcast *Total Athlete*, Herbie interviews prominent professional and elite members of sport to discuss their journeys. "There are multiple types of fitness which contribute to becoming a total athlete when all are aligned. This is a balance I strive for in my life and one I try to help others find," he shares.

HERBIE'S CAUSE-AND-EFFECT FORMULA

Herbie considers his ministry a privilege and a tremendous responsibility. Helping a young pro athlete appreciate the many dimensions that impact individual and team performance is serious work. He begins by building trust with the athletes. The common denominator at this level is the desire to win. Herbie appeals to this shared priority, drawing attention to the cause-and-effect relationship of the decisions players make in preparation for game day. "My encouragement to any of my athletes is to get them to understand that if they are lacking in terms of emotional stability or spiritual fitness, or making poor social choices, that when they line up across from their opponent, they will not be at their best. Simply getting an athlete to see the direct effect people in their inner circle have on their health and performance can be very powerful." For some players, the light goes on after a single conversation with Herbie. For others, the conversation may take an entire season to complete. Herbie himself is blessed with many talents. It appears patience and holding up a mirror are two of them.

Players are drawn to Herbie. He brings all of the characteristics one would expect from a chaplain who ministers to up-and-coming and pro athletes. He is professional, supportive, and nurturing. But he is also real. It is this authenticity that endears him to his community. Bear Woods, Grey Cup Champion and CFL All-Star linebacker, shares that "Within professional football, there are highs and lows, successes and failures, wins and losses that are experienced daily, just like in life. Herbie's guidance and challenging encouragement through the teaching of Biblical truths maximized my personal preparation to fight these daily battles mentally, emotionally, physically, and most importantly, spiritually."

When former NBA player Anthony Parker was asked about Herbie's influence on his career, he offered, "There is so much pressure to consistently perform at your best in professional sports. In addition, there are the push and pulls of everyday life added to these demands. Chapel and Bible study with Herbie provided me with the daily peace of mind and focus I required to not only perform at the highest level, but to have an impact on all those who witnessed it."

HERBIE OWNS UP TO HIS OWN TRUTH

Herbie openly shares his stumbles in life, as gifted mentors are inclined to do. Missteps present excellent teaching opportunities.

Sharing drops an athlete's guard and makes Herbie more relatable. He holds himself to the same standard that he asks his athletes to strive toward and makes no attempt to hide from the truth of his habits.

> **I would never pretend to have it all figured out. I still have a pulse, so my life is still a work in progress too."**

In the spring of 2020, Herbie found himself practicing habits that had led him down a path further from his definition of a "total athlete" than he had ever been. He was not living a balanced life, and his health was paying the price. His weight had crept up to 236 pounds, and back pain stood firmly between him and his ability to play with his son. "At the time, we had just brought a new puppy home. I remember having to stop to catch my breath as I walked the dog around the block." As a former athlete, strength, balance, and power had always come easily to Herbie. Suddenly, bending down to tie up his shoes or throwing a football to his son in the backyard tested his limits. "I remember thinking to myself, 'This is absolutely ridiculous. There is no excuse or need for me to continue to live like this. I need to change physically, mentally, and emotionally.'"

In the spring of 2020, he recalls life feeling "draining" and "life sucking." Independent of the pandemic, the disappointment he felt in himself and the impact his declining health was starting to have on his performance had become a tremendous burden to carry. His physical, emotional, and mental energy to fulfill his ministry's requirements and day-to-day responsibilities was waning. In his chaplaincy, he needed to bring his A-game to every performance. After years of holding up the mirror for others, it was time for him to take a look in the mirror too. How could he possibly mentor athletes toward the balanced life of a "total athlete" if he himself could not find the motivation to do so? This realization hit Herbie the hardest, hurting his confidence and undermining his authenticity. "When you are serving athletes, you want to be able to say, 'I can empathize with what you are going through.' At this point in my life, I wasn't able to do that — at least not in the present."

In 2012, he fell into a similar trap and was diagnosed with clinical depression. He had to shut everything down, from his announcing and preaching to his email inbox for some time. His psychiatrist at the time helped him recognize his tendency to redline. The extent of his generosity and kindness left him exposed to burnout. With a heart too big for his chest, he had poured every ounce of energy he could muster into his familial and professional commitments. Exhausted, he hit the wall. In his recovery, he became more aware of his personal tachometer. His working speed was too fast, and his formula did not appropriately account for the rest and recovery he needed to perform at his best.

SELF-CARE REFLECTION #14

Herbie's kind heart left him vulnerable as he continued to prioritize the needs of others ahead of his well-being. Recognizing he was falling short of the "total athlete" standard that he encourages his athletes to strive for was a defining moment in his life.In crafting your own formula for health, strength, and hope, consider your physical, emotional, mental, social, and spiritual fitness. If you are feeling burnt out, explore how your daily choices are influencing each of these lifestyle factors.

HERBIE'S CALL TO ACTION

Recognizing that a similar pattern may be repeating itself, Herbie knew he needed to make significant changes in his life. The spark that ignited his action was found in the early days of the COVID-19 pandemic. Athletes-in-Action put out a challenge to mobilize the idle time afforded by the quarantine toward personal growth and development. For Herbie, it was the call to action he had been looking for. The path forward revealed itself shortly after, when a fundraising event was opened up to his church. His congregation was encouraged to log into Facebook simultaneously on a particular Saturday and together, complete a virtual warm up before heading outdoors for physical activity. Some members committed to a walk around the block, others a two-kilometer walk-jog, and a few, a half marathon. The distance did not matter. A community united in movement was the goal.

Herbie leans toward big dreams. His initial commitment to complete a five-kilometer walk quickly became ten kilometers. By stating this goal, it awoke the athlete within him. Slowly, he took the first few steps toward reclaiming his health. As Herbie describes it,

"There were times where I wondered what it would feel like if I started jogging for a few hundred meters. And so, I did." This was the beginning of an incredible transformation.

A week later, a copy of *Runner's World* magazine landed in Herbie's mailbox. The cover featured a running streak challenge, encouraging readers to run one mile every day for forty-one days. "When that *Runner's World* showed up, I remember thinking, 'There is no way. This is not for me. It's not happening.' As the week progressed, I kept glancing over at the cover of the magazine. It was like it was calling to me, like God was using each day to tell me, 'This is possible. Herbie, this is possible.'" Trusting his faith, he considered the challenge and worked up the courage to approach his family for support.

After establishing some ground rules with his wife, she wrapped Herbie and his new goal in a loving embrace.

He had a green light if he could agree with the following:

1. Promise to progress with caution.
2. Set realistic expectations of his body's performance and response to the challenge.
3. Treat himself kindly if an injury were to arise or he fell short of the forty-one-day target.

The next day, he ran a mile. Surviving, he did it again the following day, then again, and again. By the tenth day in a row, everything hurt, but he persisted. By the forty-second day, with his streak still alive, his attention had turned to his diet. In earnest, he was placing importance on making healthy choices and portion control. "Instead of having dessert every night, I'd maybe only have dessert twice a week. Instead of jumping into a second helping, I'd sit content with one and observe how far it could take me. I started swapping rice out for a salad."

Having been involved in sport and surrounded by world-class athletes most of his adult life, Herbie knows how to fuel the body. He also knows himself. To move through his world with authenticity, he needed to make lasting changes to his lifestyle. The strength of his spiritual fitness fueled this pursuit. A fad diet that quickly brought his weight down with unsustainable eating habits would leave him short of his goal to become a "total athlete." He committed to a common-sense framework for nutrition. "I do not deprive myself. I know that some trainers out there do not like to hear that, but it works for me. I am much smarter with my food choices now." As a Canadian with German heritage, he also had to address his love of beer. "I'll enjoy a single cold Ontario craft beer with my dinner four or five nights a week, and I have no problem with that." A second beer now represents an indulgence not worth the calories.

With the streak still alive and a renewed awareness of how and why he was eating, the bathroom scale's needle started to move for Herbie. The movement was slow but undeniably steady. Herbie's clothes began fitting differently. Suddenly, he could bounce up the stairs two at a time without a second thought. At fifty-two years of age, he felt a rejuvenation that brought energy to his family, athletes, and community.

On the morning Herbie and I sat down for an interview, he had just completed his 314th consecutive day running. Somewhere along the way, he increased his minimal daily distance to two kilometers. He has run over 1,300 kilometers during his streak and never missed a day. In a month, he is scheduled to complete a half marathon. He has lost over fifty pounds. Now, at 183 pounds, he sees himself once again as a "total athlete." His transformation is marked by "before and after" photos and a sticker from a new pair of pants that he pasted into his running journal. The sticker reads "Size Medium - 32 Width."

HERBIE'S FORMULA FOR HEALTH, STRENGTH & HOPE

HOW HERBIE MAINTAINS HIS HEALTH GAINS

Herbie's story now punches with even greater weight. There is no denying the importance of life experience in setting a winning formula."Even now, at fifty-two, I still don't feel like I have arrived yet. There are times when I continue to push the envelope too hard. That is my nature. The difference is that now I am much more aware of when I am redlining. I am finally mature enough to acknowledge that if I do push the boundaries for too long, that it will be to my detriment."

USE A HEALTH DASHBOARD

Herbie has worked very hard to get his health back. His body's response is a testament to the healing potential and capacity for biological forgiveness that is encoded in our DNA.

Determined to stay on track, his resiliency is now supported by four levels of protection. For starters, he keeps a close eye on his dashboard. "I have a built-in internal warning light that goes off when I know I am off-kilter." It is a feeling or quiet inner voice that he has learned to listen to for warning signs of danger. If his emotional response feels out of step or he is tempted with an unhealthy snack, he now takes a minute, disengages, and evaluates before moving forward. "Sometimes it is as easy as just taking an extra minute or two for a deep breath."

> **❝I am finally mature enough to acknowledge that if I do push the boundaries for too long, that it will be to my detriment."**

SET AN EXPIRY DATE ON NEGATIVITY

Herbie now gives any lingering negative emotions seeded in frustration or disappointment an expiry date. Turning back to the mirror, Herbie is actively practicing the advice he has provided athletes his whole career. "I give myself permission to feel the frustration, then move on, knowing I cannot perform at my peak if the voice in my head is telling me I screwed up. If you do not have a settled mind and a settled spirit — if you are not prepared to go out into life to have fun because you are so stressed out about what the result is going to be, you are not going to be at your best."

SELF-CARE REFLECTION #15

Setting an expiry date on negative self-talk is a powerful tool. As Herbie shared, "If you do not have a settled mind and a settled spirit, you are not going to be at your best." Begin listening to the track playing in your head. Are you kind to yourself? Create space in your reflections for gratitude. In your journal, list ten things in your life that bring you joy and fuel your purpose.

DRAW INSPIRATION FROM THOSE AROUND YOU AND FROM WITHIN

He draws energy from internal and external motivators. "A quick look back at pictures of me in the early spring of 2020, bursting out of my clothes, looking decidedly obese, is a great motivation to stay on purpose." Encouragement from friends, family, athletes, and members of his healthcare team also lift him up. "I appreciate the external motivation. They are all good and have their place to be sure, but at the end of the day, if the motivation does not come from within, there is no amount of external energy that will get you to your goal." To find internal motivation, Herbie turned to the strength of his faith. "I confess to you that I have not done a good job taking care of my one body. But I have decided I am now going to do that. My decision has a direct correlation with the husband and dad that I want to be. I am choosing to honor my Lord by being fit."

FIND SOLACE IN SOLITUDE

For Herbie to be at his best, he has to find peace in the quiet before the storm.

> 66 **Part of my process now is solo time and making sure that, amid all the noise, I find my quiet time."**

On Raptors game days, his pre-game ritual includes a peaceful dinner by himself. It provides him with twenty to thirty minutes of uninterrupted time to calm his mind. Then right before the lights go down and the player introductions begin, he drops his head in a prayer that expresses personal gratitude and asks for the players' health and protection. The excitement of the game then plays out through Herbie's iconic voice.

FIND INSPIRATION IN MUSIC

Herbie's final level of protection is found in music. The *1812 Overture* may be the theme song for his life, but Herbie also likes to rock out to the Canadian band Triumph. You will also find gospel artist Kirk Franklin, Christian hip hop artist TobyMac, and singer-songwriter Bob Seger at the top of his playlist. Music features as a big player in Herbie's formula. He calls it "part of my survival mechanism." Kicking back in a comfortable position and putting on his favorite playlist brings him tremendous joy and helps him unpack any emotional burden he may be carrying. Music unlocks a door that allows him to Play with Purpose (see Wellness Ritual #7).

Enjoying the best health of his life, Herbie has joined the Life-Starts-After-Fifty movement. He sees the world and his role in it with a renewed enthusiasm captured perfectly in the opening verse of one of his favorite Triumph hits, "Follow Your Heart," and like the lyric says, he will never stop running to keep his dreams alive.

FRANCOIS OLIVIER

Former President and CEO of Transcontinental

> ❝When you watch someone who is good at something, and you study what makes them good, you realize that it comes down to work. Most of the time, successful people do a lot more than their peers or competitors; they are excessive in their work, their training, and how they apply their smarts. It is very rare that they became good because they were lazy and lucky. Hard work is part of the success equation, but ultimately, human beings are looking to be happy, and to be happy is about living in equilibrium. Too much of one thing for too long is often not healthy.❞

These words were my introduction to Francois. He was at his chalet in Mont-Tremblant, Quebec, and I was in my clinic in Mississauga, Ontario. A first encounter can be awkward over video. This was not the case with Francois. He had just finished a run before our call and was fully present during our conversation. I was immediately drawn in by his wisdom and calm confidence. With the equanimity of a Grandmaster, he shared his views on success and leadership as we took a deep dive into his routine.

In his fifties, Francois is the former president and CEO of TC Transcontinental, a North American leader in flexible packaging, Canada's largest printer, and a French-language academic publisher. Under his guidance, TC Transcontinental's story has been one of innovation and transformation, and the company's success is a product of strong family values, entrepreneurial spirit, and long-term vision.

Francois holds a Bachelor of Science degree from McGill University and is a graduate of the Program for Management Development at Harvard Business School. He also serves on the boards of directors of CAE, The Conference Board of Canada, the Flexible Packaging Association, and the Montreal Heart Institute Foundation. Considered a force in his industry, Francois is a triple threat: handsome, thoughtful, and intelligent.

SUCCESS IS LIFE IN EQUAL MEASURES

At 6'3" and 210 pounds, his chiseled, athletic frame reflects the value and pride he places on hard work and discipline. As a talented hockey player in the Quebec Hockey League in his youth, he was drafted by the Boston Bruins. When his father passed away early in his life, Francois took up the responsibility of providing for his family. Chasing success as a pro hockey player seemed like too big of a risk, so he decided to hang up his skates, complete his degree, and pursue a career in business instead. In doing so, he discovered the thrill of competition in business was every bit as compelling as it is in sport.

Francois believes that success is intimately linked to the art of finding an equilibrium or balance in life, so he possesses an amazing capacity for work and fun in equal measure.

Francois' formula has an elegant structure with two seasons, winter and summer. The structure is deliberate and based on what he has learned from years of experience, adversity, and the dangers of an obsessive and singular focus. He has become acutely aware of the influence his daily practices have on his overall happiness. The seasonality of his approach brings variety to his life and helps him prioritize fun.

THE THREE DISCIPLINES

Sleep Discipline

Sleep, exercise, and play are the key components to his formula that exist in both seasons. For starters, Francois gets eight hours of sleep almost every night. For a man that spends more than fifty percent of his time away from home, traveling throughout Canada, the US, and South America, this is impressive. Airports, hotels, and different time zones all present a test to healthy sleep hygiene. "I have this ability to disconnect from the challenges of the day. Sleep is not a problem for me. My philosophy is that I put a tremendous effort into my work, so after thirteen or fourteen hours on an issue, I know I've done my best. I'll go to sleep and start over again tomorrow. The day has an end — no one died, and it is only money."

Francois' ability to quiet his mind on-demand with such precision stands out as a remarkable talent. Some leaders can develop this skill through the practice of meditation and deliberate mindfulness or stress resiliency training. Francois' commitment to his sleep ritual helps him keep his energy where he wants it.

For most leaders, creating time and space for sleep, rest, and recovery at the end of a day is a common and serious challenge. As the oppressive force of fatigue mounts, mental health often deteriorates and performance lags. Francois sees this pattern as a trap and skillfully avoids it by dropping his mental luggage at the front door and choosing to walk away.

Unburdened, he frees up this mental capacity for things that bring him joy and allow him to recharge. When it is time to sleep, his attention has shifted from the challenges at work, and he is capable of finding peace. This is a special talent. To understand it, Francois and I spent some time discussing the ease of his transition to sleep.

It appears to be as simple as placing trust in the following four absolutes:

1. The day only has twenty-four hours.
2. He gave the day his best effort.
3. He will perform better tomorrow if he prioritizes his sleep today.
4. A rested mind often presents a new perspective.

Most nights, he tries to be in bed by 10 p.m. If he feels his energy declining, he will adjust to 9:30 p.m. "I can get by with seven hours; six is an absolute minimum, but I perform better and strive for eight." On a typical workday, he is up and on the move by 6:30 a.m. When at home in Montreal, most days finish sometime between 6 and 7 p.m. When he is on the road, days are much longer. He is often not back to the hotel until as late as 10 p.m. Dinners with his team, customers, or business partners demand his best performance and stretch his endurance. On weekends, his day may start a little later, but not by much. The only time he appears to waver from his sleep ritual is in response to the occasional emotional tug of a family concern.

Exercise Discipline

The second featured component of his formula is physical activity. Francois is a multi-sport athlete whose seasons are defined by which sports he can indulge in. He craves the outdoors and is an avid runner. On average, he will run 800 kilometers a year, accumulating the bulk of his mileage in his summer season. "There are some days it is hard for me to get outdoors. My driver picks me up in my garage and drops me off at the garage at the office. I then go to work for the day. He may pick me up again later that afternoon and take me to the airport, and off I go. On days like that, I'm indoors all day." For this reason, a run first thing in the morning holds great appeal for Francois. Early exercise primes his motivation for the day ahead and gives him a chance to connect with nature.

"I had a friend who I didn't see as an athlete who ran marathons. I thought, 'If this guy can run a marathon, anybody can run a marathon,' and so I started to train and realized just how tough it is." The endorphin kick and solitude of running grabbed hold of Francois profoundly. For the first three to four years he ran, he pushed himself hard, driven to run further and faster. He started passionately tracking his performance and running metrics and training even harder. With his competitive standard positioned just slightly out of reach, his pursuit of excellence eventually throttled his enjoyment of the activity. After a short break, he found his way back, recognizing that "no one cares if my running split times were five- or six-minute kilometers. I still keep a running journal, but I no longer push my performance as hard."

Play Discipline

The third component to his formula is play. As Francois shared the details of his daily rituals, he frequently referenced the key to finding happiness in his life has been his ability to live in balance. "Leadership jobs can consume you if you are not careful. Early in your career, you are eager for experience, want to learn, and want to prove to yourself and others you can perform. This is good, but you don't know how to manage the demands that come with opportunity and responsibility. You don't know yet how to perform under pressure, how to protect sleep, how to eat well — you just don't understand all of these things until you head down the wrong path a few times and fall down."

SELF-CARE REFLECTION #16

Sleep, exercise, and play. These are all important Wellness Rituals to help you be better. In your journal, over the course of a week, write down how your day is divided among these three rituals. On Day 8, review your notes. Where can you make improvements to bring more balance and energy to each day? Where are the trouble spots in your week?

HARDER AND FASTER LED TO BAD OUTCOMES

When Francois stumbled in the past, it was because he pushed to excess with a singular focus for an extended period, leaving little to no time for fun. He calls it a "negative spiral," and it plays out like this: "You stress, you sleep less, you work more, and then you become less and less efficient with every passing hour. Days get longer at the office and shorter at home. Exercise falls away. Your diet suffers. Many times, you are blind to the spiral and your declining performance because all you can see is the business issue in front of you."

> 66 **When you run too fast and spend too much time focused on one thing, you usually end up alone. People stop following you. This is a good indication you are off track."**

Twice Francois has fallen down such a spiral. His tendency to seek perfection can get him into trouble. He has experienced this temptation in hockey, running, and business at various times in his life and has come to understand that when his drive to succeed is overplayed, his joy is lost, and equilibrium is not possible. A mentor helped him to pull out of his first spiral. The second time, recognizing the trap himself, he found his own way out. "I asked myself, 'What am I doing? What am I chasing?' and started to listen to the good people around me who were holding up a mirror and telling me I was working too hard."

Realizing the push to go harder, faster, and higher was coming from within, he started to become more aware of the choices he was making and learned to leverage his off switch.

"When you run too fast and spend too much time focused on one thing, you usually end up alone. People stop following you. This is a good indication you are off track." By honoring the things that brought him joy, he found he could maintain the high standard and competitive drive that had always anchored his success.

To prevent another negative spiral, he has established a series of mental alarm bells that trigger his awareness of dangerous behaviors or tendencies. "There are times when work demands your full attention, and you need to devote more time to a business file if you are going to make it happen, but you have got to have performance balance warning bells that ring when you push off track. They keep you sleeping, eating, and exercising to support your high standard." When he oversaw forty-four plants in seven different countries, Francois managed to make site visits to each one every two to three years. "I cannot have a bad day. I need to be on, funny, cool, and engaged at every visit." On autopilot, this would not be possible.

Francois now encourages leaders on his team to invest time into understanding what makes them happy and what brings balance to their lives and then make choices to seek these things out. Expecting to find happiness waiting for you around the corner is for the lazy and the lucky.

FRANCOIS' FORMULA FOR HEALTH, STRENGTH & HOPE

MAKE HEALTHY FOOD CHOICES

Francois' nutritional rituals are also closely monitored in his formula. To ensure he fuels his fast-paced day with healthy food options, he put his family doctor in direct contact with his executive assistant. The doctor coached her on power foods and healthy choices for Francois' diet, and Francois empowered her to make all the food decisions in support of his performance. "She handles all decisions related to food when I am on the road, from meal selections on the plane to dinner reservations with customers, to where we will stop for food as I travel between sites."

His EA has also re-stocked Francois' fridge in his office with healthy snacks for a quick meal on the go and will order in his lunch from a set menu of healthy choices. On the odd cheat day, she will authorize a pizza or poutine order, but not often. This action completely changed his eating patterns throughout the day. Upon opening his office fridge and pantry, you will find bottles of water, various nuts, low-sugar granola bars, low-fat cheese, blueberries, raspberries, yogurt, and dark chocolate. Popcorn is a favorite mid-afternoon snack that he offers to guests meeting in-person in his office. He does not drink coffee.

When pressed to reveal his dietary vices, he admitted to butter being his kryptonite. "I put it on everything." He keeps a mental log of his food choices and evaluates his discipline daily on the bathroom scale. He makes micro-adjustments to keep to his desired weight of 210. Techniques that work for him include portion control, passing on dessert, avoiding after dinner or bedtime snacks, and drinking water, not juice.

A LIFESTYLE OF TWO SEASONS

The final common component to his seasonal formulas is one of solitude in nature. Francois needs time alone outdoors. As CEO, the demands on his attention and time are extensive. His team presents directly to him, and he is actively engaged as they do. These meetings are scheduled in between his extensive travel itinerary. As such, he has little time for reflection. "When I exercise, I don't have to talk to anybody. I don't have to negotiate with anybody. I am just alone, and this time is especially important to me. The more this time can be outside, the better." The fresh air clears his head. "A friend once told me that the reason I love being in nature is that the trees just give; they ask for nothing in return." Fresh ideas come to him when he is exercising outdoors, and he loses himself in the physical performance and landscape.

The Winter Season

Francois' winter season is the shorter of the two and extends from December until late March. The season plays out with time spent at their family mountainside chalet at Mont-Tremblant. The mountain offers some of the best skiing in eastern Canada, with a peak of 2,871 ft. and over 630 acres of skiable terrain. Weekends on the mountain are structured to push his body physically and spend as much time outdoors as he can, skiing, hiking, and playing ice hockey. Up at 7 a.m., he will be on the mountain to ski first tracks at 7:45 a.m. The ski resort opens early for members on the mountain, and the early runs provide the solitude he craves after a full work week. He skis until late morning and then meets with his wife for an hour's hike up the mountain before returning to the chalet for lunch. After lunch, he may have a power nap, which helps him regulate his sleep cycle after a week of corporate travel or hours of video conferences. The late afternoons are often spent playing ice hockey with friends at a local rink.

Saturday evening offers a time for social connections, whether that be time alone with his wife and family or in the company of friends. As a collector of red wine, he likes sharing and introducing wines to friends and colleagues that they might not otherwise try. He enjoys hosting and draws great pleasure from telling stories about wine and the vineyards that produce it. "I try to make a link between my guests, the occasion for our meeting or gathering, our meal, and the wine selected."

Sunday mornings, he is back on the mountain skiing until lunch. In the afternoon, he slows things down, spends time resting in the chalet with his wife, and prepares for the week ahead. While skiing, hiking, and hockey are his preferred winter sports, he continues to run at least once a week throughout the winter, keeping his winter mileage above fifty kilometers a month.

The Summer Season

Summer weekends are spent in the Eastern townships south of Montreal. Known for breathtaking panoramas overlooking impressive mountains, time here offers Francois and his wife a beautiful respite. Running is his primary athletic focus in the summer, but he also enjoys golfing and cycling. His mileage significantly increases once the ski season comes to a close. Francois runs regardless of where he is in the world. Most hotels have treadmills or know of safe local trails he can run. He completes two half marathons annually, one in September and one in October.

During the pandemic, with more time available, he topped 1,200 km a year. "I've done marathons, but I've found it requires a lot of training. As I'm getting older, too much of the same type of training is hard on the body." Cross-training makes him a better runner and supports his efforts to gradually increase his mileage from April to September in preparation for his half marathons in the fall.

He tracks distance, pace, split times, and notes related to performance in his running journal. Manual note-taking has become an essential part of his discipline for his Move to Stay Young Wellness Ritual. It provides him with an interesting insight into his performance and is another important warning bell. Should his weekly distance or pace start to drop off or his energy levels dip, he knows his professional schedule is beginning to infringe and bad habits are creeping back in.

Weight training is often the first activity he drops when pressed for time. After a full day on video calls, he would choose an outdoor activity over lifting weights in the basement. At the time of our interview, he was working on incorporating push-ups, chin-ups, and pull-ups into his outdoor workouts.

SELF-CARE REFLECTION #17

Francois' two-season approach to life keeps his movements varied. In your journal, reflect on whether a seasonal approach to exercise would help you make healthy activity choices with greater consistency.

EQUILIBRIUM AND ACCOUNTABILITY

"With life experience, there comes a point when the challenge of proving you can do the job falls away. You have made it happen and are doing the work simply because you enjoy it." To keep this spark alive, Francois does not subscribe to going it alone. "You need a lot of people and good practices to help you along your way." He relies on family, his running journal, mentors, a Pilates instructor, a massage therapist, his family doctor, and his EA to keep him in equilibrium while his system of warning bells hold him accountable. It is clear that the challenge and thrill of performing at a high level still excites Francois and brings purpose to his day. His approach is a good reminder of the value of play. The cadence of his voice, the words he chooses, and his body language reveal a rhythm that suggests he is a man who has found his balance and the formula to maintain it.

Francois tracks distance, pace, splittimes, and notes related to performance in his **running journal**. Manual note-taking has become an **essential part of his discipline** for his *Move to Stay Young* Wellness Ritual.

PATTIE LOVETT-REID

Best-selling Author, Financial Commentator

*A*t the time of my interview with Pattie, she was the chief financial commentator for CTV News Channel. She has since left that role, but I know that some, perhaps many, of the readers of this book will be interested to learn the routine she followed to achieve her best on and off camera.

While at CTV, Pattie's day started at 3:30 a.m. Her signature on-air enthusiasm and energy that fans grew to love was present, even at this time of day. Rising well before the sun, she woke with eager anticipation and often proclaimed to her husband, Jim, "Something really special is going to happen today." To keep pace, Jim was up at 3:30 a.m. as well to start their morning ritual together.

In her role with CTV News Channel, she was responsible for discussing current economic, market, and personal financial planning trends to help Canadians take control of their financial health. She provided weekday financial updates for CTV News Channel, CP24, and regional CTV *Morning Live* broadcasts across the country. Pattie also contributed analysis on market-moving business stories to CTV *National News* and guested regularly on BNN Bloomberg, CTV's *Your Morning*, *The Social*, NewsTalk1010, and other Bell Media channels. She became a dynamic force in media and remains one of Canada's most trusted and respected financial experts.

By 4:45 a.m., Pattie was hard at work, reading financial reports, researching trends, and writing blogs. From here, she determined her top four business stories of the day and began to craft a crisp narrative to bring to Canadians as they started their day. By 6:40 a.m., Pattie had already completed her first live on-air financial updates for radio and television. Appearances typically continued on various forms of media until 12:30 p.m., at which point, she bowed out of the spotlight.

While Pattie has stepped away from CTV, she has not stepped away from her profession as a renowned journalist or the health rituals that became integral to her life.

PATTIE'S FORMULA FOR HEALTH, STRENGTH & HOPE

FOLLOW A SLEEP DISCIPLINE

Pattie's ability to succinctly bring clarity to the complex financial and business stories of the day demands she approach each day with a clear mind and laser-sharp focus. Seven hours of sleep makes this possible for her. The discipline Pattie brings to this aspect of her life is second to none. She could offer a masterclass on the subject. Her class would highlight the importance of sleep hygiene principles, discipline, and the art of living a large life. She understands sleep deficits cannot be repaid with a weekend sleep-in and appreciates the on-demand access to her peak performance that is afforded by her formula. "We have built our lives around this need."

 Rituals are important to us from a lifestyle and family perspective, and also from a health perspective."

Nine in the evening is considered a late night for Pattie and Jim. "I am not the life of the party past eight-thirty," she admits. To help keep her on track, she wears a Whoop Strap (*whoop.com*). Drawn to numbers, she likes poring over the data the smart device tracks, including the daily monitoring of strain, sleep, and recovery. The device provides an evaluation of sleep quality, measuring not only how long she sleeps but also the time she spends in each stage of sleep. It uses heart rate variability, average resting heart rate, and sleep patterns to give her a sense of how her body has recovered overnight and her capacity to push to her peak the next day. Pattie's husband, a former fighter pilot, author, and newly minted entrepreneur, no doubt benefits from her discipline. Pattie shares, "Rituals are important to us from a lifestyle and family perspective, and also from a health perspective."

Pattie is keenly aware of where she falls on the stress response curve, which is why rituals are so important. There is no compromise in her workday to meet a schedule that is unforgiving. "I do take ridicule from my friends. They will say, 'Let's get on a Zoom call,' and I'll say, 'Okay, how about 5:30 p.m.?' They know I won't waver from it because I can't."

By 7:30 p.m., she begins to wind things down. Her evening script is every bit as predictable as her morning one. Time after dinner is spent with a glass of wine in hand in Jim's company. After twenty-six years of marriage, Pattie still looks forward to closing her day with her husband. They value this time together and are one other's sounding board, champion, and best friend. When her head hits the pillow, she is out cold. Sleep is welcomed and comes easily. "There has been a book on my bedside for months. I think our cleaning lady thought it was a prop. And it is a romantic novel; it is nothing serious." After a couple of paragraphs, Pattie is gone.

SELF-CARE REFLECTION #18

Reflect on this sentence: "There is no compromise in her workday to meet a schedule that is unforgiving." Pattie made a conscious effort to maintain her health in the face of an unforgiving schedule. What steps are you taking to disengage from work and practice self-care? Are the steps "just enough," or could you do better?

EAT WELL AND BE PHYSICALLY FIT

Breakfast consists of a protein, yogurt mixed with flaxseed, and coffee. The protein is typically a low-fat cottage cheese or an egg white omelet. "It fills me up. I like it. So there is not a lot of variation there for me." Mid-morning, she will eat again. Favorite choices include almonds, cheese, oat bran pancakes, yogurt, natural peanut butter, and apples. As a general rule, she will have something to eat every two and a half hours, spreading out her daily calorie intake to maintain her energy. Her choices are strong on protein and light on carbs, nothing processed. Lunch and dinner are virtually identical, with variations in the vegetable and protein choices. JuJube candies appear to be her one weakness.

Prior to her second career in media, Pattie enjoyed a very successful thirty-three-year career as an executive for TD bank, retiring as a senior VP. Transitioning from behind her desk to in front of the camera came with pressure to look a certain way. However, Pattie was immune to it. She is refreshingly proud and confident in her appearance, and for a good reason.

Pattie prioritizes her physical fitness much the same way she does her sleep. Wellness Ritual #4: Move to Stay Young is the second foundational ritual in her formula. For three decades, she has worn a size six. "I feel good at my weight. I like the way I look. I'm never going to be tiny, tiny, tiny, but my frame is good for mobility, strength, and flexibility, and all of those things matter to me."

Pattie runs, boxes, lifts weights, walks, practices yoga, balance, and flexibility, and plays with her grandchildren. "I am a cardio junky. I want to get my heart rate up. I love it. I want it." Most recently, she has added circuit training on her Peloton bike to this list of activities. She is quick to hop on for a short twenty-minute cardio workout mid-afternoon with a bike at home or at the cottage. Her Instagram account provides evidence of her passion for exercise. She also makes time to train with a personal trainer twice a week for an hour at a time. "My trainer will force me to hold a plank a little longer or bang out a few more push-ups than I would without her watchful eye."

Scheduling time for exercise at the last minute means it does not happen with any consistency, so Pattie will map out her exercise time in advance. "It is like paying yourself first." Life quickly fills the gaps when you travel at her pace. Given the early-morning demands of her role, she has found mid-afternoon to be the best time to exercise. Her sweet spot for fitness and self-care typically falls between 2 and 4 p.m. The premature death of her father fuels her motivation for fitness. Tragically, he died at the age of thirty-six from a massive heart attack. He smoked and was overweight. He pushed hard with little regard for the consequences. Pattie was only nine at the time of his passing. On her thirty-sixth birthday, she realized just how short her dad's life had been. With her life immeasurably influenced by his, she has vowed to do everything within her power to live a healthy and balanced lifestyle and enjoy the longevity that he did not.

FAMILY IS HER NORTH STAR

The third fundamental ritual in Pattie's formula is the art of nurturing mental fitness.

Pattie draws mental strength and deep resiliency from her family, which anchors her in a profound way. Leveraging her positivity with their love, Pattie is a force in this world. Her family is her True North, and her heart beats in sync with theirs.

> **66 Success is your kid calling you in the middle of the day just to see how you are doing."**

Pattie and Jim each brought two children from their first marriages to their relationship. All four kids feature prominently in their lives, as do their four young grandsons. Listening to Pattie share family stories, it sounds like her energy amazes even them. She offered, "Let me explain it to you this way. Our son has two dogs — a Vizsla and a Pointer. The Vizsla is a lovely, low-spirited, good dog. The Pointer, whose name is Hugo, is nuts. He is literally insane and goes all day, from the minute he wakes up to the end of the day, tearing up the place. The family's nickname for me is Hugo. I'm not so sure it is very flattering, but I do wake up ready to go. I'm like the family camp counselor."

During one of our discussions, two of her four adult children called, simply to check in. Their calls were not received as interruptions or distractions pushed to the sidelines. The expression on Pattie's face and the tone of her voice as she answered their calls revealed how her priorities stack up. When needed, her family has her undivided attention. After a quick exchange to ensure they were okay, she agreed to call them back. Later, I would ask Pattie how she defines success. She responded, "Success is your kid calling you in the middle of the day just to see how you are doing."

SOME DAYS NEED A RESET

Pattie models a mentor lifestyle through her actions and sets an example as a professional, wife, mother, and grandmother who also happens to be fit, active, fun, and attractive. Wired as an optimist, Pattie's mindset is best defined by the Stockdale Paradox, a concept developed in Jim Collins' book *Good to Great.* The paradox posits that productive change begins when you confront the brutal facts. "I am on camera. There is a healthy dose of narcissism going on here, but I don't have regrets. I have learning moments."

She is sincere and kind to herself and appears to be able to reset adversity proficiently.

A couple of days before one of our calls, she shared that she was feeling off. It was one of those days that feel like you are swimming against the current. Yes, even Pattie Lovett-Reid has such days. "Everything I seemed to touch that morning was harder than it should have been. I just wasn't grasping the day and delivering like I usually do. I stood up, went outside, and said out loud, 'This is ridiculous — snap out of it. Put on a hot red lipstick and a pop of color, and the day starts again right here, right now.'" And with that, she turned it around, determined not to let a rough start ruin a perfectly good day.

SELF-CARE REFLECTION #19

Next time you find yourself in a rut, try giving yourself permission to re-start your day. Choosing to reframe your mindset can be a powerful performance tool. As we will discuss in Wellness Ritual #6: Nurture Mental Fitness, our thoughts control our emotional response.

OVERCOMING DYSLEXIA

Pattie has dyslexia. She struggles to read a teleprompter, and despite her financial genius, she never completed a university degree. Earlier in her life, she doubted she had the smarts to pursue formal education because traditional approaches to teaching made school difficult.

Years later, Jim recognized a few of her tendencies and arranged for her to have a proper assessment, confirming the diagnosis. Through sheer determination and trial-and-error, she developed strategies that set her up for success, resulting in two high-profile careers and several best-selling books on financial health. "The best way for me to deal with my dyslexia is to work without distraction. I don't multitask, I complete what I start, and I reread complex data. I will imprint my material by reading it over and paraphrasing in my mind. It may sound strange, but I have to understand what I'm talking about and visualize it completely. When I work, I need to do so in silence — no music or TV. Silence helps me concentrate."

When Pattie goes quiet, her family notices, especially Jim. It is during these times that she says she is generating new thoughts. Her daily walks provide her with this opportunity, and like most mentors profiled in this book, she prefers to walk alone.

Pattie is a goal-setter who holds herself accountable and thrives on knocking down the high bar she sets for herself. One such goal for 2021 was to complete 2,000,000 steps walking outdoors. She can micro-adjust her routine without losing ground, whether that be getting to bed earlier, dialing back a workout, or carving out additional time for one of her kids because she is so in tune with her formula. She accepts the input and guidance from experts as well and has cultivated a team of professionals who support her performance.

In addition to her personal trainer, the Peloton trainers, and her chiropractor, she also has an annual executive health examination at Cleveland Clinic Canada. Her trainers push her and keep her focused on her mobility. Her chiropractor keeps her aligned. "I have a rib that pops out from boxing from time to time that my chiropractor helps put back in." The clinical team at Cleveland Clinic provides a reference guidepost and contributes to Pattie's health dashboard. She knows her numbers and actively monitors her blood work and comparative fitness metrics, including her daily step count, Whoop score, and body mass index. If extra encouragement or incentive is ever required, she turns to her daughter Jane.

BE A POSITIVE ROLE MODEL

With over 23,000 Instagram followers, Pattie's profile provides a genuine glimpse into her life and her five Fs: Fun, Family, Friends, Fitness, and Finance. The majority of her followers are females empowered by the example she sets. "Many women at a certain age begin to feel like they no longer have a presence, that they have become a forgotten part of society. I do not subscribe to that thinking."

Taking an active role on social media over the last five years, Pattie has expanded her influence as a positive role model. Whenever asked about her age, she responds that it doesn't matter. "I have a chronological age, a financial age, a biological age; I know that. But I will not throw my age out there because that is not how I choose to live my life. The minute I do, I start to put limiting beliefs in place."

To be clear, Pattie is not embarrassed by aging. She is clear-minded about its reality but intends to have it play out on her terms. She does not define her life by the candles on her cake. She is fit. She is healthy. She looks good, and age has nothing to do with that. The discipline of her formula does. Tapping into the power it provides, she lives with purpose.

If you lack the energy to hold a sustained peak effort, have a closet full of clothes that no longer fit, or are just frustrated with your track record of weight management false starts, then **you are not alone.** Fad diets and lifestyle strategies that prey on our desire for quick weight loss fail to provide sustainable results and contribute to unhealthy relationships with food and body image.

WELLNESS RITUAL #3

FIGHT FOR YOUR WAISTLINE

7 WELLNESS RITUALS
FOR HEALTH, STRENGTH & HOPE

WELLNESS RITUAL #3: THE SCIENCE

Evolution favored those with the reserves to weather unexpected adversity; in other words, in a cold climate with food scarcity, having fat to burn meant living to see another day. In our climate-controlled and sedentary world, stored-up fat is difficult to get rid of. Attempts to out-burn a daily energy surplus to achieve a healthy waistline is a fool's errand. Losing weight is only possible if we consume fewer calories than we burn. There is no magic pill or shortcut to make this happen. Formulas that support this state that by eating less, choosing nutrient-dense foods, limiting processed calories, and getting active produce sustainable results.

The indulgence of extra calories is easily rationalized with the promise of a future sacrifice. A commitment to hit the treadmill a little longer or harder tomorrow in exchange for another glass of wine or second slice of apple pie seems like an equitable eye-for-an-eye transaction. The guilt of overconsumption can motivate even the most apathetic from a couch's warm embrace. Unfortunately, the belief that a calorie consumed can be intentionally spent some time down the road in a fair and equal, open-market energy exchange is flawed. Attempts to out-burn a daily energy surplus is a fool's errand — even for those faithful to their treadmill promises.

We have been taught to believe that the number on our bathroom scale is based on simple math. On paper, it is. For our waistline to hold, calories consumed must equal calories burned. However, the rules are much more complex in the real world, and the rising rates of obesity bear this out. Obesity is now an epidemic. The vast majority of well-intentioned dieters fail in repeated attempts to lose weight.

Unfortunately, short-term weight loss at any cost gets more clicks than commonsensical, long-term strategies that promote good health. Regardless of your approach, the truth is that losing weight is hard to do, and keeping it off is even harder. But hard is not impossible. The objective is to get your weight down to a healthy level and keep it there. This path is a slow burn, but fighting for your waistline is worth the effort.

Our metabolism has evolved to protect our energy as a precious resource. When we burn calories, we do so wisely and with a hint of reluctance. A calorie stored is not easily released because human evolution has rewarded those who conserve their energy supply. With over sixty-three percent of adult Canadians at increased health risk due to excess weight,[1] our metabolisms are struggling to find their way in the modern world. Any combination of habits that favor calorie consumption over calorie expenditure, played out over time, does not end well.

We cannot walk, run, swim, jump, box, lift, skate, or sweat our way out of a poor diet. To achieve optimal body weight and enjoy metabolic health, we need to take a fresh look at the science of human energetics and our tendency to over-consume, and we need to do so with a sense of urgency.

If you lack the energy to hold a sustained peak effort, have a closet full of clothes that no longer fit, or are just frustrated with your track record of weight management false starts, then you are not alone. Fad diets and lifestyle strategies that prey on our desire for quick weight loss fail to provide sustainable results and contribute to unhealthy relationships with food and body image.

At the heart of this Wellness Ritual is the understanding of how humans consume, store, and transform energy. Applying this knowledge will help you appreciate the "why" behind your specific struggle and offer an alternative path forward. To prepare for the journey ahead, we must explore both sides of your energy equation — consumption and expenditure. The creation of an energy deficit needed to lose weight requires a command of both. However, greater emphasis will be given to consumption, as this is where the biggest battles against obesity must be fought. An honest look at the obstacles standing in our way, and a review of evidence-based strategies to overcome them, will give you a running start.

Welcome to Wellness Ritual #3: Fight for Your Waistline.

Let's get to work.

HOW DO OUR BODIES CONSUME ENERGY?

When we eat, we take in calories that contain energy. This energy powers our ability to breathe, think, move, reproduce, heal, laugh, and love. Within the chemical bonds of your morning toast is enough energy to power your first 2,000 steps.

This is the magic of metabolism.

It is a game of energy transfer, and it has life and death consequences. By harnessing the energy stored in the foods we choose to eat, we are capable of powering the chemical processes that sustain our lives. The trick is to discover the specific rules of the game that your body is programmed to play.

This discovery requires a working knowledge of how your metabolic engine operates. The last time you were encouraged to look under the hood was probably back in your high school biology class, when the very idea of human energy having limits seemed either abstract or irrelevant. The Krebs cycle may as well have been an undiscovered universe in a galaxy far, far away. The value of cellular energy and desire for more is earned with age.

If you could travel back in time with your adult mind still intact to attend a single high school class, the day you were taught about the digestive tract, metabolism, and the brilliance of ATP would be the one to choose. This knowledge is fundamental to human performance and cannot be ignored if you hope to command your biological potential. So if you missed that class years ago, were distracted by the haze of pheromones that filled the classroom, or were hung up on the truth that Darth Vader was Luke's father, here is an updated version of what you missed.

WHAT IS A CALORIE?

By definition, 1,000 calories are equivalent to the energy required to raise the temperature of one kilogram (2.2 pounds) of water by one degree Celsius. This definition doesn't invite a lot of clarity, but it is how the energy value of food is measured, which makes it important to your metabolic health and waistline.

If your daily caloric intake is a complete unknown, start reading food labels. The goal here is not precision. Counting calories is far from an exact science. Maintaining an accurate count of incoming calories is challenging, even for those with a talent for numbers. Food labels tend to be based on averages. How a meal is prepared will alter calorie loads, and significant variations in how individuals absorb calories and mark portions make a true count difficult. But there is still value in the practice.

Becoming familiar with food labels will help you understand your consumption patterns. If you are new to tracking calories, start by building an appreciation for where your calories are coming from and a rough estimate of your daily intake. A mid-afternoon stop at a local Tim Horton's to treat yourself to a medium iced cappuccino delivers 360 calories.

While acknowledging that we all have unique energy needs, Health Canada states that a daily intake of between 2,000 to 2,400 calories is a decent benchmark for most adults. Dr. Herman Pontzer, one of the foremost researchers in human metabolism, disagrees. In his recent book, *Burn — New Research Blows the Lid Off How We Really Burn Calories, Stay Healthy, and Lose Weight,* he shares that "every nutrition label in the supermarket will tell you that the standard American diet is 2,000 calories a day, and every label is wrong. Nine-year-olds burn 2,000 calories; for adults, it is closer to 3,000, depending on how much you weigh and how much fat you carry."[31] When leading experts can't agree, it is no wonder most of us either ignore this metric or downplay its significance. However, continuing to do so would be a mistake.

Your energy needs will depend on your gender, age, stage of life, weight, body composition, genetic predisposition, medical history, and activity level. This mixed bag of tricks makes your calorie requirements unique. A standard, one-size-fits-all recommendation from a national food guide won't cut it.

The National Institute of Diabetes and Digestive and Kidney Diseases offers a reliable calorie calculator online that will get you close to defining your specific requirements. *Note:* You can find links to my recommended calorie calculators at **7WellnessRituals. com.**

Define your target intake and share it with your healthcare team, tweak it if necessary, and obtain their endorsement before making any radical changes to how and what you eat. With their approval, begin aligning your daily consumption with this calorie load or just short of it. A qualified nutritionist, dietitian, or naturopath can help you draft a meal plan that will act as a guidepost, restricting your intake to healthy choices without leaving you feeling deprived.

Calories can quickly add up when you are not paying attention. And generally speaking, Canadians are not. Our trend is to over-consume. Making matters worse, just under half of our total daily energy consumption comes from ultra-processed foods.[2] This is a problem. These calories are nutrient-poor, and their consumption directly contributes to our weight crisis and the diseases that follow.

The idea that a calorie consumed can be selectively spent is an over-simplification and insult to evolution. Once packed away in long-term storage, a calorie is difficult to burn.

Consider the energy delivered from the following popular processed foods:

- three strips of bacon provide 120 calories
- a chocolate chip muffin, 420 calories
- a slice of pepperoni pizza, 315 calories
- a Big Mac, 550 calories

A 155-pound person would need to take a thirty-minute brisk walk to burn roughly half of the calories consumed from a single slice of pizza. To burn the full 315 calories in the same amount of time, they would need to work a lot harder. Trading the walk for a thirty-minute, full-body HIIT (high-intensity interval training) workout would get them close.

And therein lies the rub: *As long as we continue to stack incoming calories at a pace that demands an unrealistic level of physical activity to keep our daily energy equation balanced, we will lose this fight and continue to gain weight.*

The calories we eat and drink must be either used or stored. This truth holds regardless of the combination of carbohydrates, fats, or proteins that we consume. It also means that every fat cell currently in our bodies contains energy stored from the excess calories consumed in a previous meal. As discussed in the second Wellness Ritual, we are what we eat.

While the number of fat cells we have remains fairly constant throughout life, their size varies. Research shows that patients who successfully lose a significant amount of weight still maintain the same number of fat cells; the cells are just smaller.[3] In other words, dieting does not eliminate our fat cell count. New fat cells that are produced to replace those that eventually die off want to be filled up.[3,4] That is their purpose. In times of abundance, any fuel left over is spent on non-essential biological processes and ensuring our fat cells are well stocked.

Genetics has a role to play here too, which may explain why certain nutritional strategies work for some and not for others. When the DNA code of an individual calls on the production and maintenance of a higher fat cell count, it is not a personal failure or character flaw. It is simply genetics. To date, more than 400 different genes have been implicated in obesity, influencing everything from appetite and satiety to stress-eating and body-fat distribution.[5] To fight for a healthy waistline, you must learn to play the hand you have been dealt. Your fat cell count may be out of your control, but the excess fuel you make available to them is not.

If weight loss is your goal, it is only achievable if you change your state from abundance to adversity by consuming less than you burn. Diets and lifestyle practices that successfully reduce weight trigger the body to mobilize fat reserves in response to an energy deficit. The laws of physics dictate that this is the only way we shed pounds. Our fuel stores are monitored closely and given a high priority, so to lead your body down this path, you must outduel human nature and the evolutionary forces that have shaped human metabolism, neither of which will release their fat reserves willingly. This is what makes this fight so difficult.

The complexity of weight management and metabolic health extends well beyond the simple counting and balancing of calories. Understanding how digestion works and how the body stores the excess energy we consume will help you change how you eat and drink.

DIGESTION 101

There are four basic stages to food digestion.

1. Digestion begins with the first bite. Chewing and a wash in the digestive enzymes found in our salvia gets the process started. From the mouth, the food then makes its way down the esophagus into the acidic environment of the stomach and then moves into the small intestine. This is where the bulk of digestion occurs.
2. Nutrients released as food is broken down get absorbed into our bloodstream and transported throughout the body.
3. Remaining undigested food is passed along into the large intestine where water and additional nutrients are absorbed.
4. Whatever is left forms our stool and is excreted.

We fuel our body from three main macronutrients found in the foods we consume: carbohydrates, fats, and proteins. All three provide energy, measured in calories, but at different levels and speeds. One gram of carbohydrates or proteins will supply four calories, whereas a gram of fat delivers nine.

Incoming Calories: Digestion of Carbohydrates

Life forms have a long evolutionary history of relying on carbohydrates as a primary fuel source, and they come in three forms: sugar, starch, and fiber. Most nutrition experts recommend that fifty to fifty-five percent of our total daily calories come from carbohydrates, with the bulk drawn from fruits, vegetables, beans, legumes, and unrefined grains. As carbohydrates are digested, they are set on one of three paths. They are used to a) power our cells; b) satisfy future, quick energy demands by transforming into glycogen; or c) combat future famine by converting into fat for long-term storage. For this discussion, we will set fiber aside. Fiber plays a crucial role in helping to regulate digestion and feed our gut microbiome (see Wellness Ritual #2) but does not provide a ton of energy.

The end product of carbohydrate digestion is glucose, which is the body's fuel of choice. Once absorbed into the bloodstream, the presence of glucose raises our blood sugar levels and triggers insulin secretion from the pancreas. Insulin is essential to our survival and provides the body with real-time direct control over blood sugar levels. Sugar levels need to be controlled because the presence of too much sugar can lead to hyperglycemia.

TYPE II DIABETES

Type II Diabetes occurs when the body can't make enough insulin or can't properly use the insulin it does make. It usually develops gradually over a number of years, beginning when muscle and other cells stop responding to insulin. This condition, known as insulin resistance, causes blood sugar and insulin levels to stay high long after eating. Over time, the heavy demands on the insulin-making cells wear them out, and insulin production eventually stops.

This is a condition where damage to blood vessels occurs, which can lead to heart attack or stroke. Some carbohydrates require a stronger insulin response to keep our sugar levels within an optimal range. Simple carbs found in fruit juices, syrups, soft drinks, or processed foods with added sugar spike blood glucose quickly. In contrast, complex carbs found in whole plant foods maintain their natural fiber, slow down digestion, and elevate energy levels for a longer period of time.

A highly processed meal with lots of sugar that causes a massive spike in blood glucose will demand an equally strong counter-response from the pancreas. Insulin surges from these food choices can swing the energy pendulum in the opposite direction and leave you feeling hungry, struggling to concentrate, and prone to mood swings. This isn't a pleasant state to be in and triggers many to return to the kitchen because they feel hungry. But these feelings of hunger are not due to an energy shortfall. The body has all the calories it needs and more. This pattern of eating can promote a behavioral loop of overconsumption that leads to weight gain.

The best way to avoid this rollercoaster is to slow down digestion by fueling the body with nutrient-dense foods rich in complex carbohydrates, protein, and fiber. These foods take longer to digest and consequently result in a slower and more manageable rise in post-meal blood sugar levels.[6] Nuts, carrots, apples, bran cereals, beans, and lentils all make this list.[7,8] Processed, pre-packaged treats do not.

Incoming Calories: Digestion of Fat

The end goal of fat digestion is to break it down into smaller fatty acids and glycerol. Most of this action occurs in the small intestine, where the liver, gallbladder, and pancreas combine to attack the fat we consume. Once digested, the fat molecules are passed through the lymph system and then transported throughout the body via the bloodstream to be either used or stored as energy or recruited to support cell repair, growth, hormone production, and nervous system function.

Fats are available in our foods as monounsaturated, polyunsaturated, or saturated. This last group is the one to watch out for. Foods like butter, palm and coconut oils, cheese, and red meat have higher saturated fat levels. When featured prominently, diets high in saturated fats are linked to increased cholesterol and risk of atherosclerosis.[9] Fats from plants typically provide monounsaturated or polyunsaturated fatty acids and are healthier alternatives. To help you distinguish between healthy and unhealthy fats, saturated fats are solid at room temperature whereas mono and polyunsaturated are liquid.

Another fat to be closely monitored are trans fats. Artificially made, they are added to many commercially prepared foods to prolong shelf life and give foods a desirable taste and texture but have been linked to increased risk of heart disease.[10] When you see "partially hydrogenated oils" on the food label, it means the product contains trans fats. Make an effort to limit consumption of trans fats.

Dietary recommendations suggest our fat consumption be kept to less than 28% of our daily caloric intake, with less than 6% coming from saturated fats.[11] Nutrition experts recommend that we make a strong effort to reduce the amount of saturated fats in our diets, replacing them with foods that contain a healthy dose of essential omega-3 and omega-6 fatty acids. These fats are both beneficial for heart health and are found in vegetable oils (like olive oil, sesame oil, and canola oil), nuts, avocados, natural peanut butter or almond butter, tofu, fatty fish (like salmon, sardines, herring, or trout), and sunflower, sesame, or pumpkin seeds.

Incoming Calories: Digestion of Protein

The primary role of protein is not fuel. Proteins are needed for cellular construction and maintenance. Their digestion supports hormone, muscle, and specific protein production. Because proteins are large nutrients composed of smaller amino acids linked together in complex arrangements, they take time to unpack and digest. This makes proteins a much slower and longer-lasting source of energy than carbohydrates.

In total, there are twenty different amino acids. Our bodies are capable of synthesizing all but nine. These nine, which are considered essential amino acids, must be consumed in our diet. High-quality protein sources, such as meat, fish, eggs, and dairy products, contain all nine. As such, they are known as complete proteins. Other protein sources can be combined to ensure all nine are consumed in a meal. It is possible to get all essential amino acids from a plant-based diet.

Adults need to ingest roughly 0.8 to 1.2 grams of protein per kilogram of body weight per day. Growing children and those looking to bulk up may need more. If weight loss is your goal, protein consumption continues to be essential to ensure that the energy deficiency you are working hard to create does not result in muscle loss. Not only is muscle loss serious, but it also slows down your metabolism. As a bonus, protein consumption is also more satiating, which helps prevent overeating. This isn't a free pass at the all-you-can-eat protein buffet, though, as excess calories, regardless of the source, will still expand your waistline.

WHAT HAPPENS TO THE EXTRA CALORIES WE CONSUME?

When we overindulge, the extra calories have to go somewhere. Digested sugar, fat, and protein can't remain in the blood, so it gets packed away in one of two storage bins as either glycogen or fat. This fork in the metabolic pathway has a massive impact on whether you are on track to lose weight, gain weight, or hold steady. The glycogen option is built for quick, easy access, but has a limited capacity. Its ability to rapidly fuel short bursts, power moves, and first steps make it a precious resource. When glycogen burns, it burns brightly, but not for long. On the other hand, fat is built to satisfy our long-term energy needs and helps bridge unexpected periods of scarcity. It is a very rich, dense energy that is essential for life, but unlike glycogen, fat capacity knows no limits.

Think of your glycogen storage like the battery on your smartphone. It can fuel the better part of a typical day's activity if fully charged. Glycogen is packed away in our liver and large muscles and stands at the ready. Since each gram of glycogen requires three grams of water for storage, it is heavy and bulky, which is why its storage is limited. As our glycogen tank is emptied, our body will make a point of filling it back up from the next available delivery of calories. We turn to our fat stores for fuel for the long haul or sustained peak efforts that extend beyond what our glycogen capacity has to offer us.

Early and quick weight loss in diets with inadequate carbohydrate content occurs when muscle glycogen is broken down and the associated water molecules that accompany it in storage are excreted in urine. This initial weight loss success can be exciting for those who do not understand where it is coming from and so set unrealistic expectations for the rate of their future weight loss. These losses quickly plateau, and weight is regained as glycogen reserves are restored. As a rough estimate, our whole-body glycogen content is about 600 grams, although this amount varies widely based on body mass, diet, fitness, and amount of recent exercise.[12]

Sedentary individuals that barely scratch the surface of their glycogen reserves will have only one option for their energy surplus. The body moves excess calories to fat production when glycogen stores are full. This is the fat we see on our belly, between our thighs, back of arms, or on our backside. When consumed calories are stored, the body is programmed to protect them.

Roughly ninety percent of body fat is subcutaneous. The balance, known as visceral fat, is stored in your abdominal cavity in the spaces surrounding the liver, intestines, and other organs. While a certain amount of visceral fat is normal and provides a degree of internal insulation and protection, excessive amounts can be deadly. Research has shown that visceral fat cells are actually biologically active and function as an endocrine organ, secreting hormones and other molecules that have far-reaching effects on health and performance.[13] They have been shown to make proteins called cytokines that can trigger low-level inflammation and are linked to an elevated risk of heart disease. They have also been shown to release a precursor to angiotensin, a protein that causes blood vessels to constrict and contributes to increased blood pressure.[13]

By restricting calorie intake to a healthy target, the gravy train of extra calories filling our fat cells comes to an abrupt end, and access to the rich fuel they protect becomes available. It is here that your waistline will begin to retreat and healthy weight loss occurs.

However, consumption is only half the story. To understand the full picture and gain even more momentum, the other side of the energy equation must also be explored.

HOW DO WE BURN ENERGY?

The energy required to power a human body in good health is considerable. With our incoming nutritional requirements met, we convert our stored fuel into a cellular power known as Adenosine Triphosphate or ATP. ATP is our biological ticket to ride. It is the principal molecule for storing and transferring energy at a cellular level. Thanks to our mitochondria and the magic of the Krebs cycle, we can ramp up its production to meet our needs on demand.

The bulk of the energy we burn gets spent unconsciously to fuel our bodies' most basic life support systems. Our specific energy needs to keep our nervous system, respiration, circulation, digestion, immune response, and the regulation of our core temperature on point are unique, much like a fingerprint. Known as our Basal Metabolic Rate (BMR), this baseline energy requirement accounts for roughly 60% of the calories we burn on any given day.

Our BMR is influenced by several factors, including our body composition, gender, and age. Larger bodies or individuals with more muscle mass burn more calories, even at rest. Our metabolism adapts as we mature, and our bodies shift their physiological priority from growth to reproduction. Through puberty, a female body composition changes as it begins to gain more body fat. Fat does not expend as much energy as other tissues, so the average calories burned per pound is typically lower for women than it is for men.

As for the impact of aging, a recent landmark study suggests that metabolism does not fall off with age as we once believed it did.[14] This study found that metabolism peaks around age one, when babies burn calories at a rate 50% faster than adults, and then gradually declines at roughly 3% a year until the age of twenty. At this stage, it appears we enter a metabolic plateau that holds until the age of sixty, when it starts to slowly decline again by less than 1% a year. Life-stage metabolic peaks and valleys believed to accompany adolescence, pregnancy, and menopause were not observed. After the age of sixty, BMR decline is related to the loss of muscle mass and increased body fat that commonly accompanies aging. In Wellness Ritual #5: Protect Your Strength, we will review how resistance training after age sixty helps slow this decline.

By introducing critical thinking and movement to the day, our energy expenditure increases above and beyond BMR demands, but by how much fluctuates from person to person. Scientists refer to a typical day's activity that is not deliberate exercise as Non-Exercise Activity Thermogenesis or NEAT. Your NEAT burn rate powers all basic daily movement patterns and accounts for about 100 to 800 calories a day.[15] Any intentional exercise costs additional calories and gets added to your daily expenditure. With a quick Google search, you can easily define the energy cost of performing your exercise of choice. But to give you a sense of your activity burn rate, a moderately paced walk of sixty minutes will burn only 200 to 300 calories, depending on your weight. Hit the 10,000 steps a day target, and the average person will burn closer to 500 calories.

Intentional exercise will burn calories, but its impact on total energy expenditure is not as significant as most people think.

METABOLISM AND BODY WEIGHT

Metabolism and body weight are commonly linked but misunderstood. A slower metabolism is rarely the cause of weight gain. Our BMR and NEAT do not waver a whole lot. Our metabolism is heavily regulated by complex systems designed to protect our survival above all else. Strategies claiming to boost metabolic burn rates or dial up your BMR belong in the magazine rack at your local grocery store checkout, not in your wellness formula. Ice water, chili peppers, caffeinated beverages, or body-sculpting lotions will not drop your waist size. Your focus must be directed to the quality of what you eat and drink and how active you are if you hope to shift the balance of your energy equation.

Weight gain is influenced by genetics, hormonal controls, mental health, and various lifestyle choices, including diet, sleep, and physical activity. The sustained combination of these factors will tip your equation into an energy deficit. That is the sweet spot. Finding it takes patience, focus, and trust in your body's ability to respond.

The key take away from biology class many years ago is this: Our body weight is a reflection of our energy management. Evolution favored our ability to take advantage of periods of calorie abundance, so our metabolisms covet a daily energy surplus and skillfully convert it into long-term storage. This talent provided our ancestors with a bridge to survive adversity that most of us have never known. Our lives are playing out in times of abundance, when patterns of overconsumption offer no survival advantage and result only in obesity. To break free from this trend, we must make choices that curb consumption and promote access to the rich fuel found in our fat stores. The science is straightforward; unfortunately, its application is not.

MODERN-DAY OBSTACLES TO WEIGHT MANAGEMENT

Metabolic experts continue to explore how to manipulate biology to our advantage. Can lifestyle actions alter the energy we make available or change the way our bodies store or mobilize fat? Can we influence our metabolic rate or energy expenditure to burn more calories, helping to offset our overconsumption tendencies? And most importantly, how do we bring an end to the obesity epidemic?

While the answers to these questions are not yet entirely understood, considerable progress is being made to unearth them. Dr. Pontzer's research is challenging how we think about metabolism. In his groundbreaking studies of modern hunter-gatherer tribes, like the Hazda of northern Tanzania, he argues that our bodies are skilled at maintaining our calorie burn to a very narrow window of 3,000 calories a day, no matter our activity level. In a new model of human energetics he calls Constrained Energy Expenditure, Pontzer suggests the old Additive Model of the more we move, the more we burn, was wrong.

He believes the body works on a fixed energy budget, re-routing available energy away from nonessential tasks to keep our burn rate within the desired narrow window and account for increased energy spent on physical activity. In *Burn,* he states, "What was once a life-saving evolutionary strategy to survive hardship now seems to be what is behind the wave of obesity. Weight loss is clearly possible, but through calorie restriction, not attempts to increase expenditure."[32]

Pontzer's position has created a stir in both academic circles and the fitness industry, with critics questioning some of the assumptions in his theory. While more research is required, his work is pushing the fight against obesity toward calorie restriction.

Researchers are studying calorie restriction as a pathway to rewiring many metabolic and immune responses that boost lifespan and health. In a recent 2022 study published in the journal Science, calorie restriction improved both metabolic and immune responses.[16] The study found that people who cut their calorie intake by about 14% over two years were able to reprogram the pathways in their fat cells, helping them regulate the way mitochondria generate energy, improve the body's anti-inflammatory responses, and potentially increase longevity.

The focus on calorie restriction has brought three obstacles to the surface that must be overcome for this Wellness Ritual to find its place in your formula.

OBSTACLE 1: STRESS-EATING

Weight management is as much psychological as it is physical. If eating were just about hunger, we would eat when hungry and stop when full. For a few of our mentors, this is the case; for most, it is not. Many people will need to learn how to disrupt unhealthy, entrenched habits that extend well beyond the body's need for fuel if they are to successfully manage their weight.

The field of behavioral and cognitive psychology points to a number of psychological mechanisms that account for our overconsumption and resulting obesity.[17] Studies measuring the impact of prolonged periods of chronic stress have shown subjects demonstrate elevated cortisol levels, amplified hunger, and increased cravings for sugary, salty, and fatty foods.[17] To dampen stress-related emotions, many turn to "stress-eating" for some form of temporary relief.

Research highlights that the best approach for stress-eaters is rooted in an integrative, multi-disciplinary, customized model of care that features the following:

1. A strong emphasis on health literacy through health coaching designed to improve attitudes and beliefs regarding weight management and body image;
2. Behavioral therapy that targets unhealthy habits and teaches healthy coping strategies;
3. Cognitive-behavioral therapy for depression to enhance resiliency skills and improve mood levels.[17]

Having a talented mental health expert on your team to help you develop a strategy for overcoming stress-eating, and hold you accountable to it, is essential. Self-directed tough love and a firm resolve provide a distinct advantage, but to think of this ritual as a test of individual will or discipline would be a mistake.

I'll save you the hardship and disappointment. Convincing yourself that discipline alone will be your strategy to eating well will not work. In the long run, our desire to consume will defeat a "discipline" mindset or deprivation diet the same way a full house beats a pair of aces. The comfort and reward of the path of abundance are too tempting, and eventually we simply tire of holding back and return to old patterns. Finding the motivation to make the behavioral changes necessary hinges on your ability to redefine your relationship with food. This requires you to put in the work and invest in your mental health.

OBSTACLE 2: THE REWARDS OF VARIETY

There was a time when overeating impulses had survival value, but when caloric overload is possible on a daily basis, this tendency is dangerous. Countless delicious options are readily available in fast-food restaurants, expansive grocery stores, and speedy delivery services. This temptation is proving too much for our metabolic commands and our neural control center — the hypothalamus.

Located at the base of the brain, just above the pituitary gland, the hypothalamus has evolved to play an essential role in regulating our body temperature, maintaining healthy sleep hygiene, and converting our emotions into a physical response. It is also charged with the responsibility of controlling appetite. As the stomach fills up and our energy needs are met, the hypothalamus triggers a feeling of fullness designed to suppress our desire to eat. At least, that is how evolution has drawn it up.

Unfortunately, the rewarding properties of calorie-rich foods loaded with sugar, salt, and fat override the basic hunger control signals governed by our metabolisms.[18] The foods we crave reward our brains in such a way that we continue to eat even when our energy requirements have been met.

In animal studies, biological factors that act to match energy intake with energy expenditure to precisely control body weight over long periods have been identified.[19] Humans seem indifferent to these controls, suggesting that our anxiety, pursuit of pleasure, and prior social experiences may be more influential than any cry to stop eating from the hypothalamus.[18] Efforts to explore our tendency to eat beyond our metabolic needs have become a priority in the fight against obesity.

The abundance of energy-dense, tasty foods loaded with sugar, salt, and fat trigger our dopamine reward mechanism (we will explore our dopamine reward in greater detail with Wellness Ritual #7: Play with Purpose) and override the biological controls that help us maintain a stable weight. Input from our taste buds to dopamine-secreting neurons in the brain, coupled with various hormonal responses to the foods we eat, keep us at the dinner table. This vulnerability hits some of us harder than others, as individual life experiences, environmental influences, and our genetic code determine our responses to the rewarding properties of different foods.[18]

To convey the struggles of our hypothalamus, researchers offer two explanations. Firstly, our ability to judge intake has become distorted by the variety of foods we eat and the different neurological rewards they offer. Even after a satisfying, filling main course, most can still find room for dessert, and that is because sweets trigger a different neurological reward.

Secondly, modern foods have been designed to be overeaten. Pontzer describes this well in *Burn*:

"Much of the food we buy at the supermarket, the canned and packaged foods have been engineered beyond anything our ancestors would have recognized. Fiber, protein and anything else that will make you feel full is removed. Sugar, fat and salt, and other things to tickle your reward system are added. Our evolved reward systems are unprepared for the intensity and breadth of reward signals that these processed foods provide. Our hypothalamus is too slow to shut down our appetite, and we overconsume." [33]

There is no easy way around this obstacle. Limiting temptations by following a structured meal plan that offers a variety of healthy choices, limits processed foods, and doesn't leave you feeling deprived is the path many of our mentors have taken. Note that while their formulas possess structure, they are not rigid. By trial and error, they learn to manipulate their metabolic responses to the energy balance their lifestyles promote.

OBSTACLE 3: SEDENTARY HABITS

The time and effort required to out-exercise a poor diet does not offer a great ROI. Of course, there are exceptions to this rule. Those able to find the time and motivation to burn 400 to 500 calories per workout five or more days a week will prove me wrong.[20] To this group, I say, "All the power to you." Again, if what you are doing is working, stick with it. However, this is not actionable advice for most.

According to Statistics Canada, on average, Canadians employed in full-time work are sedentary for as much as 9.6 hours a day.[21] The evidence that increased sedentary behavior significantly elevates the risk for diabetes, cardiovascular disease, cancer, and premature mortality is strong.[21] Yet only 18.5% of us are meeting the Canadian Physical Activity Guidelines. Office and desk workers have been found to get the lowest number of steps per day, the lowest amount of light-intensity physical activity, and the greatest amount of sedentary time. Large volumes of moderate to vigorous physical activity (sixty to seventy-five minutes a day) are needed to offset the risks associated with prolonged sitting.[22] Those chained to a desk are falling well short of this requirement.

As more and more evidence demonstrates that meaningful changes in your daily energy balance are extremely difficult to achieve through exercise alone, it is crucial not to lose sight of the importance of staying active. Regular exercise is a vital component of good health. There is no shortcut where it doesn't feature prominently. Finding time in your waking hours to move with a purpose unlocks a force of health-boosting advantages that extend the quality and quantity of your life.

Regular physical activity has a vital role to play in preventing weight gain, supporting mental health, and improving body image and physical performance.[22] In addition, if Pontzer's theory proves to be accurate and our bodies do regulate how and when they spend their fuel to keep expenditure within their targeted, narrow range, then burning calories through exercise will leave less fuel available for processes that potentially take away from our performance.

Studies are now looking at how the body responds to calorie restriction to determine whether large energy investments in nonessential processes, like inflammation or the stress response, still occur when resources are limited. A reduction in fat mass and adipose tissue inflammation, both of which are known to contribute to systemic inflammation, have been documented in response to regular exercise.[23] Another group of researchers exposed athletes and sedentary individuals to the stress of public speaking and then tracked their stress response and recovery rates.[24] While both groups demonstrated elevated cortisol and heart rate, the athletes recovered quicker and appeared to invest less energy in the stress response.

Finding opportunities to move throughout the day and avoid prolonged periods of sitting is a must. The damage done by sitting for more than seven hours a day cannot be undone with exercise at either end of your day. It is important to not only limit the total time you sit each day but also to introduce frequent movement to interrupt the time spent sitting. Research has linked sitting for long periods (more than eight hours per day) with a number of health concerns, including obesity, elevated blood pressure, high blood sugar and cholesterol levels, and cancer.[25] Frequent micro-breaks to stand, stretch, or simply change your posture every forty-five minutes is a valuable practice to adopt.

CHAPIN CLINICAL CORNER

LEARN THE RULES OF YOUR GAME

Healthy weight loss looks like one to two pounds (0.5 kg to 1 kg) a week.[26] At this pace, people are more successful at keeping the lost weight off. Anything faster is typically hard to maintain. Healthy eating is about finding a new relationship with food and eating behaviors that will fuel your best self. Even modest weight loss of 5% to 10% of your total body weight can result in significant positive changes in blood pressure, blood cholesterol, and blood sugars.[27]

TikTok and Instagram offer endless reels promoting products that boost metabolism and accelerate weight loss. Unfortunately, very few foods are shown to have any measurable impact on metabolism beyond the normal costs of digestion. Those that do register a small metabolic boost are, at best, minimal and are more than likely offset by increased hunger and food intake. There is no generic, magical mix of carbohydrates, fats, and proteins to accelerate weight loss. Diets that work do so because calorie intake has been reduced.

Here are some of the most common dietary and lifestyle pitfalls to watch out for:

- calorie-laden late dinners
- between-meal and end-of-day stress-eating
- hidden liquid calories found in alcohol, fruit juice, and soda pop
- meals loaded with simple carbs, such as white rice, white pasta, and white bread
- processed snacks high in sugar

TRACK YOUR CRAVINGS

When you begin paying attention to your food intake, cravings make more sense. Following an event that demands your best performance, it is normal to experience an energy drop and crave sugar. Anticipate and counteract this response by ensuring you have a healthy snack waiting for you. A small handful of nuts, yogurt, a few veggie sticks with hummus, blueberries, or an apple can prevent an energy crash and will help you avoid poor food choices made down the road as hunger takes over. If the energy deficit of a calorie-restricted diet leaves you with insatiable hunger, keep a bottle of water close. Sipping water throughout the day helps keep hunger down, and the extra trips to the washroom will introduce more movement to your day.

CUT PORTION SIZE

Using a smaller plate or bowl can trick your mind into thinking you are still enjoying a full-size meal. Eating slowly gives your body and mind a chance to switch off the hunger signal and enjoy the meal. Stepping away from the table after a modest meal and shifting gears to an activity that distracts your mind from food also helps hunger pass.

REMOVE TEMPTATIONS

Clear your pantry and fridge of all unhealthy options. Try serving food in the kitchen and not from larger dishes on the table. Keep tasty, healthy options easily accessible so you don't feel guilty or deprived when you do snack.

MONITOR YOUR EMOTIONAL HEALTH

If you snack out of boredom or eat when you need some emotional support, don't let the behavior go unnoticed. Recognize your desire to eat outside of regular meals and try finding another channel for these emotions. Going for a walk would be ideal, but listening to a ten-minute guided meditation, making a phone call to a friend, reading, or listening to music are other options to consider. Engaging with a creative DIY project, exercise, or volunteer work are also great distractions. If you are having trouble breaking a stress-eating habit or pattern of emotional eating, seek the assistance of a mental health expert. Help is available, and asking for it is a sign of strength.

CREATE A COMMUNITY

This journey can be lonely if you charge ahead on a solo expedition. Find or build a community to join you and share your experiences along the way. Clearly stating your goals and setting accountability standards will help you through plateaus or low points. Supporting another person's journey can also help strengthen your resolve.

Centenarians make healthy food choices, but they are also committed to sharing their meal times with loved ones. Social connections boost health for everyone at the table.

GET ACTIVE

Put the powerful action of walking to work. This easy and cost-effective form of physical activity will reduce the risk of depression, aid in weight management, and improve brain, bone, muscle, and heart health.[28] Prioritize movement by finding 150 minutes (2.5 hours) to dedicate to moderate-intensity activity each week. (More on this in Wellness Ritual #4: Move to Stay Young.)

TRACK YOUR PROGRESS

The Heart and Stroke Foundation promotes two methods of self-assessment that can give you a clearer picture of how your weight may be affecting your health and the progress you are making.

Waistline Measurement

Here is how to measure your waist correctly:

1. Stand upright, facing a mirror with your feet shoulder-width apart and stomach relaxed.
2. Wrap a tape measure around your waist, just above the high point of the crest of your pelvis.
3. Take two normal breaths and after the second breath out, with your stomach relaxed, tighten the tape around your waist so it is snug but not pressing into your skin, and record the measurement.

Males more than 94 cm (37 inches) are at increased health risk; more than 102 cm (40 inches), and you have a substantially increased risk.[29] Females more than 80 cm (31.5 inches) are at increased health risk, and those with a waist measurement of more than 88 cm (35 inches) have a substantially increased risk.[29]

A study completed by Mayo Clinic that looked at data from 650,000 adults showed that men with a waist circumference of 110 cm (43 inches) had more than a 50% greater risk of death than men with a 94-cm (37-inch) waist. For women, those with a 94-cm (37-inch) waist had an 80% higher risk of death than did women with a 70-cm (27.5-inch) waist.[30]

Start with a small goal of reducing your waist circumference by a single centimeter, then two. A drop of 4 cm has been shown to have massive benefits to your health risk profile.[29]

Body Mass Index (BMI)

BMI is the ratio of your height to weight. It is used to measure health for people between the ages of eighteen and sixty-five. BMI calculators can be found online. For those who like mental math, divide your weight in kilograms by the square of your height in meters. Individuals with a BMI between 25 and 25.9 are considered overweight. Scores over thirty are considered obese. Scores between 18.5 and 24.9 are at low risk of health complications.[29]

Individuals who learn how to control the balance of their energy equation are more successful at reaching their goals and maintaining the progress they have made.

Tip: You can find recommended BMI calculators at **7WellnessRituals.com**

RITUAL ACTIVATION

TAKE THESE STEPS:

- **Practice Wellness Ritual #1.** Sleep deprivation promotes the production of visceral fat and drives over-consumption.

- **Practice Wellness Ritual #2.** Build your diet around filling, nutrient-rich foods without packing in a lot of calories. Choose whole foods and track what you eat. The short-term pleasure and convenience processed foods offer are not worth the hit to your health. Play the smart, long game. Foods with more fiber, more protein, and fewer calories per bite will be the most filling. Foods loaded with sugar, salt, and fat are way too easy to overeat.

- **Plan your meals.** Decide in advance what you're going to cook, then shop for only those choices. This will help limit temptations at home and in the grocery store.

- **Keep healthy snacks handy.** Stock your workspace and kitchen with various healthy, fresh fruits, vegetables, and nuts.

- **Avoid added sugar where possible.** Start reading food labels and make an effort to reduce consumption of corn sweetener or corn syrup, dextrose, fructose, or maltose. Ketchup, white pasta, bagels, fruit juices, energy bars, sports drinks, and energy drinks will spike blood sugar. Foods with natural sugars tend to be low in calories and salt and high in water, fiber, and essential vitamins and minerals, like blueberries.

- **Avoid eating when bored.** By recognizing and stopping this habit, you can significantly reduce your calorie intake. Eliminating this habit will jump start your weight-loss.

- **Practice stress resiliency strategies (see Wellness Ritual #6).** Our brains will substitute food rewards for the emotional and psychological rewards we crave when feeling isolated, fearful, or sad. To help regulate your reward systems and sharpen your resistance to overeating, speak to a mental health expert. Walking, starting a yoga practice, or completing a short, daily guided meditation can help reduce daily stress.

- **Divert negative self-talk.** Be kind to yourself. Recognize self-criticism and work at redirecting these thoughts and staying positive. Read happiness expert and author Shawn Achor's book *The Happiness Advantage*.[34] The practice of identifying three new things you are grateful for and why every day can help you reframe your mindset.

- **Spend more time in motion**, preferably outdoors (see Wellness Ritual #4). Avoid long periods of sitting. Prolonged inactivity is linked to poor eating habits and unhealthy weight gain. Buy a raincoat and a good pair of running shoes, and make an effort to walk 10,000 steps per day, every day.

- **Stay Strong (see Wellness Ritual #5: Protect Your Strength).** Hardwire time in your calendar for resistance training every week. Increasing your lean muscle mass and keeping your muscles toned will accelerate weight loss and help you achieve and maintain a healthy waistline.

IN SUMMARY

To master this Wellness Ritual, you must learn how to control your energy equation. A formula designed to lose weight and keep it off will require you to eat less, choose nutrient-dense foods, limit processed calories, and get active. This journey will demand patience, structure, and attention to your relationship with food and your mental health. Through the creation of an energy deficit and the support of your community and team of health professionals, it is possible to achieve a healthy waistline.

Dr. Andy Smith turns to a hockey analogy to help explain his drive to excel in life: **"I like to play in the blue paint.** I'm just drawn to the challenges and competition you find in front of the net." Playing in the blue paint takes **courage**, something that is not in short supply within him.

MENTOR PROFILES

———

DR. ANDY SMITH
PHILLIP CRAWLEY
MICHAEL "PINBALL" CLEMONS

DR. ANDY SMITH

President and CEO of Sunnybrook Health Sciences Centre

*A*ndy Smith, MD, MSc, FRCSC, FACS, is the President and Chief Executive Officer (CEO) of Sunnybrook Health Sciences Centre, one of Canada's largest academic health institutions. At fifty-five, he views age as simply a number. It does not limit or define him.

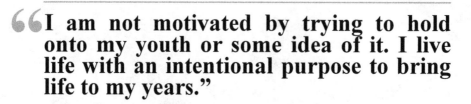

> ❝I am not motivated by trying to hold onto my youth or some idea of it. I live life with an intentional purpose to bring life to my years.❞

In fact, like a fine wine — or, in Andy's case, a smooth, complex-flavored, oak-aged bourbon — his game improves with each year. I asked him for a mid-decade health status report, and his response was: "I am not obsessed with staying young, turning gray, or the passing of the clock. I am not motivated by trying to hold onto my youth or some idea of it. I live life with an intentional purpose to bring life to my years."

A GRATITUDE RITUAL BEGINS THE DAY

The notion of "intentional purpose" was grounded in Andy's early years. His dad, John, born in Jamaica, his mum, Susan, in England, were both loving but firm. As a young boy, he shared a single bedroom with his four brothers in what they referred to as The Barracks. His dad would enter The Barracks with an early-morning greeting: "Boys, you are second to none. It is time to get up." The wake-up call would frequently trigger a 5 a.m. start to Andy's day. Shortly afterward, he would be out the door, delivering *The Globe and Mail* newspaper to neighbors' front doorsteps. If a doubt or hesitation to embrace the day were ever revealed, his mum would remind the boys that "life is not lost in dying. Rather, it is lost in all of the days you do not live."

Andy made his mark as a surgeon and leader in the management of colorectal cancer. Clinical experience in this discipline comes with a sobering appreciation for the gift of health and the value of the day in front of you. This clarity is ever-present for Andy. He starts each day with an expression of gratitude for his ability to move freely without restriction and the strength to charge into the day. These precious few minutes are the quietest moments of Andy's day. He says a short prayer his mum taught him and reflects on the blessings and opportunities afforded to him. A positive energy takes shape in this moment that sparks his motivation and purpose. Ten thousand steps a day mark his daily, minimal, acceptable standard for movement. Like a good friend, this ritual greets him and provides a trusted hand of support in his 24/7, full-court press, professional role.

SELF-CARE REFLECTION #20

Susan A. Smith's words, "Life is not lost in dying. Rather, it is lost in all of the days you do not live" are profound. Andy begins each day with an expression of gratitude for the blessings of the day ahead. Do you begin your day with quiet time through meditation, prayer, or reading? If not, consider giving it a try. For Andy, it centers and prepares him for the day ahead.

FROM RUPTURE TO RECOVERY

At six foot, two inches and 210 pounds, Andy has an athletic build that reflects his commitment to an active lifestyle. Ten years earlier and fifteen pounds lighter, running was his passion. At his peak, he was capable of posting thirty-four-minute 10 km race times. To be clear, this is really fast. You are not posting 10 km times under thirty-five minutes as a weekend jogger. This accomplishment requires punishing hill training, 800 m speed work, and a strong obligation to performance excellence.

Andy turns to a hockey analogy to help explain his drive to excel in life: "I like to play in the blue paint. I'm just drawn to the challenges and competition you find in front of the net." Playing in the blue paint takes courage, something that is not in short supply within him. His character also reveals a healthy sense of competitiveness and an unquenchable passion to succeed. These traits shine through Andy's accomplishments and are likely a combination of his DNA and years spent competing hard in The Barracks' arena. Growing up with four brothers undeniably helped shape Andy's approach to work and play. The bond of the Smith brotherhood is strong.

He is proud of his twenty-five and two, head-to-head record against a younger brother who is also a runner. Unfortunately, one of these two losses cost Andy the Smith family race record by only eight seconds. The memory of the loss now brings a smile to his face, but I'm guessing it also still stings a little. Despite being a man who does not live in the past, these are eight seconds he would like back.

He completed one marathon in 1984, and the experience gave him the permission to check that box and accept that his frame was not built for ultra-long distances. Ten kilometers was his race. Andy knows his lane and how to stay in it.

As a surgeon, running became a way to decompress after a long shift at the hospital. The run would provide Andy with a therapeutic distraction from the life and death decisions that dominated his day in the operating room. However, the true value of this ritual would not be fully realized until Andy suffered an injury that marked the end of his days as a runner. At the age of forty-five, running home after a long day of surgery, he ruptured a tendon in the back of his leg. Lying in the street, Andy knew the injury was severe. He remembers feeling a sudden disappointment for ignoring his flat feet. The injury was likely an acute tear of a chronic condition that he later realized could have possibly been avoided with custom orthotics, better shoes, and closer attention to his movement quality. A surgeon at St. Michael's Hospital in Toronto gave him two options: fusion or reconstruction. He went with the second option, hoping to preserve his ability to move, even though this procedure, at the time, was not as common of a practice.

Reconstructive surgery proved to be the correct path for Andy, and to this day, he still expresses tremendous appreciation for his surgeon's advice and skill. His pace has had to change, but his commitment to movement has not wavered. He now walks home from the hospital, but his gait is unencumbered, and he is pain-free. His flat feet are now happily supported with hiking boots and orthotics.

While Andy misses running, he expresses no frustration. "My running days are in the past, and I'm okay with that." He has found the same mental and physical enjoyment walking that running once provided. True to form, his walking pace is also aggressive, with a fast-paced cadence that most who try to keep up describe as uncomfortable. Unapologetic, Andy warns walking companions, "I like it quick enough to work up a sweat and feel the surge of adrenaline."

THE LINK BETWEEN MOVEMENT AND PERFORMANCE

In my experience, when runners are told their running days are over, most find it hard to accept their truth. Not Andy. As he adapted his routine to walking, he quickly realized that his love for movement and the way it made him think, feel, and perform, not the act of running itself, made this ritual come alive. From this point forward, Andy would look to movement as the key to sustaining his high performance level. As he made the significant career change from surgeon to hospital executive, he would need this support.

His transition from a successful colorectal surgeon to his leadership role with Sunnybrook Health Sciences Centre took "blue-paint" courage. "I love my job. It is amazing, but walking away from the operating room was a big-time risk." When asked where the courage to make the career pivot came from, he again cited his upbringing and *carpe diem* philosophy of life. Before making the move, Andy demonstrated strong leadership skills in roles within the hospital and at the University of Toronto, including Head of the Division of General Surgery at Sunnybrook; Chair of the Division of General Surgery at the University of Toronto; Chief of the Odette Cancer Program; and Regional Vice President for Cancer Care Ontario. However, he remembers when he was first tapped on the shoulder for the role of Executive Vice President and Chief Medical Executive at Sunnybrook, feeling as though a door to a new career path had just presented itself. This particular crossroad had snuck up on him and hit him squarely in the chest.

The executive position would require him to give up his role as a surgeon for less money and longer hours. Truth be told, the "ask" by the president at the time, Dr. Barry McLellan, was more of a call to action by someone who saw tremendous potential in Andy. After his fourth interview and discussion with family, Andy took the road less traveled and accepted the position. He called Barry and said, "I'm in. Let's go for it."

He would spend the next four years in the VP position, receiving extensive executive training and seeking out mentorship at every opportunity. Two years into the role and loving his work, Andy came to realize that if he were successful in landing the CEO position, he would need to work at a maniacal pace for the next ten to fifteen years to have the impact he desired. He must then be prepared to pass it on to the following custodian.

And that is exactly what he set out to do. He walked the fine line, applying discipline to his training and focus to his steep learning curve; this was necessary in order to position himself as a candidate for the CEO job while preventing the pace and demands from clouding his appreciation for the blessings of the present day. His mum's voice remained always in his ear: "Do not live for tomorrow."

On July 1, 2017, he was officially welcomed as the new Sunnybrook Health Sciences Centre President and CEO. He was now responsible for leading one of Canada's largest academic health sciences centers with 11,000 staff and physicians, 1,300 beds, and an annual budget of more than $1.1 billion.

ANDY'S FORMULA FOR HEALTH, STRENGTH & HOPE

STRESS RELIEF AND MENTAL RESILIENCY

The enormous weight of his new responsibility would require nothing short of his best effort, and so he doubled down on his commitment to movement. Door-to-door, his home is 7.5 km from the hospital. He takes an Uber to work in the morning and walks home every day. On occasion, he can also be found power-walking the grounds of Sunnybrook's campus, working through a mid-day challenge toward a solution.

Walking does not just give Andy a physical boost; it sharpens his mental acuity too. Practicing daily movement presents numerous biomechanical advantages to human physical performance, but it is also essential to mental health and stress resiliency. Knowing this, Andy learned to leverage his movement to elevate his mental performance. Some of his best ideas come to him during his commute home.

He chooses to walk to music, audible books, or scheduled phone calls and rarely walks in silence. He does not appear to crave silence as other mentors profiled in this book do. I was surprised by this, expecting to hear that his walks were reserved for solitude, and took the opportunity to discuss the benefits of introducing quiet meditation to his walking ritual. He said he would give it a try.

> ❝**Honestly, after fifty-five years of life, you had better know yourself well enough to recognize your tendencies.**❞

Some days push Andy's limits. As he laces his boots up for the walk home on such a day, the walk's ritual provides confidence and clarity. With each step forward, his resolve strengthens. On occasion, if he reaches home with the burdens of the day still on his mind, his wife is quick to detect his "stress monster." In this state, Andy can be short on patience, irritable, and may raise his voice if provoked. Stress monsters are nasty that way and tend to show up at home when your guard is down and fatigue from a tough day exposes a few cracks in your armor. Thanks to the love and support he receives at home, stress monster sightings are becoming rarer in Andy's life and are quickly exterminated with an after-dinner walk.

As an executive, Andy has learned to become acutely aware of his position on his stress-performance curve and has developed an "monster alarm" of his own. "Honestly, after fifty-five years of life, you had better know yourself well enough to recognize your tendencies," he states.

As an example, he offered this short illustration. During the pandemic, he began washing the dinner dishes by hand, finding the practice soothing. According to Andy, his wife, who is also a brilliant surgeon, sets a high bar for quality control inspection of the pots and pans he washes. If a failed pot inspection triggers even the slightest sensation of his stress monster, he knows another walk is in the cards. "Really, with everything on our plate, is rewashing a pot that big of a deal? No! So if it bothers me, I know I'm not where I want to be mentally."

The adrenaline surge from a fast-paced walk reduces his stress level, and Andy finds peace. He brings considerable enthusiasm to all aspects of his life, including maintaining positivity and seeking happiness in his professional and personal life. He will turn to his chiropractor and personal trainer or book the odd massage at a spa with his wife to keep his body in shape and moving optimally. Those few words, "I'm in. Let's go for it," are a simple yet profound insight into Andy's commitment and drive to meet the challenges of his day head-on, from within. "I may work seven days a week, but my life is fun."

WALKING WITH ANDY

One of our discussions for this book was at 8 a.m. on a rainy Saturday morning in February. While many were still curled up in bed, Andy was already out embracing the day. Truthfully, as a runner myself, I woke the day of our call disappointed with the cold, damp weather and felt a fruitless resentment toward February. I considered whether I would skip my scheduled long run outdoors for a shorter indoor run on the basement treadmill. But after listening to Andy describe the beauty of the day and share his enjoyment of walking outside regardless of Mother Nature's mood, it inspired me to lace up my running shoes and head outdoors following our call.

During my run, I replayed our conversation in my mind and was struck by his influence. One of the more remarkable things about Andy is that he invites you into his world with open arms, and through his lens, the world seems a degree or two more positive and full of opportunity. Spending time with him has a lasting impact.

Do not let stress continue to negatively impact your health. Ask your healthcare team for help and find out what resources are available to you in your workplace. Healthy organizations provide third-party support and encourage their employees to take advantage of it.

SELF-CARE REFLECTION #21

There are days when Andy's limits are stretched. Can you imagine the challenges he must have faced leading one of Canada's largest hospitals through the early days of the pandemic? To survive, he leaned on his awareness and self-care skills to quickly course-correct if he felt his mindset drifting toward negativity. Undoubtedly, there have been days in the last few years that you felt your capacity was being tested. Stress, when constant and left unchecked, is dangerous. What are the early warning signs that your stress monster is emerging?

PHILLIP CRAWLEY

Publisher and CEO of The Globe and Mail

*F*or many years, Phillip's routine followed a predictable rhythm — in bed by midnight, up at 5:30 a.m. at the latest, and in the gym by 6 a.m. on most mornings. With his workout complete, he would head to the office sharply dressed, physically and mentally alert, and with his game face on. At seventy-six, he still holds himself to a remarkable and inspiring personal standard of excellence. Having spent fifty-five years in the newsroom, his instincts are astute, his skin thick, and his stamina legendary. As Publisher and CEO of *The Globe and Mail*, heralded as Canada's national newspaper, Phillip's first thought every day is news.

On waking, he is quick to grab his smartphone. "What is the *Telegraph* in the UK reporting? What is the *New York Times* saying? What are we covering, and how does it compare?" I have witnessed Phillip's leadership for the better part of fifteen years as the onsite chiropractor for employees of *The Globe and Mail*. It is a unique vantage point from which to observe their work culture. Tasked with supporting Phillip's physical performance, I help keep him moving. Our doctor-patient relationship has evolved over the years, and Phillip has become a trusted mentor of mine. We enjoy discussing biomechanics, sport, politics, family life, and the headlines of the day. I know him to be generous, quick-witted, and kind.

To step into his professional world and watch his team navigate a breaking story or creatively deliver the news to Canadians in an ever-changing digital landscape is fascinating. Here, Phillip is phlegmatic, deliberate, and strategic. His competitive spirit, work ethic, and commitment to excellence are woven deeply within *The Globe and Mail* brand. A newsroom does not suffer fools. The adrenaline rush of a big story can be intoxicating and set in motion a ripple effect that plays out across the news organization. In an industry that has seen few survivors, Phillip's healthy lifestyle rituals profoundly influence his leadership. How he manages his stress, when he exercises, and what he eats all became essential points of focus as he crafted a health formula that would sustain him at a high level.

SELF-CARE REFLECTION #22

As the leader of a national newspaper, Phillip Crawley prepares himself physically and mentally to be a role model to his team. Managing his stress, exercise, and diet support his endurance and cognitive edge. As you read Phillip's profile, note which steps you deliberately take to be at your best for the day. What aspects of your formula need attention?

PRIORITIZING PHYSICAL EXCELLENCE

Phillip is a keen athlete. At 5'6" and 137 pounds, he must rely on speed and mobility in sport. "I'm very competitive by nature. Whether on the soccer pitch, tennis court, or wherever, to be physically fit gave me an advantage. I may not be the most skilled player, but if I brought a higher level of fitness to my game, I could beat a better player."

Soccer was his early passion. Later in life, it became running and tennis. In athletics, he recognized that his determination and competitive nature would give him an advantage in the business world.

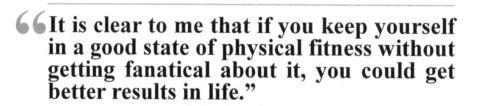

> **It is clear to me that if you keep yourself in a good state of physical fitness without getting fanatical about it, you could get better results in life."**

His chosen profession demands a high level of resiliency. The prevalence of post-traumatic stress disorder in journalism is known to be higher than it is in the general population. Aware of this risk, Phillip found mental and physical refuge in Wellness Ritual #5: Protect Your Strength. "I knew I could count on being more determined. I could be a terrier, snapping at the heels of my opponents, bringing bigger players down. This has always been my approach. It is clear to me that if you keep yourself in a good state of physical fitness without getting fanatical about it, you could get better results in life."

Setting physical excellence as the central pillar to his formula has served Phillip well. In many respects, he is stronger and healthier now, in his mid-seventies, than a significant number of executives in their mid-forties. Maintaining a high level of physical fitness has enabled him to continue to lead in a very competitive industry. His body is so well trained to respond to movement that the ritual operates on autopilot. There is no hesitation or even a hint of reluctance to carve time out for exercise. Driven by data and goals, he reverse engineers his training schedule to achieve a targeted outcome.

STEPPING UP THE CN TOWER

When *The Globe and Mail* got behind the United Way fundraiser to climb the 1,776 steps to the top of the CN Tower, Phillip was in his early sixties. It would not be enough for Phillip to just register and complete the climb. "I wanted to know what the best possible times were." For months in advance, he left work at lunchtime, crossed the street to a local gym, and trained on a step machine. "People would ask 'why?' I would answer, 'Because I had a purpose.'" He knew the concrete stairwell of the CN Tower was narrow, dark, dusty, and offered poor air quality. He also knew that many tackle the challenge ill-prepared and fall short of the finish line. Not Phillip — he was determined to lay down a time that would be difficult to beat and would raise eyebrows. With his reputation, and by extension, the reputation of *The Globe and Mail* on the line, he would deliver. On the day of the event, he had put in the work and was prepared, completing his first attempt in seventeen minutes and four seconds. As a reference point, the fastest official recorded time for a male over fifty is fourteen minutes and six seconds. The average climber completes it in thirty to forty minutes.

A PASSION FOR RUNNING

As a runner in his sixties, Phillip brought the same intensity to training for local 5 km and 10 km races. At his peak, he could complete a half marathon in an hour and a half. This is fast. He found a thrill in competition that continued to encourage his motivation to run.

He also saw running as a way to help others get active and played an instrumental role in supporting the launch of community-based fun runs in the UK during the early

1980s. Brendan Foster, a British long-distance runner and bronze medal winner in the 1976 Summer Olympics, approached Phillip while working for a Thomson newspaper. He was looking for media and marketing support for what would become the Great North Run. The event is now the largest half marathon in the world and takes place annually in north-east England each September. Phillip's love for community fun runs persisted years later in Toronto. His annual commitment to an early-spring race in High Park kept him training all winter long. Dressed in winter thermal gear with spikes on his shoes, January's snow and ice did not slow him down. In between races, an easy 5 km or 8 km run through a ravine or along a wooded trail offered something even more rewarding than the excitement of race day.

The solitude of running also provides Phillip with the time and space to do some of his best thinking. "My mind is free to wander when I run." Wherever Phillip lived in the world for the better part of thirty years, the ritual of a forty-five-minute run became a treasured time to process the week's challenges and problem-solve. The workout could be easily scheduled around the demands of the day in ways a tennis match or fitness class could not.

> 66 **Running was my release. It was the way I cleared my head, de-stressed, and relaxed."**

PHILLIP'S FORMULA FOR HEALTH, STRENGTH & HOPE

NEVER SURRENDER

In early 2016, thirty years of running and a lifetime of sport had caught up with Phillip. Persistent hip pain following a snow-shoeing expedition led to a diagnosis of hip osteoarthritis. "I limped along for a bit, but eventually, this marked the end of running for me." He had one hip replaced that year and the other three years later. "It is worth reflecting how you adjust with age to a different set of expectations for yourself — you have to recalibrate your capabilities in terms of what you are now able to do compared to what you thought you might be able to do. In my early sixties, I thought I would be running until I dropped." No longer able to maintain his fitness standards as a runner, he joined a gym and turned his attention to flexibility, strength training, and dynamic movement. Recovery from his second hip operation came twice as quickly, and he was back on the tennis court inside three months.

Phillip tackles aging head on. Recognizing that one of the realities of getting older is the need for more clinical support to maintain functional abilities, he leans on chiropractic, acupuncture, physiotherapy, and guidance from his personal trainer to keep his body moving to its full potential. "I make sure that I stay on top of my aches and pains with regular treatment." During the summer of 2020, he returned to playing singles tennis with renewed mobility.

> ❝If I am not physically fit, I'm simply not going to be able to do the job as well as I should be doing it."

He is in the gym by 6 a.m. to train hard for forty-five minutes three days a week and continues to play tennis weekly to keep his physical and mental edge sharp. "I recognized that I was getting older and needed to set some new targets to make sure I was not falling off the physical standards I had set for myself. I do not accept that getting older means that you have to give up." Even at the peak of Phillip's hip pain, his determination to move was not diminished. In fact, the decision to have the surgery was not about reducing pain. It was about maintaining his ability to move. "If I am not physically fit, I'm simply not going to be able to do the job as well as I should be doing it."

MAINTAINING MENTAL ACUITY

Studying the arc of Phillip's career, it is apparent that his lifelong bond with exercise has allowed him to tap into an energy reserve uninfluenced by age or circumstance. It has elevated his performance in immeasurable ways, allowing him to maximize his physical abilities. While this is impressive, it is the mental confidence he draws from his fitness dominance that is perhaps even more unique and fascinating. Time to second guess is not a luxury Phillip's professional role affords. Decisions must be made precisely on cue or even slightly in advance. To do this effectively takes a special kind of confidence and courage. "In high-pressure times, faced with cross-road decisions, you must be able to draw on inner strength. Sometimes, big moments in your life come down to a binary decision. You can go this way or that. Making the wrong decision can have serious consequences."

Phillip made several bold decisions to advance his career by drawing on this confidence. Before joining *The Globe and Mail*, he held various senior executive positions with some of the world's leading media companies in Europe, Asia, and New Zealand. "Uprooting our home and moving from the UK to Hong Kong was a big family decision. With teenagers in tow, I was asking my wife and family to move to a place they had never even visited." The enormity of this decision struck me. Getting the teenagers in my home to agree on a movie for family movie night can feel significant. Acknowledging the importance of such small wins, he offered me a smile, but to really understand Phillip's process, we discussed big choices.

"I find that people underestimate just how limiting it can be if you wait and do not act while you are in your peak physical health. At forty-eight, I was living in Hong Kong. I wanted to move into management from being an editor-in-chief. Moving back to the UK at fifty, relocating my family again, took courage. But when presented with the opportunity, I took it while I could."

His family would face another big decision when they moved from New Zealand to Canada. Phillip was once again in a job he was enjoying. The family was settled and happy, but the opportunity in Canada was too compelling to turn down, despite having to endure two winters in one year. He shared that internally there is always some doubt when making a big decision, but by maintaining peak physical and mental health, he has been able to consider opportunities with a clear head and not miss out. "Many decide to stay put and not take chances in life, avoiding risk and settling for where they are. This lack of ambition will limit you."

THE NEWSPAPER WAR: BLACK VS. CRAWLEY

Arriving in Canada in 1998 to lead *The Globe and Mail*, Phillip's confidence, standards of excellence, and ambition would be tested. His team was counting down to the launch of Conrad Black's *National Post*, only three weeks away. *The Globe and Mail* was preparing for a fight. Phillip told me, "I was arriving very late on the scene to lead a business that needed a change in leadership style and a cultural renewal. For the first time, we were facing a challenge of our supremacy as the national newspaper." His major concern was complacency. "After a quick scan of the staff, my sense was that half thought that we were impregnable; we have been here since 1844; no upstart is going to knock us from our perch. The other half was thinking Conrad Black is a global force who usually gets what he wants, that his record of being a successful newspaper publisher was a threat to the future of the *Globe*."

Phillip's approach was to ensure everyone was on the edge of their seats, ready to go full throttle, prepared for the fight. "It was extremely competitive for about two years, the impact of which was very disruptive in value right across the industry as prices dropped and papers were being given away." It was a high-stress match as the media giants exchanged blows over content and talent. "If you were not sleeping, you were doing nothing else." Phillip and the *Globe* held their ground.

NEW BEGINNINGS

Following his own advice to live life full throttle, Phillip fell in love and remarried. His second wife, a professional, brilliant, strategic thinker in her own right, brought love back into his life. Her tender support seems to soften Phillip's corners. When he speaks of his wife, the importance and impact of their relationship are evident. She is someone he can confide in, providing him with a trusted, nurturing sounding board away from the pressures at work. While he admits to not always liking the advice she gives, he always appreciates it. "She will tell me like it is."

With the rhythm of life disrupted during the COVID-19 pandemic, Phillip, like many, was presented with more time on his hands. Business travel had stopped entirely, and most days were spent in front of a screen on back-to-back video conference calls. He missed the human contact, the buzz of the newsroom, and the cadence of his pre-pandemic life. When gyms were closed, he went for daily walks with his wife and their two dogs. He now aims to get 7 to 7.5 hours of sleep a night, although he is not convinced the increased time in bed translates to more quality sleep.

As for nutritional rituals, Phillip maintains a healthy diet. His weight has held within ten pounds his entire adult life. He will enjoy a glass of wine with a meal, but avoids heavy drinking. He steers clear of junk food and makes healthy choices at virtually every meal. His discipline, again, allows him to avoid poor choices. It helps that his wife is an exceptional cook. Together they are mindful of the significant influence diet has on health and performance. "The meals my wife prepares are healthy, creative, flavorful, and beautifully presented." The odd night, they might cheat with an order of fish and chips from a local shop, but otherwise their diet is extremely clean. Healthy eating is an easy choice for Phillip.

Phillip's pursuit of excellence is not measured by a bucket-list, checklist, or cabinet full of awards. He appears indifferent to the good opinion of others, internally motivated by the challenge that lies over the next hill. His path is principled and guided by the discipline of his routine. Whether competing in a local race, representing the business in a corporate fitness challenge, or training to beat a personal best one-mile pace, Phillip has successfully set and maintained a high standard for physical performance his entire life. This commitment has provided mental confidence and steadied determination that have elevated his impact. Phillip has left nothing on the table and continues to live, compete, and lead at an elite level.

SELF-CARE REFLECTION #23

For this exercise, think about Phillip's words, "I do not accept that getting older means you have to give up." This is a powerful sentiment, and within these words is the core of the 7 Wellness Rituals mindset. While our bodies change physiologically due to age, this does not mean the wrinkles and gray hair are signs of diminishing physical strength or mental clarity. Where do you fall along the spectrum of "giving up"? Does your mindset need to shift? Think about Phillip's resolve and how he sustains his well-being in his mid-seventies.

MICHAEL "PINBALL" CLEMONS

GM of the Toronto Argonauts & Co-Founder of Pinball Clemons Foundation

"*I* remember having one game as a kid where I was just running crazy. I was only ten or eleven at the time, playing minor football in Florida. I already had four touchdowns in the first half when I broke loose and was on my way again. As I'm sprinting down the field with a clear path to the end zone, I see my coach running along the sideline screaming, 'Get out of bounds! Get out of bounds!' Thankfully, I clued in before scoring and stepped out just short of the goal line.

66 I was raised to believe that to be human is to deserve dignity."

"Coach didn't want to run up the score any more than we already had. With the game in hand he told me I was done for the day and would sit out the rest of the game. Selfishly, I wanted back in the action. From the stands, my mom saw me hanging my head despite the team's success. She came down at halftime, marched on the field, looked me straight in the eye and said, 'Your teammates love you, and every week they cheer for you. You are on the field all the time. Right? I want you to know that if you don't become the best cheerleader on this field in the second half, you will never play football again.'

"I was raised to believe that to be human is to deserve dignity. This was the calling that resonated in our home. My mom taught me an appreciation for humanity that is so much a part of who I am today. So I can't take any credit for my life other than to say, at some point, the work belongs to you. If you want to show me a truly great person, don't tell me about records or awards, money or power. If you want to show me a truly great person, show me what that person has done for someone else. Therein lies true greatness."

SELF-CARE REFLECTION #24

For this exercise, think about Michael Clemons' words, "The work belongs to you." The "work" he is talking about is what you have done or what you are doing to make someone else's life better. As you read Michael's story, think about your accountability to others. Are you a role model for those aspiring to live a healthier life?

HOW DO WE FRAME SUCCESS?

Michael is American by birth but Canadian by choice. While small of stature at a touch over 5'6" and 165 pounds, he was a giant on the football field. He moved with the speed, agility, and balance of a finely-tuned Porsche 911 Turbo S. With lightning-quick reflexes, the running back and return specialist became known as "Pinball" for his ability to bounce off would-be tacklers and aggressively gain field position. In 1999, he passed the 5,000-yard mark in four separate categories: rushing (5,341), receiving (7,015), kick-off returns (6,349), and punt returns (6,025) — the only athlete in pro-football to do this north or south of the border. At the time of his retirement from the Canadian Football League (CFL) in 2000, he held the pro-football record for the most combined yards in a season, with 3,840, and most career combined yards, with 25,438.[1] Jerry Rice, the San Francisco 49ers Hall-of-Fame receiver, still sits at the top of the NFL, with 23,546 total, all-purpose yards before he called it a career in 2005.[2] That is 1,892 fewer yards than Michael.

Humble and quick to downplay his accomplishments, the record books do not hold his focus or elevate his ego. As the keynote speaker at the 2010 Mental Fitness Summit hosted at the Centre for Health and Safety Innovation in Mississauga, Ontario, he shared, "I spent my pro-career carrying a leather ball chased by guys twice my size. It was my job to move that ball forward as far as I could at every opportunity. I was literally evaluated by this distance — yard by yard. It took me eleven years to carry that ball just over 23 kms. Eleven years! An experienced marathon runner could cover this distance in less than two hours. How we frame success is essential. Those 23 kms don't define me. I measure success by the lives I've helped, not the yards I've run."

"YOUR FOCUS WILL BECOME YOUR FACT"

Studying the formula of an altruistic, Hall-of-Fame professional athlete turned sports executive and philanthropist offers a unique perspective. The burning question in my mind was, "How does someone so selfless prioritize and practice self-care in the privacy of their own life?" At fifty-six years of age, having suffered over a decade of physical abuse as a pro-football player, I assumed pain management would be one of the guideposts holding his attention. However, this was not the case. Pain did not enter our conversation. Framing his story, he shared, "Let me start with this — I believe that excellence comes from being layered."

Self-care for Michael is rooted in gratitude. He credits his mother for making him aware of the delicate beauty of humanity. She was his superhero and taught him to work hard and look for opportunities to make the world a better place. I would go so far as to suggest that Michael continues to see this calling as his primary responsibility, second only to the care and protection of his family.

As the first person of color to work in an administrative position for the city of Dunedin, Florida, Michael's mother, Anna O'Neal, led by example. Michael's birth marked the end of Anna's dream to pursue a career in nursing. However, she leveraged a clerical job with the city to work her way up to a management position in the city's utility department.

"Things were not plentiful in the Clemons home, but I've never lacked," Michael told me. He charged into the world, wanting to do right by his mom, sensitive to the sacrifices she had made for him as a single parent. From a distance, his father had an influence. However, he was not involved in their day-to-day lives. When he failed to show up as promised, Michael hid his disappointment from his mother, never wanting her to feel as though she weren't more than enough.

> **My mom would say, 'You focus on what you don't have, and that's where you're going to end up. Your focus will become your fact.'"**

Michael was a gifted athlete and student, but the focus was never "I'm the best," even though his minor football league retired his jersey in honor of his accomplishments. His mother's love was directed toward the future, ensuring Michael understood that he could grow up to do anything or be anyone he desired. "I could have been a dentist or doctor. I could have been a school teacher. I could have driven a bus. I didn't feel bound by a list of things I was told I couldn't do. Now, there are some limits one must face. The Argonauts would not have wanted me to play on their offensive line. I couldn't be a center, but I grew up with such freedom of possibility. And so, I think my greatest physical asset, in terms of my self-care, was the mental fortitude, capacity, and freedom to do and to be."

Along the way, there were stop signs. One of those was his size, and the other was the color of his skin.

"I didn't see people who looked like me on television. As I got past third, fourth, fifth grade, I ended up being the only Black student in many of those classes. There was great discontent around that, but I still grew up with such gratitude for my life. My mom would say, 'You focus on what you don't have, and that's where you're going to end up. Your focus will become your fact.'"

These six words, "your focus will become your fact," had a significant impact on the direction of Michael's life and laid the foundation for his influence on the world. To this day, they continue to guide his decisions and have provided him with the creative flexibility to adapt his daily approach to support his ongoing health and performance.

SELF-CARE REFLECTION #25

There is a small recurring theme in the stories of our mentors, which is the wise words of parents. Michael's mom told him, "Your focus will become your fact." Michael faced various kinds of discrimination: being Black in a predominately white school, being the smallest player on the football field, being the object of envy for his natural athletic abilities. By keeping your focus as your fact, you shut out the distractions. You shut out the negative energy. You focus on positivity and train harder and never deviate from your values. How would you assess your focus? Is your focus your fact?

CREATE SPACE FOR OTHERS TO GROW: THE PINBALL CLEMONS FOUNDATION

Michael's smile and positive presence alone can carry a room. Whether he is on stage speaking to a large corporate audience; in the locker room delivering a pre-game motivational speech; on one knee, eye-to-eye, inspiring a young child; or lending a hand to someone less fortunate, he is honest, genuine, and kind. Regardless of the age or position in life of those who cross his path, he graciously invests in every encounter, creating space for others to grow, share, or find a reason to smile. There is energy exchanged in Michael's presence that is undeniable. He possesses a unique ability to help others block distractions and draw focus. He listens with his soul and leaves you wanting to be better.

While Michael is too humble to say this, his true talent extends well beyond the sport of football and lies in his ability to bring kindness to the world. Through the Pinball Clemons Foundation, he is drawn to play an even bigger game with higher stakes — providing marginalized and racialized youth with educational resources and options to integrate into mainstream society. "With a big smile and hello, you can turn a person's day around and help make that person's day a little better. I am a loving guy who wants to build bridges, not fences."

With the implementation of a customized mentorship program and financial support, the Pinball Clemons Foundation acts to remove barriers that hinder success. The foundation's goal extends beyond continued education and is dedicated to assisting youth with finding an entry point into the workforce and earning gainful employment in their chosen careers.

MICHAEL'S FORMULA FOR HEALTH, STRENGTH & HOPE

WHEN A PRO ATHLETE RETIRES...

An athlete of Michael's caliber must perfect the lifestyle required to optimize athletic talent. There is only one way to do this cleanly, and it is through discipline and hard work. As a pro-athlete, accountability is built-in. The infrastructure to support healthy decisions and receive necessary treatment is hard-wired into a professional team's operations. When

Michael hung up his cleats, this support fell away. Without it, he felt his standards slipping. Michael had to learn how to prioritize his health without the watchful eye of the team of clinicians, coaches, and support staff he had come to rely on.

> ❝ **I've learned to turn to others to help keep me motivated and in the game.**❞

Stepping off the field, he continued to place a high value on maintaining his peak performance. For a brief period following his retirement, he would jump in on a recreational pick-up game of soccer or basketball but now rarely participates in team sport. Instead, he looks to exercising as a daily requirement, much like sleeping or breathing, making time for it every day. His wife and a young man named Dallas are his accountability partners.

"I've learned to turn to others to help keep me motivated and in the game. I'm in a push-up challenge with a young friend of mine named Dallas and his dad. Every Monday, Wednesday, and Friday, we get on a video call and do 100 push-ups and 100 sit-ups. It's a fun way to build accountability. Dallas is thirteen years old. I know he will be there. I won't be late for him. By making this commitment, we are helping each other. His confidence is growing, and I'm getting my reps in."

MICHAEL'S KEEP-FIT FORMULA

Michael strives to keep within five pounds of his playing weight. During the peak of the COVID-19 pandemic, that five-pound buffer stretched to fifteen pounds, much to his disappointment. He found his way back with daily power walks, light resistance training in his home gym, and tighter portion control at mealtime. "I would never have considered walking as exercise, but I now walk with the intention of completing a certain number of steps every day."

Michael fasts intermittently and typically eats only two meals a day. He finds his body operates more efficiently on this diet and is drawn to the benefits it offers brain health and longevity. His wife, Diane, is an excellent cook, and their family food choices are made from lean protein and a variety of fruits and vegetables. A slice of her sweet potato pie occasionally tests his willpower. Sugar is his weakness.

If he starts to feel sluggish, notices any irregularity in his bowel habits, or gains weight, he completes a four or five-day fast or cleanse. He drinks a ton of water and does not drink alcohol. He supports his health goals with mini weight-loss or sugar-free challenges with friends or family. When a competition triggers his motivation, he is tough to beat.

Wired for movement, he continues to live up to his nickname. He sleeps from 2 to 7:30 a.m. and takes power naps when needed. On weekends outside of the football season, he tries to sleep in a little longer. Nine in the morning is a real stretch. "My body wakes up excited. I'm ready to roll. If I try to get to bed any earlier, I'll be up at three in the morning, staring at the ceiling. While playing pro ball, I could sleep for twelve hours straight, no problem. At that level, there was a lot more sleep required. My body now seems to get by with five or six hours." His evenings provide a window to prepare for the business of the day ahead, read, watch his favorite shows, or work on Sudoku puzzles.

FAITH, POSITIVITY, AND PURPOSE

Michael begins and ends his day with prayer. Prayer is his meditation. "Diane and I have a couple's prayer we do together to keep our marriage fresh." He sees prayer as an intentional tool that brings clarity to his purpose in life. "When you give love and positivity to others, when you show interest and enthusiasm in their life, what I have learned is that they give it back. And the key is this: I'm not looking for it back. I'm doing it because it is how I feel and what I believe is the right way to treat people."

When asked about his mental fitness and how he responds to leadership pressure, he paused and offered me one of his trademark smiles. He then shared, "I believe that if the pressure from the outside world ever creeps inside, becoming the pressure I put on myself, then I know they have got the wrong guy. Responding to external pressures can be a valuable tool to elevate your performance as a leader. The design of pressure is to make us better. I look to embrace that opportunity, not shy away from it. Pressure is only relieved when the process is completed, and the process begins by setting a pathway to success that is both reasonable and probable. I told my players that their best was always good enough. But with experience, their best should continue to get better."

In unpacking his formula, Michael revealed the layers in his approach through stories of gratitude, love, kindness, determination, faith, and hard work. His life stands as an example of excellence and the power of positivity. "We all must suffer one of two pains in life — the pain of discipline or the pain of regret. The path you choose defines your life."

...let's begin by reframing the value of movement and dropping the word "exercise." It is a loaded word that immediately pivots some into retreat. As you will see from the evidence presented, the regular practice of **movement with intention** has the power to dramatically improve your health and performance and **extend your life**.

MOVE TO STAY YOUNG

7 WELLNESS RITUALS
FOR HEALTH, STRENGTH & HOPE

WELLNESS RITUAL #4: THE SCIENCE

A typical day in my clinic involves helping patients recover their mobility. There are the usual tweaked backs and necks, sprained ankles, pulled muscles, and well-used body parts that seem to have stiffened overnight. Most of these common injuries are functional in nature and can be fixed. But there are also patients with more debilitating structural issues or chronic conditions that require on-going supportive care to maintain their mobility. Both groups, functional and structural, must practice healthy movement to maximize their recovery. What we all need to bear in mind is that sleeping posture, time spent sitting, diet, dehydration, body composition, exercise patterns, general flexibility, repetitive movements, and how we manage stress all affect our ability to move freely. Time waits for no one. Aging requires sensible activity to remain mobile.

To better understand a patient's attitude toward movement and fitness, I like to ask them about the activities or sports they enjoyed playing while growing up. Memories of high school Phys-Ed class can also be particularly revealing. The fragile interactions of early adolescence can have a ripple effect that influences the relationship we form with physical activity and the priority we place on movement later in life. With remarkable clarity, people can recall school locker rooms, grade nine aerobic fitness tests, competitive games of high school dodgeball, and athletic battles against rival schools. These early memories often evoke strong emotions and are remembered as either distinctly positive or borderline torturous.

The social pressure to look and move a certain way can be all-consuming for a young teenager.

For the strong, confident, and physically mature adolescent, PE and participation in organized sports present an opportunity to test the limits of their developing body, make friends, advance leadership skills, build confidence, gain social influence, and lean into competition. Success here plants a distinct incentive to prioritize exercise down the road. For the less athletically inclined, these early experiences can play out more like the victimized in *Lord of the Flies* and are not particularly fun or rewarding. Body shaming, bullying, and discrimination are also never forgotten. Escaping the humiliation of getting picked last or walking away from that dodgeball game injury-free is the extent of some kids' athletic highlight reel. When exercise feels more like a punishment in your youth, it can be challenging to develop a passion for it later in life.

People bring all kinds of emotional baggage to exercise and allow small barriers to grow into what feel like insurmountable obstacles. Doubt in your body's ability to move well can position you in the fast lane to a sedentary lifestyle. I have heard thousands of reasons why patients can't, won't, or don't want to get active. Some of the more common excuses include:

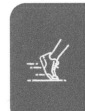

- I'm too stiff, fat, old, or tired.
- It hurts.
- I can't find the motivation.
- I have no time.
- I have an old injury.
- I have a new injury, and
- I'm just no longer comfortable going to a gym.

But the weather, old shoes, burst pipes, car trouble, work trouble, hair trouble, laundry days, relationship angst, or the endless list of the needs of others also keeps people from staying active. The patients who really pull at my heartstrings, though, are the ones who reluctantly admit that they "just don't enjoy exercise." There are many reasons someone may end up here, but none of them offer an exemption from the health costs related to inactivity. Regular movement is essential to good health, and Wellness Ritual #4: Move to Stay Young is structured to ensure you understand its value and find joy in its regular practice.

To provide a friendly entry to an emotionally charged topic, let's begin by reframing the value of movement and dropping the word "exercise." It is a loaded word that immediately pivots some into retreat. As you will see from the evidence presented, the regular practice of movement with intention has the power to dramatically improve your health and performance and extend your life.

The Move to Stay Young ritual aims to integrate a variety of movements into your daily routine designed to interrupt your sedentary postures and challenge the physical capacity of your body. The regular stimulus of movement drives a favorable adaptation that expands our potential and ability to move well.

Establishing specific movement goals and targets that are aligned with your current fitness level, health goals, and age is crucial to finding success. Let's get you up to speed on the most current movement research and help you create a framework for this practice. Welcome to Wellness Ritual #4: Move to Stay Young — your fountain of youth.

3 GROUND RULES

This Wellness Ritual is built on three ground rules:

1. Our bodies are made to move.
2. We perform better and slow the aging process when we bring movement to every day.
3. To make movement a priority, it must be enjoyable, celebrated, and rewarded.

GROUND RULE #1: OUR BODIES ARE MADE TO MOVE.

An inactive lifestyle will diminish the quality and quantity of days you have to live. Current evidence exposes the danger of sedentary behavior, linking an elevated risk of several chronic conditions, including diabetes, cardiovascular disease, cancer, and premature all-cause mortality with a lack of movement.[1] On the flip side, a daily routine that incorporates regular physical activity has been shown to provide significant protection against all of the above.[2]

We know this, yet we continue to sit for close to ten hours a day.[2]

Accumulate 150 minutes or more a week of moderate-to-vigorous physical activity in blocks greater than ten minutes at a time, and your health changes for the better. A daily sixty-minute walk can be enough to offset the risks of prolonged sitting.[3] It appears most of us know this too, yet over 82% of adults are not meeting current activity guidelines.

Changing behavior is hard. But as I mentioned earlier, hard is not impossible. Your incremental effort will be rewarded. Any belief that you are too old or too out of shape to embrace this Wellness Ritual must be left behind.

No matter what your starting point, as you begin to weave more therapeutic, purposeful movement into your formula, your body will become more capable of doing what you need it to do, and this freedom is inspiring.

Some of those reading this book will rely on this Wellness Ritual and others to fight back against a chronic disease, cast off a decline in health brought on by the pandemic, or simply maintain their independence. Those in elite physical condition may approach this ritual with the intention of hiking to the base camp of Mount Everest or completing another Ironman. Others may be looking for an advantage on the golf course, an extra gear in the executive board room, or another hour in their garden. Regardless of your situation, I am asking you to make a personal promise to move every day.

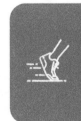

Finding the motivation to prioritize movement and get started is where most people struggle. Life gets busy, and it is easy to lose sight of the importance of staying active, especially if physical activity never felt like much of a reward. Learning how to proactively work on movement quality is not a skill set people spend much time on until pain, injury, or some type of dysfunction shows up. To help reverse this trend, behavioral scientists have shown clinicians that health recommendations, lifestyle modifications, and treatment strategies are more widely accepted and adopted if they are personalized.

So let's go there. What gets you off the couch?

Put on Your Walking Shoes

Some people respond more favorably to health objectives that are broken down into smaller, more easily achieved wins. This technique is called *delay discounting*, and it leverages the value of smaller rewards now over a larger reward in the future. Others who need to see and understand the end goal in order to find the motivation to successfully change behavior require an intervention called *episodic future thinking,* which focuses on thinking in specific ways about a future event. Given the option, would you take $500 now or $1,000 four weeks from now? Are you more inclined to commit to a regular after-dinner walk to help lower your cholesterol and improve your heart health because you enjoy the satisfaction of completing a daily activity and keeping your walking streak alive, or is it the vision of a healthy heart and longer life that will get you to put your walking shoes on?

There is no right or wrong answer to this question, but knowing which camp you are in will make the commitment I'm asking for easier. Understanding the trigger of your motivation is essential to turning this practice into a ritual and reaping the benefits offered through the science of movement.

Fear and pain can also be good motivators. I move because I love how it makes my body feel and my mind work, but my family history of heart disease also keeps me engaged in my commitment to move. In the section below, you will find the top ten dangers of a sedentary lifestyle. If this list elicits any fear or touches on a weakness in your family's medical history, use it to your advantage as extra motivation.

Sedentary behavior science is still emerging; however, the evidence to date is compelling. A variety of studies warn that sedentary lifestyles are likely to cause as many deaths as smoking. Population-based studies have found that more than half of an average person's waking day is spent sitting in front of a screen.[4] This lifestyle trend is particularly worrisome because evidence suggests that long periods of sitting have serious health effects independent of adults meeting the recommended physical activity guidelines.[5,6,7] In other words, not only is our time spent in motion falling short, but we also are not moving frequently enough.

The Costs of Choosing an Inactive Lifestyle

- You will be more prone to having poor blood circulation, elevated cholesterol levels, and high blood pressure, all of which contribute to cardiovascular disease.[8,9] Sedentary behavior is believed to alter blood flow and modify key inflammatory and metabolic processes, resulting in poor arterial health and the development of cardiovascular disease.[10] Physical inactivity, defined as not reaching the global physical activity guidelines of 150 minutes of moderate-to-vigorous activity in bouts of ten minutes or more each week, causes 6% of the global cardiovascular disease burden and has overtaken smoking as the primary cause of all-cause mortality.[11]

- You will burn fewer calories, which will tip the energy balance discussed in Wellness Ritual #3: Fight for Your Waistline toward weight gain and increase your chances of acquiring illnesses associated with obesity. Researchers have found a positive association between prolonged sitting and body composition, heart fat, liver fat, visceral fat, and waist circumference independent of physical activity.[12]

- Your ability to break down fats and sugars, regulate blood sugar, and maintain metabolic health will be adversely affected, increasing your risk of type 2 diabetes. A recent systematic review of the literature published in the *Journal of the American Medical Association* (JAMA) reported that people who watch television for more than two hours a day had a 20% increased risk of type 2 diabetes.[13]

- You will accelerate the loss of muscle mass, strength, and endurance. Use it or lose it. We will cover this topic in greater detail in Wellness Ritual #5: Protect Your Strength.

- Your bone mineral density will decline, increasing your risk of osteoporosis and making you more prone to fractures, chronic pain, and disability. The evidence here suggests that the longer your periods of sitting, the higher the harmful effects on bone mineral density.[14] Prolonged episodes of uninterrupted sitting appear to be more damaging to bone health than total time spent sitting.

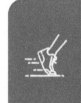

- Your risk of stroke will be higher. Evidence supports regular physical activity in primary and secondary stroke prevention and stroke rehabilitation. The Interstroke Study (a large case-control study across thirty-two countries that sought to quantify the importance of modifiable risk factors for stroke in different regions worldwide) lists inactivity as one of the ten key factors associated with about 90% of stroke risk.[15]

- Your body will be in a pro-inflammatory state and at increased risk of cancer. Evidence has linked sedentary behavior with cancer mortality risk.[16] Cancer is the leading cause of adult death in Canada and the US, although more than 50% of cancer deaths are preventable through healthy lifestyle choices.[17] Being physically active is a key lifestyle behavior associated with reductions in the risk of incident cancer and the risk of death from cancer.[18] Adults (aged fifty to seventy-one) who watch TV for at least seven hours a day had a 22% increased risk of cancer mortality relative to those who watched TV less than one hour a day.[19]

- Your mental health will suffer. High amounts of sitting are linked to psychological distress.[20] The evidence suggests a positive association between prolonged sitting and depressive symptoms in children, teenagers, and adults. Overweight and obese adults who gradually decrease their sedentary time and increase their moderate-to-vigorous physical activity have a reduced risk of depression.[21]

- You will have back pain. Low back pain is the number one cause of disability and one of the leading causes of lost-time at work.[22] According to the Canadian Chiropractic Association (CCA), more than 11,000,000 Canadians suffer from an injury or disorder that affects their movement, with one in eight reporting a chronic back problem and almost one third citing activity limitations due to back pain. A daily movement strategy that combines muscular strength, flexibility, and aerobic fitness is beneficial for rehabilitation of non-specific, chronic, low back pain.

- You may literally be cutting your life short. Sedentary behavior has been associated with an increased risk of all-cause mortality of up to 24% to 49%.[9] Replacing one hour of sitting with low-intensity activities such as household chores, garden

WHY DO I FEEL STIFF IN THE MORNING?

As we age, the mobility in a joint can gradually diminish due to changes in connective tissue, loss of muscle mass, altered biomechanics, or arthritis. Changes in the health of joint cartilage and a decrease in the lubricating synovial fluid secreted by the soft tissues surrounding our joints account for your morning stiffness. Macroscopically, these changes result in cracking and fissuring of our cartilage and ultimately, erosion of its ability to act as a shock absorber that cushions our bones against impact.[24] This change accompanies aging and is common. However, your routine will influence its severity. Review the Chapin Clinical Corner and Ritual Activation sections of this book for strategies to improve your morning mobility. For those who draw greater motivation from positive performance outcomes than they do from fear, let's turn our attention to the second ground rule of Wellness Ritual #4.

work, and daily walking has been shown to reduce all-cause mortality by as much as 30%.[23]

Are you still sitting down? If so, now would be a good time to stand up and move.

GROUND RULE #2: WE PERFORM BETTER AND SLOW THE AGING PROCESS WHEN WE BRING MOVEMENT TO EVERY DAY.

Our greatest weapon to fight chronic disease and age-related decline is not found in a prescription bottle; it is movement. A well-crafted movement strategy provides an effective defense against all ten health risks of inactivity. The very idea that a simple brisk walk holds the power to significantly reduce your risk of cardiovascular disease, obesity, diabetes, age-related muscle loss, osteoporosis, stroke, cancer, mental illness, back pain, and all-cause mortality seems like a fantasy — but it is not.

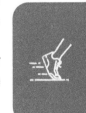

Our biological response to healthy movement holds a tremendous influence over our ability to heal, adapt, and excel. However, this biological potential will continue to lie dormant if you remain sedentary.

Key performance boosts unlocked through daily movement:

BETTER Movement Quality

When you can consistently rely on your body to move well, you feel strong, youthful, and confident. The opposite is true when you fall into a rut of inactivity or are limited because of pain. It is tempting to blame poor movement quality or an achy body on aging. This is seldom exclusively the case. Make movement your objective when crafting your formula.

Whenever possible, limit periods of uninterrupted sitting to sixty minutes. Take a micro-stretch break, change your posture, grab a glass of water, march on the spot, dance, take a phone call standing up, use voice-to-text software and dictate emails while walking around your office, or walk up and down a flight of stairs. Find a reason to move every hour and experiment with different types of movement that incorporate a variety of body parts.

Changing your posture allows the mechanical receptors in your joints and the muscles in your body to reset, and this helps to limit the physical punishment of sitting.

Consider introducing a sit-stand workstation, and limit your sedentary time by alternating between sitting and standing throughout the day. Complete five mini-squats every morning as you get out of bed, or try brushing your teeth while standing on one leg or while doing calf raises. The point is to explore different ranges of motion in as many joints as you can throughout the day, every day, without exception.

Elevate your heart rate for ten minutes or more periodically throughout your week until you have accumulated the recommended 150 minutes of moderate-to-vigorous activity. Banking this effort pays off in a big way. For those new to fitness or unfamiliar with this intensity of movement, it is imperative to begin slowly and engage your healthcare team to help you set an appropriate program for your age and ability before getting started. Brisk walking provides the easiest, most convenient, and most cost-effective approach to reaching this target.

For those interested in and capable of advanced training, progressing to interval training or establishing heart-rate performance and VO2 max targets (the maximum rate of oxygen consumption attainable during physical exertion) to expand aerobic capacity is an excellent way to keep this Wellness Ritual dynamic and hold your interest. Many of the mentors enjoy this physical challenge. Finding an experienced personal trainer or workout buddy with similar health goals will help you do this safely and hold yourself accountable.

MOVEMENT HELPS ALLEVIATE ARTHRITIC PAIN

Even though movement can be painful and difficult for people with arthritis, evidence suggests that increased physical activity can mitigate arthritis symptoms by 40%.[25]
Arthritis is typically treated with non-steroidal, anti-inflammatory drugs and analgesics. However, current chronic, non-cancer pain and opioid prescription guidelines recommend conservative therapies and physical activity as the first line of defense.[26]

Meet these two movement goals, and you will maintain adequate physical strength, balance, coordination, and functional range of motion to promote good health while significantly reducing the risks of inactivity.

BETTER Sleep

Engaging in frequent moderate-to-vigorous activity during the day will help you fall asleep quicker and improve sleep quality. Aerobic training has been shown to increase the amount of time we spend in deep sleep. This is when and where the body pours its resources into repair and rejuvenation, as discussed in Wellness Ritual #1. Daily activity also stabilizes your mood and decompresses the mind, which can help you unwind at the end of the day and transition into a healthy sleep routine. Additionally, this Wellness Ritual can help alleviate daytime sleepiness, decrease symptoms of obstructive sleep apnea, and for some people, reduce the need for sleep medications.

People who engage in thirty minutes of moderate aerobic activity report a difference in sleep quality that same night. This is not a benefit that you have to wait to pay dividends. The benefit is typically felt immediately.

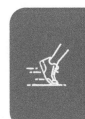

When deciding where to fit higher-intensity activity into your day, it is best to avoid evening workouts, as it may interfere with your sleep quality. Physical activity releases endorphins that stimulate the brain and elevate your core body temperature, which signals the body clock that it's time to be awake.

BETTER Mental Health and Mental Acuity

The endorphin release from activity that improves sleep also supports your mental well-being. Numerous studies support the link between physical activity and brain health. Regular movement stimulates chemical changes in the brain that enhance learning, mood, memory, and thinking.[27]

Studies show that physical activity can treat mild to moderate depression as effectively as antidepressant medication. Research conducted by the Harvard T.H. Chan School of Public Health showed that running for fifteen minutes a day or walking for an hour reduces the risk of major depression by as much as 26%.[27] The current available evidence suggests that all movement counts when it comes to mental health; piecing together smaller movement breaks can be an effective strategy to keep depression at bay. In other words, you don't have to become an elite runner to reach some magical therapeutic threshold. Movement benefits are cumulative. Every extra step you take helps to support brain health.

BETTER Longevity

The practice of this Wellness Ritual elevates our performance by:

- reducing the levels of circulating stress hormones
- improving blood flow
- slowing down our resting heart rate and blood pressure
- increasing our high-density lipoprotein (HDL) or "good cholesterol" and helping to control triglycerides

PHYSICAL ACTIVITY CAN FIGHT AGE-RELATED MEMORY DECLINE

Aerobic activity and weight training also appear to slow age-related decline in memory. Recent studies have indicated that vigorous aerobic activity can improve memory and reasoning in people with mild cognitive impairment, which is often a precursor to dementia.

One recent study randomly split a group of seniors with mild cognitive impairment into one of two groups. The first group did weight training twice a week for six months, lifting 80% of the maximum amount they could. The second group completed a set of stretching exercises.

As reported by Harvard Health Publishing, both groups were given cognitive tests at the beginning and end of the study, and then again as a follow-up twelve months later. The weight training group scored significantly higher at the end of the study than at the beginning and retained that gain at twelve months. The increase in test scores was most significant for those who made the greatest strength gains. The scores of the group who performed only stretching exercises declined somewhat.[28]

- reducing inflammation in the body
- improving cardiorespiratory endurance and energy levels
- increasing our strength
- altering our blood chemistry through the secretion of endorphins, serotonin, and dopamine, which promotes a feeling of well-being, makes us happier, and suppresses hormones that cause stress and anxiety.

As impressive as this list is, movement also influences how we age at the cellular level. Researchers are studying the telomeres in blood cells of adults with different fitness habits and finding a striking disparity between them. Telomeres are the caps found at the ends of our DNA strands that protect our chromosomes from deterioration. Think of them as the plastic tips on the end of your shoelaces. Our telomere length naturally shortens with age, but it appears that unhealthy lifestyle factors — such as obesity, smoking, and inactivity — accelerate this process. Progressive shortening of telomeres leads to cell death and is associated with cardiovascular disease, diabetes, and major cancers. As a hallmark of aging, telomeres provide a window to assess one's lifespan.

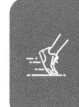

Evidence shows that the telomeres of those who maintain healthy physical fitness levels are longer, suggesting that movement slows down cellular aging and supports longevity. In a recent study funded by the Centers for Disease Control and Prevention, 6,000 men and women who engage in high activity levels were estimated to have a biological aging advantage of nine years over sedentary adults.[29] Researchers reported that the individuals who moved more — the equivalent of at least a half-hour of jogging five days a week — had telomeres that appeared to be nearly a decade younger than those who live a more sedentary lifestyle.

There is no denying our biological need to move. Let's now discuss practical strategies to make it happen.

GROUND RULE #3: TO MAKE MOVEMENT A PRIORITY, IT MUST BE ENJOYABLE, CELEBRATED, AND REWARDED.

Patients who consistently practice Wellness Ritual #4: Move to Stay Young, keep a keen eye on the third and final ground rule. Maintaining a log or tracking a movement streak will help you lock this behavior down. Sharing your intention to move more and capture your 150 activity minutes with someone in your inner circle also helps hold you accountable. If this person joins you, you get the added advantage of having a workout buddy to share the experience with. There will be days that you will need each other's encouragement.

Travel plans to explore a new hiking trail or city, enroll in a charity walk or bike ride, or sign up for an adventure race with friends are all great motivators. Bringing different types of movement at varying intensities into your day. Gardening, playing with kids or grandkids, doing yoga, golfing, skating, completing household chores, dancing, or just unpacking groceries all have a positive cumulative impact on your ability to move. Look for opportunities to move and keep movement fun.

When you land in a spot where the time you have dedicated to activity no longer feels like a burden but has become one of your favorite times of the day, you have reached a tipping point in converting this practice into a ritual. It is here that the science of movement reveals its true influence. The quality of life for a patient who overcomes their doubt and fear to find unexpected joy and health in movement is forever changed.

TALK TO YOUR HEALTHCARE TEAM ABOUT THE EXERCISE IS MEDICINE® INITIATIVE

Exercise is Medicine Canada (EIMC) is a movement encouraging all Canadians to live healthy, active lifestyles. Their vision is to make physical activity assessment and promotion a standard in clinical practice. Visit *exerciseismedicine.org/canada*. By connecting primary healthcare providers with evidence-based resources, they aim to help Canadians appreciate the importance of physical activity and exercise as a way to reduce the risk, prevalence, and severity of chronic diseases.

CHAPIN CLINICAL CORNER

To achieve the quantity and quality of movement required to unlock the advantages of this Wellness Ritual takes discipline. Releasing any fear, doubt, or anxiety you bring to your physical appearance, ability to move, or prior life experiences takes courage. I am asking you for both. This will undoubtedly leave some feeling exposed and uncertain about whether this Wellness Ritual is for them. Negative self-talk and the choice to continue following a path of least resistance that favors a sedentary lifestyle will not only cap your potential but is also harmful. Allow yourself the indulgence of forming a new relationship with movement, and see what your body is capable of.

Now that you are hopefully striving to get eight hours of sleep a night, you have sixteen waking hours each day to work with. Over the course of a week, that gives you 6,720 minutes. The global physical activity guidelines require 150 of these. That is less than 2.2% of the time you have available.

In addition, if you also committed to moving for at least one minute every waking hour in the time that remains, you would still have 96% of your waking hours to live your life uninterrupted. This is plenty of time. Do not let the perception of a lack of time be your excuse for remaining sedentary.

The total time commitment of this Wellness Ritual starts at 3.86% of your week.

Anyone interested in expanding their potential and living a healthier life can muster up the discipline, courage, and time management skills to lock down 3.86%.

Make this happen

Can you imagine how you would feel if you were to double this time?

HOW TO PROCEED

Each week, the 150 minutes of moderate-to-vigorous activity can be spent doing any activity that leaves you feeling challenged. In Wellness Ritual #5: Protect Your Strength, I will ask you to spend some of this time doing resistance training. To meet the requirements of this Wellness Ritual, beginners are best served spending this time in an enjoyable activity that requires 50% to 70 % of their maximum heart rate. Five thirty-minute brisk walks each week with a good friend will get you there.

This activity should increase your breathing rate but not leave you out of breath. After ten minutes, you should notice that you are starting to sweat. If you can carry on a conversation but would have trouble singing a song, you are in the correct zone.

With improvement in your fitness level, the brisk walk will no longer present the same challenge. Moving into more vigorous activity at this stage to accumulate your 150 minutes is a good idea. As your effort intensifies, your breathing will increase in rate and depth, sweat will follow after only a few minutes of activity, and speaking more than a few words without pausing will become difficult. This hypoxic response is excellent for inducing just enough stress to activate your body's response to movement without causing harm.

What Is My Maximum Heart Rate?

It is easy to find a heart rate calculator online, but here is the quick and dirty calculation.

Maximum Heart Rate (MHR) = 220–your age

If you are trying to incorporate more challenging vigorous activity into your formula, you want to elevate your heart rate between 70% to 85% of your MHR. Keep it closer to 50% to 70% for moderate activity.

The MHR for a fifty-year-old is 170. Their target heart rate zone when performing a vigorous activity is between 119 and 145 beats per minute. Training with a device capable of tracking your heart rate allows you to keep an eye on this metric. As your fitness level improves, you will need a greater physical challenge to get your heart into this target zone.

High-Intensity Interval Training (HIIT)

HIIT kick starts your body. For the time-strapped executive or busy parent looking for the most time-efficient way to work out, this is it.[30] From elite athletes to patients in cardiac rehab, interval training offers the biggest bang for your buck. I tell patients that HIIT will unleash your inner superhero.

HIIT workouts are designed to leverage the body's response to bursts of intense activity. The workout structure is simple enough: You push yourself through short bouts of high-intensity effort followed by a recovery period, and then repeat. Most workouts consist of four to ten cycles and are completed within twenty to thirty minutes.

Our physiological response to this type of training demonstrates the profound healing power of movement. Researchers have shown that HIIT burns 25% to 30% more calories than other forms of activity[31] and supports an elevated metabolic rate long after completing a workout.[32] This drives favorable changes in your body composition by burning abdominal and visceral fat while maintaining muscle mass or increasing it in less active individuals. Some studies have also shown that HIIT encourages the body to use fat as energy rather than carbohydrates and improves the body's oxygen consumption, supporting weight loss and improvements in physical endurance.[33] Overweight or obese individuals incorporating HIIT into their formula have also shown improved blood pressure, heart rate, fasting blood sugar levels, and insulin sensitivity.[34]

Some studies also show that HIIT effectively slows aging at the cellular level by improving age-related decline in muscle mitochondria (the cell powerhouse) and releasing proteins, specifically brain-derived neurotrophic factor (BDNF) that protects nerve cells. This exciting research highlights the positive impact movement choices have on learning, memory, and perhaps even how we regulate eating, drinking, and body weight.[35]

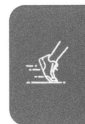

How Does It Work?

High-intensity movement forces your body to use its anaerobic system for energy once your oxygen demand outpaces your aerobic capacity. As you enter the recovery phase and your movement intensity drops, you revert to your aerobic system for fuel. Throughout the workout, this cycle repeats as you bounce between the two energy systems until, eventually, your quick-release energy sources become depleted. This forces you to power your continued movement through aerobic respiration, which burns fat. By repeatedly challenging both energy systems, you see a performance improvement in both.

Peak efforts will leave you huffing and puffing as your heart and lungs try to repay the oxygen deficit you have created. This excess, post-exercise oxygen consumption (EPOC), a hallmark feature of HIIT, burns an additional 6% to 15% more calories than continuous exercise does.[35] Over time, as the body adapts to this type of training, your energy and endurance will dramatically improve.

HIIT training can easily be modified for people of all fitness levels and can be incorporated into various activities, including cycling, walking, swimming, aqua training, elliptical cross-training, and any number of group exercise classes.

While considered safe for most when correctly practiced, an established foundational fitness level is a prerequisite. If you have been living a sedentary lifestyle or have an increased risk of coronary disease related to your family history, cigarette smoking, hypertension, diabetes (or pre-diabetes), abnormal cholesterol levels, or obesity, obtain medical clearance from a physician before starting this type of movement. I recommend patients start with six to eight weeks of continuous lower-intensity training before pushing into higher-intensity workouts. Once this hurdle is cleared and you have medical approval, you can safely begin to experiment with HIIT.

Regardless of age, gender, or fitness level, one of the keys to safe participation in HIIT is learning to modify the intensity of the work interval to an appropriate level.

HIIT kick starts your body. For the time-strapped executive or busy parent looking for the most time-efficient way to work out, **this is it.**[30] From elite athletes to patients in cardiac rehab, interval training offers the biggest bang for your buck.

SAMPLE HIIT WORKOUTS

1.   Warm up with an easy-paced, five-minute walk, and then repeat the following five-minute interval two to three times: moderately paced walk for three minutes, brisk-paced walk for one minute, fast-paced walk for one minute. Cool down with an easy-paced, five-minute walk. Total time: twenty to twenty-five minutes.

2.   Warm up with an easy, five-minute ride on a stationary bike, then complete five repetitions of the following: pedal as quickly as you can for thirty seconds followed by three minutes of slow and easy cycling with low resistance. Finish with a five-minute, easy cool down. Total time: twenty-seven minutes.

3.   Complete a five-minute, dynamic warm up. Complete as many jumping jacks as you can in thirty seconds followed by walking on the spot for sixty to ninety seconds. Repeat for ten to twenty minutes. If a regular jumping jack is too difficult, step side-to-side while raising your arms or replace jacks with squats, butt kicks, forward or side lunges. Total time: twenty-five minutes.

4.   Run at an easy pace for 1 km, and then sprint at or near peak effort for ten to fifteen seconds. End with a slow-paced jog or walk for one to two minutes. Repeat for ten to twenty minutes. Total time: twenty-five to twenty-eight minutes.

Note: Be sure to complete a dynamic warm up prior to HIIT and an appropriate cool-down. Visit **7WellnessRituals.com** for suggestions.

How to Get Started and Avoid Injury with Interval Training

- Get medical approval from your healthcare team before adding interval training to your formula.
- Start slowly, especially if this type of movement is new to you.
- Pick an activity that you enjoy and are familiar with at a low intensity, and begin to experiment with different speeds. If you are not a runner, do not start with sprints. Walking at different paces is a great place to begin.
- If you have any joint pain, choose a lower impact activity, like cycling or swimming.
- Do not rush the recovery period. Your ability to repeat the short bursts of high-intensity movement hinges on the time spent in active recovery.
- One to two interval workouts a week will do the trick. Any more than this, and you risk injury. These workouts are demanding. Spending more than thirty to forty minutes a week at 90% of your maximum heart rate can place a work load on the body that may have adverse effects. High-intensity, vigorous activity, like other forms of resistance training, causes microtears in your muscles, and those muscles need time and protein intake to repair. A healthy diet and adequate rest between workouts are essential. Allow for at least a few days between workouts.

Completing one to two interval workouts of twenty-five minutes each week leaves you with 100 to 125 minutes of moderate-to-vigorous activity to meet the weekly 150-minute target. Spend this time doing an activity that you enjoy and look forward to, keeping your heart rate between 50% and 70% of your maximum.

Hourly Movement

Having met the physical activity guidelines, you now need to introduce a minimum of one minute of activity for every sixty minutes of inactivity to limit the negative health impact of prolonged sitting. Remember, the more you move, the better your body will be at it.

Set a reminder on your phone to get up and move every hour. The intention here is not to disrupt your focus or flow. The goal of this break is simply to unpack the compressive load caused by sitting and give your body a chance to physically reset. In these movement breaks, you want to incorporate different types of movement that challenge your functional mobility. *Note*: You will find a list of easy movement breaks at **7WellnessRituals.com**.

Here are three of my favorites:

1. **Heel-to-Toe Walking:** Walk slowly along a straight line (follow a carpet edge, floorboard, or tiles) with one foot placed directly in front of the other — heel-to-toe — for twenty steps. If necessary, keep your arms out to each side for balance. Turn around and repeat.

2. **Tree Pose:** Standing next to a counter, lift one leg up and place the foot of this leg on the inner edge of the opposite leg (either at the level of your inner thigh or your shin). Concentrate on rooting the foot of your weight-bearing leg to the ground and firing the hip muscles of this leg for added balance. To help you recruit the correct muscles, try pushing hard into the ground with your stance leg. Hold the pose for thirty seconds. Repeat with the other leg.

3. **Dead Bug:** Lie on your back, lift your feet off the ground, and flex your knees and hips to ninety degrees. Raise your arms straight up toward the ceiling. Keeping your back flat and core engaged (bracing your abdomen like you are about to be punched in the stomach), lower the opposite arm and leg away from one another toward the floor. Return to the starting position and repeat with the opposite pair. Complete twenty to twenty-five reps.

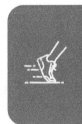

Many of the mentors start their day with a morning movement ritual before touching their phones, checking their email, reviewing their calendars, or catching up on the daily news. Dogs are always looking for a morning walking buddy and can be a great companion for those needing extra motivation first thing. A simple movement practice on a yoga mat before your morning shower is also an excellent way to prime your mind and body before jumping into the day.

Once you are north of fifty, greater effort is required to maintain your functional range of motion and flexibility. A simple fifteen to twenty minute introductory yoga routine or gentle stretching program completed two or three mornings a week will help you maintain a decent functional range of motion and prevent common musculoskeletal injuries. *Note*: You will find a video of my morning mobility practice at **7WellnessRituals.com**.

RITUAL ACTIVATION

If you are interested in becoming more active or are currently working out but want to increase your intensity, the physical activity readiness questionnaire (PAR-Q) is a good starting point.

Created by the British Columbia Ministry of Health and the Multidisciplinary Board on Exercise, the questionnaire has been endorsed by the American College of Sports Medicine (ACSM) as a simple self-screening tool to determine the safety of physical activity based on your health history, current symptoms, and risk factors.[36-37]

PAR-Q QUESTIONNAIRE:

1. Has your doctor ever said that you have a heart condition or high blood pressure?
2. Do you feel pain in your chest at rest, when doing regular day-to-day activities, or when doing physical activity?
3. Do you lose your balance because of dizziness, or have you lost consciousness in the last twelve months?
4. Have you ever been diagnosed with another chronic medical condition (other than heart disease or high blood pressure)?
5. Are you currently taking prescribed medications for a chronic medical condition?
6. Do you currently have (or have had within the last twelve months) a bone, joint, or soft tissue (muscle, ligament, or tendon) problem that could be made worse by becoming more physically active?
7. Has your doctor ever said that you should only do medically supervised physical activity?

RESULTS:

If you answer no to all PAR-Q questions, you have a low risk of incurring any medical complications from getting more active, and it is safe to begin. If you answer yes to any of the above, you should speak with your physician before increasing your activity.

TAKE THESE STEPS:

- Pain is an excellent motivator, but waiting for it to show up before seeking help can complicate a recovery and prevent you from staying active. Proactively maintain your musculoskeletal health by addressing areas of restricted range of motion, difficulty with balance, or diminishing flexibility with your healthcare team.
- Take every opportunity to bring movement to your day. Practice a morning movement ritual. Take the stairs. Use a sit-stand workstation. Schedule movement breaks and walking meetings. Go for a walk at lunch time. Park at the back of every parking lot. Perform calf raises or a yoga tree pose while washing dishes. Move during every TV commercial break. Get out of the car when you refuel during a road trip and walk for five minutes. Dance around the house when doing chores. Celebrate your ability to move.
- Accumulate 150 minutes of moderate-to-vigorous activity every week, with each workout lasting at least ten minutes.
- Introduce high-intensity interval training into your exercise routine if you are medically cleared to do so.
- Work on your flexibility.

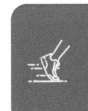

IN SUMMARY

Rekindling a joy for movement is possible at any age. Those who are physically active tend to live longer and healthier lives. Research shows that moderate physical activity, such as thirty minutes a day of brisk walking, significantly contributes to longevity and improved mental and physical health. A challenging movement strategy appropriate for your age and current physical fitness level that interrupts sedentary postures and pushes the physical capacity of your body is the goal of *moving to stay young*. Our bodies are made to move. Get to work.

Greg explains the nature of his motivation: "I didn't like my mental retreat from fear in Ecuador, so **I decided to lean into it**, get familiar with the sensation, and learn how to overcome it. **My ability** to handle stressful situations and control my performance and mindset, regardless of the challenge, is **better now than it ever has been.** I wish I had this mental skill earlier in my career, especially when I was competing in the pool."

MENTOR PROFILES

———

DR. GREG WELLS
SILKEN LAUMANN
MICHAEL GRANGE

DR. GREG WELLS

Performance Physiologist, CEO of Wells Performance, Author

*F*ive years ago, Greg found himself 400 m from the summit of Chimborazo, an ice-capped inactive volcano in Ecuador, South America. Given its location along the Earth's equator, the volcano's peak is recognized as the farthest point from the planet's center. The summit awaits at 20,548 ft. Reaching the top requires an extraordinary technical skillset, which, on this particular day, exceeded Greg's ability. He admitted, "Two members of our crew reached the summit. I did not. I was afraid to continue and decided to turn around. Looking back, I know I made the right decision that day and can live with that, but I did not love my mindset during the summit attempt when things got hard."

A world-renowned performance physiologist, scientist, best-selling author, and former member of Canada's National Youth Swim Team, Greg has dedicated his life to exploring and researching human limits, particularly under extreme conditions. He has a unique talent for making science understandable and actionable. Greg lives on the edge and applies the human truths revealed in medical performance labs at every opportunity. As an expedition adventurer, he has journeyed through every imaginable terrain and condition in over fifty countries. Bucket list experiences already checked off include the punishing Nanisvik Marathon north of the Arctic Circle, Ironman Canada, and the grueling From-Cairo-to-Cape-Town 11,000 km Tour d'Afrique. As CEO and founder of Wells Performance, he helps top performers get even better.

Greg committed himself to changing the mindset that left him short of his goal at Chimborazo. Fascinated by the mind's command over performance and the plasticity of the human nervous system, Greg set a goal of completing a challenge once a month that had an element of fear. Two weeks before our call, he set out to climb a 100 m vertical rock cliff that would challenge his physical and mental capacity. At the fifty meter mark, approximately fifteen stories above the rocks below, with his weight strategically balanced on a lip no wider than a dime, he came across the first of two difficult overhangs. Greg anticipated his physiological reaction to the stress of the endeavor, knowing his brain would activate a fear-related response to this dangerous point in the climb. As the strength in his fingers started to wane, he also knew the sustained exertion was leading to hydrogen accumulation in his tissues. Facing the overhang, his brain called for him to rappel down to the lake below and swim out. But he did not. He met and vanquished his fear and pushed through to the top.

SELF-CARE REFLECTION #26

Think of a time when you had to turn back from a challenge based on a rational decision that was the right call. Were you disappointed? In Greg's case, he decided to challenge his fear and overcome it in what he refers to as his "mental retreat" below. What challenge is keeping you from your summit, and what steps have you taken to overcome it?

PUSHING THE BOUNDARIES OF YOUR MINDSET

It is the opportunity to challenge his mental strength in an environment with consequences that drives him. Greg and his wife, Judith, and their two children moved to Western Canada during the pandemic, where nature offers tremendous risk and reward. Opportunities to push the boundaries of his comfort and performance while mountain biking, climbing, or skiing were waiting for him out the back door. Most of his monthly challenges are physical, but some are more cognitive and tied to his career as a performance scientist.

Greg explains the nature of his motivation: "I didn't like my mental retreat from fear in Ecuador, so I decided to lean into it, get familiar with the sensation, and learn how to overcome it. My ability to handle stressful situations and control my performance and mindset, regardless of the challenge, is better now than it ever has been. I wish I had this mental skill earlier in my career, especially when I was competing in the pool."

To be clear, he would never intentionally turn a blind eye to safety. He is in a harness on challenging climbs, bolted to the wall, with a guide above him. He does not free-climb or recklessly pursue risk for the sake of risk. The actual challenge of the climb, ride, or pitch of a ski run holds little significance. It is not competition or even accomplishing the task at hand that motivates Greg. It is the opportunity to practice his mental strength, achieving performance excellence with something on the line that excites him.

GREG'S FORMULA FOR HEALTH, STRENGTH & HOPE

QUALITY OF EFFORT VS. VOLUME OF EFFORT

Greg actively manages his performance stress while skillfully ignoring distractions. "I quadrupled my workout time during the pandemic given the additional time that was suddenly available.

> ❝ **My formula is skewed heavily toward recovery to support the performance demands of my life."**

Exercise is my recovery; without it, I am miserable." The adrenaline rush of a keynote address or live television appearance offers a thrilling ride, but it can also be exhausting and, at times, super stressful.

"My formula is skewed heavily toward recovery to support the performance demands of my life." On any given day, the intensity of his workout will vary according to his energy. "When tired, I will still exercise, but I may not complete intervals; I may just ride my bike. With more energy — especially in my morning workouts — I'll hit harder intervals, push higher heart rate zones, or go for a longer period. It is the consistency of this schedule that helps me dissipate my stress. Getting outdoors makes an even bigger difference; there is a clear correlation between my exercise time outdoors and my mental health. When I'm trapped inside, my mental health suffers."

Focus on the quality of performance versus the volume of work is a theme that appears to play out in Greg's life repeatedly. "It is possible to be healthy and high performing at the same time." The pandemic provided time and space for Greg to pause, evaluate his position in life, and question how sustainable and desirable his pre-pandemic pace was.

With the disappearance of business travel, no commute, and fewer external commitments, the day held greater potential for him. Seizing that opportunity, he tested recovery and rejuvenation strategies, landing on an approach that allows him to operate at his best when it counts.

FUEL FOR RESET AND RECOVERY

"For years, I focused on preparing my peak performance and did not give much attention to my reset. I remember one event when I was interviewed for a CTV television segment following Georgian luger Nodar Kumaritashvili's tragic death at the 2010 Vancouver Winter Olympic Games. It was a challenging, emotional interview. I was prepared and handled it well, but afterward, the wave of stress hit me like a truck. I was completely depleted following the interview and literally collapsed into a chair off-camera when it was done. Suddenly ABC and other networks started calling, wanting to conduct a similar interview. The accident was world news. I had to rebound quickly and find a way back to my peak. From this point, I became somewhat obsessed with recovery."

He began tweaking his formula, looking for ways to achieve his peak quicker and shorten his recovery interval. "One of my biggest challenges following a big performance is the crash. The fatigue that follows a performance event is real and immediate and leaves me feeling tremendous hunger. Evolutionary biology dictates that you get your hands on food as soon as possible in this state. This is when we are prone to making poor food choices."

Identifying this pitfall, he now preps his post-event recovery strategy. Keeping nuts, berries, and lemon water at the ready, he can stabilize his blood sugar and hydrate quickly. He then looks to get some physical exercise outdoors as close to completing the event as possible. An hour's walk at a quick pace usually provides the reset he needs. On occasion, he may also grab an extra fifteen to twenty minutes for a power nap after the walk. The combination of the post-recovery snack, walk, and nap allows him to bounce back to his peak and limits his crash's depth and length.

RESPECT YOUR TIME AS A RESOURCE

Time management is another important component to his formula for success. "I've learned not to book back-to-back performance events. I now only book one to two performance moments a day and keep them separated with an appropriate recovery time." He recently broke this rule and was talked into delivering five virtual keynote addresses in one day, hosted across India, the UK, Canada, and Australia. The effort had a negative ripple effect that lasted for days. "I will never do that again."

PROTECT YOUR SLEEP

Greg puts considerable effort and energy into prioritizing sleep. Doing so fuels his confidence, resiliency, and performance. Judith also sees the value of healthy sleep. Together they welcome rest as a reward at the end of their day. A commitment to an early bedtime of 9 p.m., asleep by 9:30 p.m., consistently delivers a minimum of seven hours of rest a night. An evening that extends past 10 p.m. would be very late for them. They might enjoy the occasional glass of wine on the weekend but otherwise avoid alcohol entirely. It disrupts Greg's sleep cycle, leaving him feeling sluggish the following day. His day starts sometime between 5 and 5:30 a.m. with optimism and energy. Greg used to wear an Oura ring to track his sleep habits and now uses a sleep app he developed with his team at Wells Performance. If his demanding schedule leaves him feeling fatigued, he will push his wake time later and pick up an extra hour in the morning. In the past, when sleep has been disrupted by travel or pace, he has had success with magnesium or melatonin supplements.

Once every week or two, usually on the weekend, he will call it a day shortly after dinner and sleep for twelve to fourteen consecutive hours. This provides a reset, allowing him to deliver his A-game with greater consistency.

"Doom scrolling as I relive a negative stress in my mind will sometimes keep me up staring at the ceiling." To limit this, he avoids reading anything related to work after dinner and exercises discipline to avoid end-of-day email checking at all costs. The day following a restless night, he will crush a workout intentionally designed to "exercise into oblivion." This will usually help recalibrate his sleep.

MENTAL WELLNESS THROUGH MEDITATION

Greg has started practicing meditation following his workouts and enjoys the Headspace App during his cool down. "There is mounting evidence supporting Mental and Physical (MAP) training, which is a clinical intervention that combines physical training through aerobic exercise immediately followed by mental training through meditation." Neuroscientific studies indicate that MAP training increases neurogenesis in the adult brain, improving mental and cognitive health outcomes and decreasing symptoms of depression. Greg looks for opportunities to embrace science and take action to keep his formula on the leading edge.

SELF-CARE REFLECTION #27

The way Greg manages his calendar and approaches recovery ensures he can access his peak performance when needed. Are you setting yourself up for success with your calendar? Do you have a recovery strategy?

FROM NEAR TRAGEDY TO NUTRITIONAL SCIENCE

As our conversation turned to his experiences as a competitive swimmer, he shared that his life story narrowly escaped a tragic end at fifteen years old. While away at a swimming training camp in Florida, Greg broke his neck. Bodysurfing with teammates on a day off from the pool, he caught a rogue wave that forcefully drove him into the ocean floor headfirst, fracturing his neck. He avoided any spinal cord trauma and made a full recovery. However, after surgery and three months in traction, he put on thirty pounds and lost his elite conditioning. True to form, Greg worked hard and smart, and with the support of his teammates, coaches, and medical professionals, he battled back to compete at the national level.

The lessons Greg learned during his recovery from this injury sparked a curiosity that led him to become the scientist he is today. Given his fascination with human performance, nutritional science is another area that continues to pique his interest. "When I was training, I don't remember having a single conversation with a sports nutritionist about vegetables, protein, or fat. The focus in the eighties and nineties was almost entirely on simple carbohydrates. We now have a much better understanding of healthy nutrition. Judith, the kids, and I now consume an anti-inflammatory diet with various healthy complex carbohydrates, proteins, and fats. We eat organic as much as we can afford to, limit processed foods, and drink lots of water. We look to build our diet around a rainbow of vegetables, berries, nuts and seeds, lean cuts of grass-fed meat, and plenty of wild-caught fish."

On performance days, he uses caffeine to his advantage. In a Vitamix blender, he blends a strong coffee with one to two tablespoons of cashew nut butter and a teaspoon of cinnamon and honey each. "It is my rocket fuel." After a couple of cups, he will transition to green tea in the afternoon. Throughout the morning, he grazes on a full pint of blueberries and blackberries. A bowl of almonds, walnuts, and macadamia nuts are also within arm's reach, providing a rich source of vitamins, minerals, fiber, antioxidants, and healthy fat. Mid-morning, he will drink a power green smoothie with green vegetables blended with forty grams of vegan protein powder, a healthy fat source, and water or almond milk. Lunches and dinners are built from a foundation of fresh veggies and lean protein.

A MOBILITY ROUTINE

Approaching his fifties, functional mobility and tissue quality has moved to the forefront of Greg's formula.

> **My movement routine, swimming, and yoga practice are no longer things that I do just because I enjoy them. They have become much more than that. I now see this focus as essential to my performance, and without it, I am in pain and can't move through life as I want to."**

Greg can evaluate his movement efficiency and self-identify biomechanical issues that require additional attention when swimming. He rolls out daily with a foam roller, uses a Thera gun to work on muscle tension, and gets a massage once a week. When in Toronto, he will head down to Lake Ontario daily right through to December for twenty minutes of cold water immersion. Clearly, his fear conditioning helps him with this routine.

TUNING MENTAL AND PHYSICAL FITNESS

Greg is a happy man who has found inspiration and motivation in the entrepreneurial freedom he has carved out in the field of human performance. He understands his weaknesses, much like Dr. Andy Smith recognizes the negative effect stress has on his well-being. In Greg's case, he knows he is prone to losing sight of his "off" switch. To address this weakness, he practices his mental fitness with what he calls his *One-Two-Three Rule*. He takes an hour a day, two days a month, and three weeks a year off, and by off, I mean entirely unplugged. This time is invested in his family, hobbies, and self-care. Getting outdoors as much as possible to push his physical and mental ability provides him with an outlet to express his gifts and balance the passion he brings to his work. Shifting toward playing for the sake of play and learning to say no have resulted in considerable peace of mind and happiness.

At one point in our conversation, Greg observed that a trend in professional sports has emerged as athletes shift from working harder to working smarter. He noted that "Sport is moving away from high-volume training. The best are no longer trying to do the most work the most often. Athletes are now training at world-class speeds for shorter durations and then applying an equal focus and intention to sport-specific movement patterns, self-care, and recovery — massage therapy, chiropractic, physiotherapy, yoga, cold water immersion, technical skills practice, and dynamic strength and conditioning are all now considered as important as traditional training. This is a completely different approach than when I was growing up as a competitive swimmer. As a result, careers are now longer, and chronic injuries are fewer."

He then paused and asked, "How can we become world-class more often?"

Always and ever the scientist looking to push the boundaries of our human potential. Sharing his curiosity, I offer this book as my response.

SILKEN LAUMANN

Olympic Rowing Athlete for Team Canada, Author, Motivational Speaker

May 27, 1992. Essen, Germany.

Canadian rower Silken Laumann's dreams of competing in the 1992 Barcelona Games were shattered. Her right leg was seriously injured when the German men's double-scull rammed her boat while training for the games, set to open on July 25. According to *Maclean's*, "In the first of four operations performed at the Essen hospital, surgeons secured one of the bone chips with a screw and removed from her leg a number of wooden slivers from her broken boat. The follow-up procedures checked for infection and any dead tissue caused by loss of blood supply; no evidence of either was found."

Commenting on Silken's prognosis, Richard Backus, medical director for Rowing Canada, said, "She is very fit and a very surprising person in terms of her healing capabilities. But even with optimal healing, it will not be sufficiently advanced for her to compete in the Olympics."

Following the surgeries to repair the horrific fracture and extensive muscle damage to her right leg, orthopedic and rehab specialists laid out a conservative road map to recovery that would close the door on her participation in the upcoming Games and cast doubt on her ability to return to world competition. In doing so, they underestimated the fire in Silken's heart. Indifferent to pain (she refused to take painkillers) and determined to compete, she was back on the water training before she had even regained the ability to walk unassisted. With time and odds stacked against her, she turned a blind eye to the distraction of doubt and channeled every thought and every action toward rowing Canada to the podium.

Determination carried her to the Olympic final in Barcelona, to the disbelief of most, after finishing second in her qualifying heat and winning her semifinal. Had her Olympics ended here, she would have earned the world's respect, but Silken's best was still yet to come. Finding another gear with just 250 m remaining in the Women's Single Sculls final, Silken would chase down American Anne Marden to capture the bronze medal by less than half a boat length. Her smile in victory suggested she may have even surprised herself on this day.

COMPETING AGAINST A MORE DANGEROUS OPPONENT

Now, at the age of fifty-seven, as she did in Barcelona, Silken has once again found another gear. Her determination and force of will have enabled her to overcome crippling emotional trauma and unlock her inner peace and self-confidence. In her memoir titled *Unsinkable,* Silken offers an honest and brave look at her struggles with body image, disordered eating, depression, and anxiety. Readers are given rare insight into the Olympic hero's world. She describes the fear she felt growing up with an abusive, erratic mother and the demons of unworthiness that accompanied her into adulthood.

Much like her performance on the water, her life story is one of courage and grit. Learning to block negative self-talk and tap into the power of self-love required hard work. Thankfully, Silken does hard work very well. By applying the focused discipline she perfected as a competitive rower to her mental health, she invested in her healing and recovery. In the time we spent together, it was clear that Silken has chosen to live her life unencumbered by self-imposed limitations.

Her approach reveals the human capacity to heal and embrace healthy daily rituals: "I am stronger now than I was ten years ago." Achieving this growth requires active listening to your body and mind.

SELF-CARE REFLECTION #28
Silken's athletic accomplishments put her in rare company. Her recovery story stands as a reminder of our capacity to overcome adversity and chase a dream. She would tell us that we are all capable of such courage. Go to *silkenlaumann.com/blog* to read her inspirational and practical advice for self-discovery and reaffirmation.

SILKEN'S FORMULA FOR HEALTH, STRENGTH & HOPE

To ride alongside Silken on a two-hour bike ride requires advanced training. To keep pace with her drive and creativity, you best lock down your sleep, rest, and recovery ritual, prioritize mindful meditation, and learn to practice self-love. To match her altruistic intellect and playfulness, your mental fitness must also feature as a prominent role in your formula. Through personal adversity and the extraordinary experience of competing with the best in the world, she has crafted a formula that honors her standard for personal excellence, holds loving respect for the influence of time, and sets realistic expectations.

FINDING RENEWAL IN A SLEEPING AND WAKING ROUTINE

In bed by 9:30 p.m., sleep is welcomed after fifteen to twenty minutes of meditative reading. She avoids caffeine after noon, limits screen time, and skips after-dinner snacks. "I take rest seriously, and I'm very protective of my sleep."

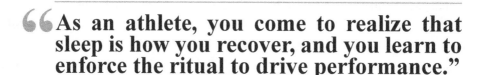

66**As an athlete, you come to realize that sleep is how you recover, and you learn to enforce the ritual to drive performance.**"

Up between 6 and 6:30 a.m., she locks in eight hours a night without exception. Her ability to prioritize sleep has come naturally. Simply put, without it, she does not function well. "As an athlete, you come to realize that sleep is how you recover, and you learn to enforce the ritual to drive performance."

Each morning, she completes a two-hour meditative practice that includes thirty to forty minutes of longhand journaling, reflective reading, and gentle yoga before she jumps into the shower and opens herself up to the world.

This period of quiet solitude is non-negotiable, and everyone in her inner circle knows to respect this space. Practiced with the intention of awakening and strengthening the connection between her mind and body, she finds this ritual offers a bridge to her spiritual health that fuels a sense of renewal.

MEDITATION AND YOGA ARE PART OF THE DAY

As she moves into her day, she works hard to stay on task and consciously removes distractions. When grinding through jobs she would rather not be doing, Silken sets a timer and commits to keeping at it until the job is done or the timer goes off. She shares that "delegating to-dos I do not enjoy or excel at gets easier with practice." To protect her creativity, she blocks a three-hour window on most days, providing her with time to think and write. No one is allowed to call or interrupt her during this time, as she deliberately steps off the grid to focus on her artistic responsibilities. A sit-stand workstation in her office affords her the ability to bring movement to this part of the day. Movement sparks ideas and her best thinking.

She enjoys recharging with her husband David "Patch" Patchell-Evans, when she comes up for air. Patch is the founder and CEO of GoodLife Fitness Clubs. He places an equally high value on health and well-being and understands what makes Silken tick. They are life partners and best friends.

Yoga and meditation show up again as a component of Silken's end-of-day, wind-down routine. Completing a short meditative yoga practice before getting into bed helps to quiet her nervous system.

Staying on point with her sleep and yoga, she eagerly begins each day, excited by the potential it offers. Checking in with this emotion every so often provides a metric to quality control her pace. If this sense of adventure ever starts to wane, she knows she is falling out of rhythm or pushing too hard. Left unchecked, her body escalates its warning signals with headaches, odd carbohydrate cravings, and a feeling of whole-body fatigue. The volume of these symptoms will continue to increase until she course-corrects her behavior.

LISTENING TO BODY ALERTS

In 2020, Silken led a small team in the production of a national television special titled *Unsinkable Youth*. The program was a springboard for a not-for-profit initiative committed to amplifying diverse voices to drive change in how young people manage their well-being and raise awareness of the current mental health crisis among Canadian youths. For twenty-seven days, Silken and her crew worked 24/7 on a shoestring budget to complete the production, bringing together musicians, performers, and athletes to send messages of hope and gratitude to young Canadians across the country. The project was a success, but on completion, Silken anticipated a personal crash. "I cleared my plate for five days once the production wrapped, knowing that I was going to have to invest heavily in my self-care to get back on track." Prior experiences have taught her that jumping right into the next challenge or trying to navigate a shortcut through recovery only ends in disappointment.

Periods of self-care following big events are now hard wired into her calendar. They are spent reconnecting with family and close friends, getting physical exercise, and enjoying solitude. During this recovery phase, she has also found that getting to bed earlier while keeping the same wake-up time helps to accelerate her bounce back.

"I am very fortunate that I have a strong body. I haven't developed disease or adrenal gland fatigue like many of my contemporaries have. My body demands what it needs, loudly. And so, I've learned how to listen and have developed a respect for rest and recovery. The cost associated with skipping this step is just too great. Early in my life, when I did, it would wreak havoc on my nervous system, and I would become impatient and irritable to the people I cared most about."

Now, when in full sprint on a project, she chooses to step off the crazy bus in time to grab her eight hours of sleep and rejoins the tour at 6 a.m. the following day, feeling recharged and sharp.

PRACTICING SELF-LOVE

Reframing the age-related changes in her body through self-love changed Silken's approach to food and provided a previously undiscovered strength. By nurturing a healthy perspective on how her body has changed and learning to celebrate its current ability, she avoids fixating on the things she can no longer do or making unrealistic comparisons to earlier versions of herself. Practicing gratitude for the body that returns her gaze in the bathroom mirror has freed her from any preconceived narrative of aging. "I now recognize the importance of holding the bigger picture surrounding health and performance. There is a fullness to my body that is new to me, but quite honestly, I love my fifty-seven-year-old self more than I did at forty-five."

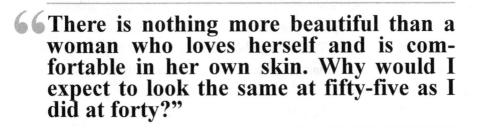

There is nothing more beautiful than a woman who loves herself and is comfortable in her own skin. Why would I expect to look the same at fifty-five as I did at forty?"

For one week, twice each year, Silken dials in her focus on the minute details of her sleep hygiene, digestion, body composition, movement quality, balance, and state of happiness. During these weeks, she will actively listen to and observe her mind and body's response to eating super clean and moving with a keen purpose. The objective is not perfection; it is a state of heightened self-awareness. Silken uses this time to recalibrate and pivot from undesirable trends that would otherwise be missed and explore small opportunities for improvements.

STAYING STRONG

No longer rowing, cycling has become one of her favorite workouts. Before hitting the road, she will fuel with a protein shake, which keeps her energy where it needs to be and prevents cramps. Post-ride, with her glycogen stores blown out, cookies have been replaced with whole-grain toast and honey. In addition to cycling, Silken practices yoga most days, lifts weights three days a week, and enjoys golfing, paddle boarding, hiking, and skiing — both downhill and backcountry. She works out with a trainer once a week, belongs to a cycling club, and swims in open water when the weather and opportunity align.

As our conversation turned to her motivation, I asked her where she keeps her medals. "Patch and I have talked about pulling them out and displaying them somehow, but just never seem to get around to it." She is proud of her accomplishments but seems to have moved on from her time on the podium. "I am either highly distractible or extremely focused. There is nothing in between."

I think we can add modesty to Silken's list of attributes. After all, Barcelona is still considered one of the most remarkable comeback stories in Canadian sports history. Inducted into the Canadian Olympic Hall of Fame, Canada's Sports Hall of Fame, and Canada's Walk of Fame, she will be forever remembered for her remarkable perseverance.

After collecting three Olympic medals and three World Championship medals, Silken retired from rowing in 1999. The rowing shell from her 1996 Atlanta Olympic Games hangs suspended from the ceiling in her home and offers a daily reminder of the work required to play with the best.

While out of the water, she continues to inspire Canadians to embrace adversity, dream big, and realize their potential through her writing, public speaking, and dedicated community service.

SELF-CARE REFLECTION #29

For this exercise, I want you to think about Silken's words: "My body demands what it needs, loudly. And so, I've learned how to listen and have developed a respect for rest and recovery. The cost associated with skipping this step is just too great."

When your body sends you messages, do you ignore them? Do you understand them? Are you finely attuned to those messages and know exactly how to respond to them?

A big takeaway from Silken's story is that her self-care routines bring peace of mind and happiness. They are her daily benchmark. When distress occurs, those signals to slow down are heard loud and clear. What routines have you put in place to achieve peace of mind and maintain the energy and outlook necessary to receive each day with excitement and optimism?

MICHAEL GRANGE

Columnist and Basketball Insider, Sportsnet

*L*ife as a journalist is stressful. Journalists have to deal with deadlines, busy work environments, schedules they have little to no control over, long hours, travel, demanding editors, the public's scrutiny, and the vulnerability that comes with the job. Such is the life of Mike Grange.

Mike is an award-winning columnist and a radio and television personality for Rogers Sportsnet. He knows basketball inside-out and is widely respected in sports media for his professionalism, talent, and work ethic. I have known him for the better part of fifteen years and can tell you without hesitation that, whether enjoying a pick-up game or facing a professional deadline with high stakes, you want Mike's leadership, demeanor, and hustle on your team. He is a team-first guy who is eager to celebrate the success of others and is comfortable leading or playing a supporting role.

A former varsity basketball player for Mount Allison University in Sackville, New Brunswick and a competitive triathlete in his late twenties, Mike knows the effort required to push his body to its peak performance. Striving to do so still invigorates him. He's had to maintain a high level of performance during his twenty-six years in the journalism business, and he is acutely aware of the grind of his trade. During the 2016 NBA playoffs, this grind reached a whole new level.

THE PLAYOFF GRIND

The NBA life is a nightlife. Mike's mental faculties and physical stamina need to be at their very best in the final few hours a day has to offer. Game times dictate his routine. In 2016, when the Toronto Raptors advanced to the NBA Eastern Conference Finals, Mike covered twenty games in forty-nine days in four different cities. During the Eastern finals, tip-off was not until 9:30 p.m. He pointed out to me that "After the game, I am not finished. People see me on the TV side, but a big part of my function is writing. And so, without an ounce of exaggeration, after the game is finished and the interviews and on-camera stuff is done, I still have to go and write another story. Many nights, I wasn't leaving the arena until 2:30 or three in the morning."

During the Raptors-Cavaliers 2016 playoff match-up, in home games, Mike would often drive home at three in the morning, then grab a few hours of sleep before getting on the road to Cleveland. Flights were hard to coordinate with his duties, so it was easier to drive. If he left Toronto by 7 a.m., he would arrive in Cleveland in time for player and coach availability around noon, and then complete his preparations for the game the next night. On the off night in the hotel, he would try to get to bed at a decent time, but this was not always easy given the pace he was pushing. The following day, the cycle would repeat.

By the end of this series, Mike was gassed. "No one wants to hear a sports reporter complain about their job. They're just not interested. So I don't do it." I was interested and persisted, wanting to understand Mike's process when he was forced to perform at his best night after night on live television. I could sense the pressure he felt when he said, "It was the first time I did a lot of live TV. The audiences were getting really big, and it was a different role for me in terms of television and what was expected of me." While he says he is grateful for the experience, it came with a cost but also with self-discovery and a higher emphasis on self-care.

SELF-CARE REFLECTION #30

Mike's success as a top-notch journalist brought with it the demand of maintaining a consistent, high level of performance. If you are accountable for maintaining a similar level of performance in your work or personal life, as you read Mike's profile, think about your routines and where they might intersect with and differ from Mike's. Note any takeaways that will benefit your own lifestyle.

BALANCING COURTSIDE LIFE AND FAMILY LIFE

When pressed, Mike leans into his fitness routine and seeks periods of solitude. These two rituals anchor his formula and keep him grounded and energized. When his schedule allows for both, he is at his very best. When it does not, he possesses an extra gear he can call on to bridge any temporary gap. A prolonged departure from his routine, however, is dangerous to his home and work life, and he knows it. "In my real life are my kids, family, and dog. And their schedule and their needs are quite present first thing in the morning." Mike's wife also has a challenging professional career that demands a high level of focus, and together they make domesticity work through compromise and shared values. "We have been together for twenty-five years — not a day has gone by where we haven't had a quick chat about our workout plans for the day."

> ❝ **I'd try to get a workout in, but sometimes you just have to let go of the rope."**

Managing schedules and coordinating family and professional commitments has been the story of their lives. Both of their kids competed in sports at a high level throughout high school. At the peak of the kids' pre-pandemic athletic seasons, the Grange family could have fifteen events, including practices, games, and tournaments, scheduled each week. During this stage of life, most weeks were a full court press on the Grange home front. "We are blessed to have busy, active, healthy kids, so we put ourselves second to that every day."

Mike made every attempt to carve out time for self-care during the 2016 playoffs, but the schedule was indifferent to his personal needs. "I'd try to get a workout in, but sometimes you just have to let go of the rope."

When the rare opportunity to catch his breath did present itself, he took it. However, literally catching his breath was really all there was time for. Cramming a workout into this time slot was not ideal. As such, his conditioning gap widened, as did the gap in his constant support — his routines. Mike called on his reserves to close the gap. He put his head down and pushed with determination toward the finish line.

The Raptors lost game six, which ended their playoff run. However, Mike's run continued — his finish line had been moved further out of reach. With two days' notice, he was asked to cover the Cleveland Cavaliers and Golden State Warriors championship series. It would become one of the greatest finals of all-time, featuring LeBron James versus Stephen Curry. Anticipating the epic battle, Mike knew the opportunity to cover it would be tremendous, but saying yes would require endurance. "I remember getting the call and thinking, 'I don't think I can do this. I'm exhausted. My wife hasn't seen me in six weeks.' And my kids were younger then and needed me more. But, I didn't feel I could say no, so I did it."

WHY HIS RESERVES RUN DEEP

Mike understands physical peaks are not meant to be maintained and must be periodically re-defined according to ability and life-stage. Respecting his limits, he works to keep his body and performance within striking distance of his peak, even now in his mid-fifties. Mike's approach to conditioning is the key to his endurance. Blessed with a responsive metabolism, his body is receptive to effort. A grassroots, old-school, put your head down and get the job done approach is how Mike rolls. At age twenty-two, in his senior year at Mount Allison, he weighed 195 pounds. His goal is to remain within ten pounds of that weight.

Sometimes you just need to suck it up and get the job done. Mike shares, "I can battle through anything professionally. There is an athletic mindset to it." He sees the ability to "suck it up" and perform at a high level as an underrated skill intimately linked to success. "Sometimes you are at mile nineteen, and you have to get to mile twenty-six. And so, you just push through it and do whatever it takes."

His routine is so well practiced that when professional demands pull him off track, it triggers an internal, automatic, immediate response to course-correct. In other words, he rarely allows slips to go unnoticed. If you've read Silken Laumann's profile, you'll see the similarities.

His family also helps keep him on track. If they recognize an edge to his tone or an uncharacteristic, diminished patience, they will call him out and suggest he gets a workout in. Exercise allows him to reboot and move forward without losing ground. Knowing his limits and keeping his health and performance high provides him with the luxury of going all in on a task without falling apart.

Heading into the 2016 Finals, he had allowed the gap between his current and desired energy levels to reach an uncomfortable distance and made a firm commitment to set a standard of self-care that he would not allow to waver. For nineteen days straight, he honored his promise and adapted his self-care routine to make it work as he bounced between Ohio and California. Starting gently and slowly, he was back in rhythm by the end of the 2016 NBA Finals and proud of both his personal victory and the quality of his work.

EXERCISE CAUTION

> "A simple twenty-minute workout can be the most important workout you will ever do."

When it has been a while since you have laced up your shoes and your reserves are depleted, finding an entry point to exercise can be hard. Mike acknowledges this truth. Feeling exhausted plus knowing how much energy it would take to cover the Finals was a real concern. This is where many leaders fail. Continuing to push from this position, with a total disregard for your depleted capacity, results in a substandard performance and high risk of injury. Aware of this pitfall, Mike suggests the re-entry is always easier when it is accompanied with kindness. "A simple twenty-minute workout can be the most important workout you will ever do.

Just an easy twenty minutes, nothing aggressive. Start with slow movement. At minute twelve, you break into a light sweat. From minutes twelve to nineteen, you get your heart rate up, and at minute twenty, you wind it down." He admits that while this workout may appear unremarkable, it will help get you back on track. Stepping through the barrier of excuses to put the twenty minutes in generates momentum, and that momentum lowers the barrier to entry tomorrow. This practice allowed Mike to replenish and recover without a drop in his performance.

VALUE PAST EXPERIENCE

Fast forward to the Raptors' 2019 playoff run. Mike was ready. The 2016 experience had taught him how to prepare and deliver at a high level. As Phil Jackson, former professional basketball player, coach, and executive, said, "In basketball — as in life — true joy comes from being fully present in each and every moment, not just when things are going your way." Mike knew the 2019 playoffs were going to be a long run, and with the Raptors likely to go the distance, his familiarity with the team would keep him in demand. The risk of things getting away from him was real. He had no intention of repeating past mistakes and adapted to avoid them. He prioritized his sleep, took power naps when needed, ate well, maintained his workout schedule, and changed how he traveled. "I no longer took early morning flights. I just decided not to catch the 6 a.m. flight to be a superman. I'll take that noon flight." The Raptors would go the distance and bring home the Larry O'Brien Championship trophy, and Mike captured their storybook victory every step of the way.

SELF-CARE REFLECTION #31

On a ten-point scale, how would you rate your current energy reserves, with ten representing your best peak effort and zero representing complete and total exhaustion?

A score less than five likely means you battle fatigue every day. The idea of finding additional time to exercise may seem impossible or maybe even offensive, but self-care is the only way to get your reserves back. Commit to trying Mike's twenty-minute workout before the end of the day tomorrow, and on completion, record how it made you feel in your journal.

MICHAEL'S FORMULA FOR HEALTH, STRENGTH & HOPE

Mike has worked closely with elite athletes his whole career and recognizes the performance advantages to fitness. Having played and competed at a high level himself, he appreciates the importance of setting physical activity as a priority and putting in the work. He is also wired with a natural interest in biomechanics, training, and athletic performance. For Mike, the immediate performance kick from exercise is found in his sleep quality and mental acuity. Motivated to monitor his athletic ability, he also engages a team of professionals to help him maintain an elite level of fitness. Along the way, his team has included a mental health expert, chiropractor, personal trainer, yoga instructor, and a few sport-specific coaches.

> ❝ **I've made great strides as I've gotten older and more mature, identifying how to kind of toggle my workout intensity back and forth, using fitness like a medication."**

As our discussion turned to his current fitness approach, it was clear that he had reached a point where he recognized the need to alter his training to align with his stage of life. He called it "maturity." Mike does not expect his fifties peak to compete with his thirties or forties peak. "I've accepted that I've got to get away from the pressure of pushing my limits and begin to use fitness as a way of nurturing a healthy body and mind as I age."

All 7 Wellness Rituals continue to remain in play in Mike's formula; however, they matter more at different times of his year or on any given day. He still enjoys the physicality of a good sweat but is starting to tap into a new benefit of exercise designed to push back against Father Time. "I've made great strides as I've gotten older and more mature, identifying how to kind of toggle my workout intensity back and forth, using fitness like a medication."

The idea of how fast he can run or how much he can lift no longer holds his interest. "As you get a bit older, how well you move is what really matters." Practicing quality movement patterns that promote a full, pain-free, active range of motion has become the framework of Mike's new approach to exercise.

"One of the most illuminating experiences I have had in all of my years of fitness and training is when I came to understand the importance of not ignoring the accumulation of nagging injuries." In Mike's early fifties, while shooting hoops, he experienced a sudden sharp pain in his thigh and knee. The injury sidelined him and left Mike questioning whether he had reached his best-before date. He saw a sports chiropractor who helped him better understand his biomechanics, treated the acute condition, and provided an exercise prescription that allowed Mike to return to his active lifestyle. "I went from thinking I'm fifty-one and totally fucked, to a month later, feeling great and moving without pain, despite having a small meniscal tear." This experience marked a fork in the road for Mike and encouraged him to adapt his formula.

His workout routine now consists of dynamic functional movements. He will incorporate some running, biking, and traditional, Olympic-style weightlifting into his routine, but his primary focus has become movement efficiency. On a day of resistance training, he might only lift for twenty to thirty minutes, but before touching a weight, he will complete twenty-five to thirty minutes of prehab. This includes yoga, Pilates, and core strengthening and conditioning exercises. On a cardio day, he will head out and run for twenty minutes, then break into side shuffles, butt kicks, walking lunges, cross-overs, and short sprints, challenging his body at different intervals and in different positions, and then jog home. Practicing varied movement patterns over the last few years has had a huge payoff in terms of his flexibility and overall athleticism. "I'm certain that a lot of people could overcome a number of mechanical issues if they went down this road with clinical guidance and a patient attention to detail."

Mike's appreciation for the link between lifestyle practices and performance is clear. When asked, he can passionately discuss the performance rewards of a healthy routine. For Mike, these would include improved sleep quality, higher energy, better mood, and elevated mental acuity. But he offered an additional consideration in our discussion, stating that he does not see the connection between fitness and performance as a linear relationship. "When I look at how fitness plays out in my life, I think of it as a signal. If I have the ability to stick to a schedule five or six days a week and get into a rhythm, that means my life is going well. It is an indication of balance." He sees exercise, and the time available to work out, not as the cause of life going well, but the effect.

MAKE THE MOST OF THE TIME YOU HAVE

"I would be perfectly happy to be in bed asleep at 10 p.m. and awake and going full bore at 5:30 to 6 a.m. in the morning. This is my default position, but that doesn't work for the job I have." The 2016 and 2019 playoff runs outline the extremes of Mike's role. In any given year, he may have to push at this pace for two to three months. The remaining 280 to 300 days a year are much more manageable, and he is able to use his schedule to his advantage. With a daughter and son in university, the level of hands-on parenting is much less demanding. Pockets of are starting to pop up. The extra time is welcomed and put to good use, but Mike gives the impression that this rediscovered freedom still feels unfamiliar.

"I probably have ten really good years and twenty pretty good years left." Looking ahead, he is likely to embrace the challenge of another triathlon or travel adventure. Nothing is off the table given his active practice and commitment to his formula.

The idea of how fast he can run or how much he can lift no longer holds his interest. **"As you get a bit older, how well you move is what really matters."** Practicing quality movement patterns that promote a full, pain-free, active range of motion has become the framework of Mike's new approach to exercise.

From birth to our early thirties, our muscles grow larger and get stronger. From this point forward, lifestyle starts to yield a more immediate and impactful influence on health. Physically inactive individuals can lose 3% to 5% of their muscle mass each decade after thirty.

WELLNESS RITUAL #5

PROTECT YOUR STRENGTH

7 WELLNESS RITUALS
FOR HEALTH, STRENGTH & HOPE

WELLNESS RITUAL #5: THE SCIENCE

The twenty-one mentors, young and old, actively challenge their bodies to stay strong. They understand the orthopedic limits of their bodies but do not willingly surrender their strength to the advance of time. By incorporating regular resistance training into their workouts, introducing variety into their activity, and surrounding themselves with friends and professionals who hold them accountable, they have fun and stay strong.

The next time you step out of the shower, take a moment and look at your naked body in a full-length mirror. Really take a good look — even at the parts you are not so proud of. It is easy to blame your body for your aches and pains and lose sight of the power you possess to change this narrative.

> Stand tall.
> Take a deep breath, slowly, in and out.
> Smile.
> Out loud, state one thing about your body that you are grateful for.
> Now ask yourself, "Am I aging well?"
> Repeat this ritual on the first day of every month.

Age-related muscle loss starts at a younger age and progresses more quickly than most people realize. Time favors fat deposits over lean muscle. The subtle physical changes of aging can occur so slowly that they may be missed if you move through life on autopilot. Suddenly, the day arrives when bending over to clip your toenails becomes difficult, and you realize you have taken your eyes off your greatest asset. Patients will embarrassingly admit being startled by an unflattering glimpse of themselves in a mirror or struggle with personal grooming and ask, "What happened to me? I feel like I got old overnight." I try to keep my response honest and discreet whenever asked to address the elephant in the room. The next two questions they ask are the ones that really matter: "What do I need to do to get my health back?" and "Is it too late?"

Aging is a complex process influenced by heredity, environment, culture, diet, exercise, leisure activities, past injuries and illnesses, and many other factors. If you allow life to play out without much consideration for your future health and performance, then by the day you hit forty, your muscular strength will already be a full decade into decline. By seventy, you will have lost close to a quarter of the strength you possessed at thirty. Accepting that this shrinking physical capacity and the diminished quality of life that accompanies it are an inevitable part of aging is one option.

Unfortunately, many select this path as a default, not knowing there is another alternative.

Thankfully, there is. Studies show it is possible to reverse this trend and gain strength as we age with a very straightforward, low-tech solution.

The previous section discussed how a commitment to regular physical activity promotes good health, reduces the risk of many chronic diseases, and supports longevity, but aerobic movement alone is not enough. An appropriately crafted fitness routine must also include resistance training. This is often overlooked, and when it is, our strength and functional ability begin to deteriorate. "Use it or lose it" is a biological certainty.

❝ You have only one body to use in this life. Do not be a passenger.

When you reach your fifties, resistance training must find a permanent spot in your formula. It is essential to preserve physical ability. With a surprisingly small investment of time, you can leverage the body's adaptability to boost muscular strength, power, speed, endurance, balance, and coordination. These metrics all have a profound effect on quality of life. Current studies contradict the common belief that muscle mass and strength decline as a function of aging alone and are drawing greater attention toward the impact of chronic disuse. Patients in their nineties have demonstrated the ability to improve in all of the above performance metrics after only twelve weeks of resistance training.[1] Other studies have shown no appreciable difference in intramuscular fat or lean muscle mass in the legs of high-level recreational athletes varying in age between forty and eighty-one.[2,3] Consider the following words the keystone of Wellness Ritual #5: Protect Your Strength... *You have only one body to use in this life. Do not be a passenger.*

WHY RESISTANCE TRAINING AND WHY NOW

If your formula currently doesn't include resistance training, you are at risk of sarcopenia. Never heard of it? You are not alone. Sadly, it does not get the attention it deserves despite its prevalence, so when you are finished reading this section, please help me educate the world and tell your loved ones what it is and how they can prevent it. Doing so will have a significant impact on how they age.

Sarcopenia, a reduction in muscle mass and muscle function, is considered a hallmark of the aging process. Current views consider it the consequence of multiple medical, behavioral, and environmental factors that characterize what it is to get old.[4] Muscle weakness, fear of falls, falls, and subsequent fractures are associated with sarcopenia and lead to restricted mobility, loss of autonomy, and reduced life expectancy.

From birth to our early thirties, our muscles grow larger and get stronger. From this point forward, lifestyle starts to yield a more immediate and impactful influence on health. Physically inactive individuals can lose 3% to 5% of their muscle mass each decade after thirty. If you aren't using your muscles regularly, you will experience faster muscle loss and increased weakness as you move past this biological milestone.[5] I know this sounds like I am stating the obvious, but most sedentary patients are genuinely surprised to learn of the serious consequences of their inaction as their bodies start to fail them. Our bodies adapt with great skill to the environments they live in. This dynamic force is constantly at work — for better or worse. Research has shown that periods of just two to three weeks of decreased activity can be enough to reduce muscle mass and strength.[6]

In addition to inactivity, the following factors can also accelerate decline:

- As we age, we experience a reduction in the nerve cells responsible for sending signals from the brain to our muscles to initiate movement. As these small neurons begin to die off, they leave the disconnected muscle fibers to shrink.
- A lower concentration of growth hormone, testosterone, and insulin-like growth factor accompanies aging.
- A poor diet that doesn't provide the nutritional building blocks for good health will interfere with physical performance at any age. Protein intake and physical activity are the main anabolic stimuli for muscle protein synthesis. Optimal dietary protein intake is approximately 1.0 – 1.2 g/kg of body weight/day.[7] Unhealthy nutritional practices, like the regular consumption of processed foods, promote inflammation in the body and negatively impact muscle health. Next time you have your blood work taken, ask about your C-reactive protein levels. As a blood inflammation marker, high levels are a strong predictor of sarcopenia.[8]
- High chronic stress levels. Evidence suggests that oxidative stress and molecular inflammation play important roles in age-related muscle atrophy. These two factors may interfere with the balance between protein synthesis and breakdown, cause mitochondrial dysfunction, and induce cell death.[9]

So what can you do to avoid an age-related decline in strength and functional ability? The most robust defense against this outcome is to make your body work.

Specifically, take Wellness Ritual #4 and add one to two fifteen- to twenty-minute resistance training workouts each week. To be clear, these workouts can be included in your weekly 150-minute movement target. There is no additional time required unless you choose to set a higher bar.

Resistance training means different things to different people, so let's clear up common myths and set the facts straight before going any further.

COMMON WATERCOOLER MYTHS ABOUT RESISTANCE TRAINING

Myth #1: Resistance training will make your body bulky.

Fact: Strength training will help you improve your body composition and leave you looking lean, not bulky. Getting big and packing on muscle in the gym takes extraordinary training and gifted genetics. The objective of resistance training is to give you a body that moves well and looks healthy with minimal time investment.

Myth #2: The weight room is a male dominated, testosterone-filled space.
Fact: The idea that only guys frequent the weight room is long outdated. More and more women of all ages are beginning to embrace the powerful benefits of weight training.

Myth #3: Resistance training makes you less flexible and is bad for your joints.
Fact: When you move through a full range of motion while performing strength training exercises, you will experience an improvement in your flexibility. Developing strength and stability in different positions and joint angles will expand your functional ability. Building muscle strength and tone helps to protect your joints and improve your posture.

Myth #4: Only work one muscle group a day.
Fact: Choosing compound movements, like squats and lunges, that work more than one muscle group at a time produces more significant results. It is possible and safe to work multiple body parts in each workout as long as you have a one to two day break between training sessions.

Myth #5: Cardio burns more fat than resistance training.
Fact: Trying to burn down unwanted fat deposits with extra time on the treadmill or elliptical doesn't work. Cardiovascular training has an essential role in your formula, but you will burn more calories by coupling the advice in the second and third Wellness Rituals with resistance training.

Myth #6: I'm too old to lift weights.
Fact: No matter your age or skill level, it is never too late to start resistance training. Research strongly supports resistance training for patients sixty and older as a strategy to increase muscle strength by increasing muscle mass and improving the recruitment and firing rate of motor units.[10]

Myth #7: I must use light weights to avoid injury. What can that achieve?
Fact: There is nothing wrong with using light weights. The foundational movements highlighted toward the end of this section can be practiced with no weight at all. What is

important is that you start with a weight you can comfortably handle and progress from there. The goal of this Wellness Ritual is to increase your lean muscle mass and make you stronger. To achieve this, you must regularly increase the weight you are lifting. When we challenge our bodies with heavier weight, we create more microtears in our muscles. It is during the repair phase of the workout recovery that you get stronger. As a general rule, if you can complete a set of twelve reps without any difficulty, it is time to increase the weight you are lifting or advance your routine.

Myth #8: Resistance training takes too much time.

Fact: Your movement commitment is 150 minutes a week. With this time already hard-wired into your weekly formula, dedicate fifteen to forty minutes of it to resistance training in one to two workouts lasting fifteen to twenty minutes each.

Myth #9: You will need access to a gym.

Fact: Resistance training can be done anywhere, with no equipment, using only bodyweight.

Myth #10: It takes a long time to see results.

Fact: It takes hard work and dedication to the practice, but meaningful results are often seen in the first four to six weeks.

GETTING STRONGER SUPPORTS WEIGHT LOSS

Resistance training builds muscle, and muscle burns more calories than fat. As discussed in Wellness Ritual #3, there continues to be considerable controversy over how much exercise influences metabolism, so it is difficult to nail down the exact impact strength gains have on weight loss. As a rough estimate, our muscles account for 20% of the total daily calories burned whereas fat tissue accounts for only 5%. For that reason, resistance training is considered a valuable weight loss tool. Maintaining muscle mass and gaining more lean tissue is often what keeps people from gaining weight as they get older.[11]

As a bonus, after completing a resistance workout, your body will burn extra calories for the next twenty-four to forty-eight hours as it works to repair stressed muscle tissues. This is known as the afterburn effect or excess post-exercise oxygen consumption (EPOC). The more oxygen you use during and after a workout, the greater the EPOC.

A study published in the journal *Obesity* found that dieters who completed strength training workouts four times a week for eighteen months lost more fat (roughly eighteen pounds) than those who didn't exercise (ten pounds) and those who did only aerobic exercise (sixteen pounds).[12]

It is not only about getting strong and lean.

The powerful vision of a stronger, leaner, and more youthful version of your body is often enough to get most patients engaged in healthful exercise. The fact that it also gives you some protection against sarcopenia adds fuel to the motivation. To seal the deal, here is a quick summary of the additional health benefits of resistance training supported in scientific literature.

Resistance training allows you to:

- Enjoy greater stamina and the ability to perform at your physical peak with greater consistency;[13]
- Increase your calorie burn rate — as you gain muscle, your body burns more energy when at rest;[14]
- Burn more visceral fat, reducing your risk of many chronic diseases, including heart disease, liver disease, type 2 diabetes, and certain cancers;[15]
- Lower your risk of falls and common musculoskeletal injuries, including low back pain;[16,17]
- Improve your cardiac health, lower blood pressure, reduce total and LDL cholesterol, and improve blood circulation;[18,19]
- Improve insulin sensitivity and reduce blood sugar levels;[20]
- Improve movement quality and increase flexibility, which can help you maintain independence later in life;[21]
- Elevate your self-confidence. There is a strong association between strength training and high self-esteem and positive body image;[22]
- Improve bone health, reducing the risk of osteoporosis and fractures;[23]
- Improve brain health, age-related cognitive decline, and reduce anxiety;[24,25]
- Improve sleep quality.[26]

This seems like a pretty good return on investment for two fifteen- to twenty-minute workouts a week. Let's now discuss the key principles to help you put this ritual in motion.

KEY PRINCIPLES OF RESISTANCE TRAINING

Resistance training is simply the practice of deliberately placing your body under a load and making it work against gravity. Our bodies are capable of six main functional movement patterns: push, pull, squat, lunge, hinge, and carry, with rotation acting as a bonus pattern that can enhance any of the other six. By performing these movements, you will be able to stimulate all of the major muscle groups in your body and improve your physical capacity for movement.

To move well and avoid injury, we must possess functional strength in every plane of motion. Work with your healthcare team to develop a customized program that mimics the movements you perform in everyday life. Your program should be challenging to complete without putting you at risk. As you can imagine, achieving this balance can be tricky, so start slowly and build intensity as you gain confidence and proficiency with the routine. You shouldn't be grinding out pistol squats if you don't possess the required functional range of motion in your hips, knees, and ankles. And unless you have built up to doing single-leg low squats, this is probably not a movement you should begin with.

Programs using bodyweight, free weights, and exercise equipment or resistance bands will all achieve results. I tell patients new to resistance training to think about increasing their "time under load," even outside of their dedicated resistance training workouts. When playing with your kids, lifting your dog, completing household chores, putting groceries away, hauling the laundry basket up and down the stairs, or washing your car, get after it. These are all opportunities to get stronger.

Most resistance programs are designed around lifting a percentage of your maximum strength. The One-Repetition Maximum test (1RM) is one of the most common measures used to find out the heaviest weight you can safely lift or press just once. Promoting significant increases in muscle mass and strength and stimulating optimal adaptive responses to reduce stiffness and improve tendon health require training loads of 70% to 85% of your 1RM.[27] Turn to Google to find a 1RM online calculator to define your starting point. Remember that each exercise has its own 1RM. Strength is specific. As a general reference, higher intensity training usually consists of three sets of six to twelve repetitions.

To get the most out of your workouts, there are four basic principles you need to follow when training:

1. **The Technique of Progressive Overload**

   By exposing your muscles to more weight, resistance, or stimulus than they receive from your normal daily activities, you will get stronger. Gradually increasing the stress or load placed on your body over time through increased reps or heavier weights drives gains in strength and endurance.

   Compound movements, like squats and deadlifts, that work multiple muscle groups and joints simultaneously, or unilateral movements, like lunges, are excellent ways to apply progressive overload. Isolation exercises, like bicep curls, are not as challenging and will not produce results as quickly.

   When selecting a starting weight, choose the heaviest weight with which you can perform a complete set while maintaining good posture and technique.

   To see results over time, you will need to continue overloading your muscles through gradual increase of your training volume by performing an extra set, introducing a new movement combination, or using more challenging weights.

2. **A Program Designed for You**

   The body's response and subsequent adaptation to how you move, the speed of your movement, your range of motion, the muscles used, and the training intensity all influence your training results. A fitness regimen must be designed to meet your goals and ability. A skilled personal trainer will take these factors into consideration to design a challenging and safe program.

3. **Bring Variety to Training**

   If you are stuck in a workout rut and have done the same routine repeatedly, your body will stop responding, and your progress will hit a plateau. This is called adaptive resistance. By creating variation in your fitness and movement practices, you will develop new stimuli for the body and leverage your tissue adaptation. Rotating between two to three variations for each muscle group or movement pattern will usually do the trick.

   Most beginners experience a rapid increase in strength when they begin a resistance training program, followed by a plateau. From this point forward, gains in muscle strength and size are hard-earned and require you to mix up your routine if you desire further improvement.

When you start resistance training, most of the initial increase in strength is due to "neural adaptation." Your nervous system responds to the demands of your workout by increasing neural activity and prompting stronger muscle contractions, recruiting more motor units (muscle fibers) to perform the desired movement. This will leave you feeling stronger even though your muscles will remain the same physical size.

In time, your muscle cells will respond to continued varied training by increasing in size (hypertrophy), so don't be discouraged if you reach a plateau; it is a sign that gains in muscle size are soon to follow.

Varying your workouts can help you push past a plateau. The theory of variation is that you can coax growth and strength from your muscles by surprising them with different stresses.

Here is a list of possible workout variations:

- Increase the number of repetitions.
- Add a set.
- Extend your workout by ten minutes or add a third workout to your week. Keep in mind that muscles need at least forty-eight hours of recovery time.
- Modify your routine. For example, add forward planks, side planks, dead bugs, and cross-crawl bird-dogs to the routine outlined below. Visit **7WellnessRituals.com** for detailed descriptions of these movements.
- Increase the weight by about 5% to 10%.
- Cross-train with other activities, such as swimming or hiking.

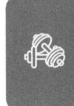

SAMPLE WORKOUT STRUCTURES

Straight Sets: Bang out a certain number of reps, rest, and repeat. Three sets of ten is a common starting point. Remember, to continue to gain benefits, you will need to push to the outer limits of your comfort zone.

Pyramid Sets: With this structure, you increase the weight and lower the reps with each subsequent set.

Supersets: Two exercises are used to work opposing muscle groups, like biceps and triceps or quadriceps and hamstrings, in each set with no rest in between. This approach keeps your heart rate elevated, involves more muscle fibers, and burns more calories.

4. Rest and Recovery

Strong muscles are not built in the gym. It is during your rest and recovery between workouts that the magic happens. By activating the overload principle, you create minor damage to your muscle fibers and trigger a growth and adaptation mechanism as your body actively repairs and reinforces the damage. This is your reward for the hard work. No rest. No reward.

It is important to note that progression is not always the primary goal of this Wellness Ritual. Once a desired body composition and strength are achieved, many mentors tailor their resistance training program to maintain their current level of fitness. Once they reach this state, they look at their resistance training as good housekeeping.

BLOOD FLOW RESTRICTION (BFR) TRAINING

Blood Flow Restriction (BFR) training is a technique that combines low-intensity exercise with blood flow occlusion to produce results similar to high-intensity training. It is a technique that has been used in the gym for many years but is starting to gain popularity with personal trainers and in clinical rehab settings. A pneumatic cuff or strap is applied around the upper or lower extremity above the muscle being trained and tightened to restrict blood flow and oxygen delivery to the working tissue. The patient is typically asked to perform a set of low intensity (approximately 20% to 30% of their 1RM) with high repetitions (fifteen to thirty reps). A short thirty-second rest between sets, with the strap or cuff removed, allows the blood flow to return to normal.

A release of hormones, hypoxia (decreased oxygen), and cell swelling occur when a muscle is placed under this type of metabolic stress, which are all believed to stimulate anabolic strength gains. BFR is an attempted hack to allow the muscles to reap the benefits of much higher intensity training and stimulate increased protein synthesis while lifting lighter loads. A 2019 study published in the Journal of Applied Physiology found that BFR, paired with low-intensity resistance training, yielded similar muscle gains when compared with high-intensity workouts in a group of adult men over a fourteen-week period.[28] Additional studies, however, are required to further investigate the potential adaptive advantages of low intensity BFR training and its use in a wider population. Individuals with elevated blood pressure or a family or personal history of blood clotting disorders should avoid BFR.

CHAPIN CLINICAL CORNER

We push, pull, squat, hinge, lunge, carry, and rotate all day. Together these actions represent our foundational movements. When training, do not let your mind wander. Fight the temptation to daydream and keep your head in the game. Block out all other external noise, distractions, demands, or to-do lists, and focus on the time you have purposefully set aside for this training.

To get the most out of each rep, focus your attention on making quality movements. Practice the 1% marginal gains rule by trying to make a 1% improvement with each workout.

Visualize the contraction and relaxation phase, maintaining a keen awareness of your postural alignment and any areas of stress or tension. Feel your muscles shorten as they contract and lengthen as they relax.

Linking your breath to your movement will give you added power and focus. Time your breathing to inhale through your nose right before the eccentric (muscle lengthening) movement and exhale through your mouth during the concentric (muscle shortening) contraction.

As an example, when performing a pushup, inhale, bend your elbows, and lower your body to the floor, then exhale as you push your body back up.

For beginners, once you have received approval from your healthcare team to begin resistance training, complete one to two sets of eight to twelve reps for each of the movements below twice a week. Delayed onset muscle soreness (DOMS) after training is normal and typically peaks twenty-four to forty-eight hours after the workout. If you experience any discomfort or pain lasting longer than five days post workout, contact your healthcare team to discuss program modifications before continuing. In four to six weeks, you will see and feel the difference and be ready to progressively increase your training intensity.

Start each workout with a short five-minute dynamic warm up to get your blood pumping and body warmed up.

TO STRETCH OR NOT TO STRETCH? HOW TO PROPERLY WARM UP AND COOL DOWN

A warm-up routine that maximizes performance and reduces the risk of injury is essential to resistance training. A decent warm up aims to increase our core body temperature, excite our nervous system and metabolic activity, and decrease joint and muscle stiffness. To achieve this, an active, dynamic warm up is preferred over passive, static stretching. Bending forward from the waist toward your toes to stretch out a tight hamstring before a workout may be putting your problem hamstring at greater risk of injury. Pre-exercise static stretching is okay if it follows some dynamic movement and is kept to less than sixty seconds per muscle group.[29]

Dynamic warm-up movements like high knees, hip circles, quarter-squats, lunges, jumping jacks, arm circles, or a few minutes on a bike or elliptical are all effective ways to prepare the body for physical activity. Moving through a warm-up routine that promotes a full range of motion primes your tissues for the demands of the workout to follow.

Set aside an additional five minutes for a post-workout cool down. This is where the bulk of your static stretching belongs. You want to hold each stretch for thirty to sixty seconds, targeting the larger muscle groups, and feel a slight pull but no pain.

BENEFITS OF FOUNDATIONAL, STRENGTH-BUILDING EXERCISES

THE PUSH & PULL

In everyday life, these movement patterns are constantly in play. We can push something away from our body or pull it closer. Pushing and pulling are further divided into two more categories — vertical and horizontal. Because pushing and pulling are functional opposites, developing balance in your up-and-down and front-to-back strength is essential.

Shoulders are especially susceptible to injury. They are built for mobility, not stability. Please proceed slowly when pushing and pulling weight, especially when pushing weight overhead. Proper form is a must. Performing arm circles or shoulder mobility drills between sets can help.

THE SQUAT

Every time you sit down or get up and off the toilet, you squat. Any change in vertical levels over your day calls on a decent squat. The squat requires a triple flexion and extension of the ankles, knees, and hips, which ideally happens in coordination as you lower and raise your body. It is a super-efficient exercise that will help to strengthen your entire lower half.

THE HINGE/DEADLIFT

The hinge is one of the most underused functional movement patterns, perhaps because we've always been told to "lift with our knees," and we are scared about hurting our backs. A bad hinge will put your lower back in real jeopardy. But if you have a strong core, hinging is arguably a safer movement pattern for lifting a heavy object from the floor than squatting. Mastering the hinge and executing it correctly can reduce or eliminate mechanical back pain.

THE LUNGE

The lunge is a single-leg cross-over between a hinge and a squat. Any movement that requires a single-leg stance (stairs, work in the garden, tennis) will call on good lunge mechanics. This movement requires a higher level of dynamic balance and control. If you feel insecure about your balance during this movement, try lightly touching (not leaning on) a chair, wall, or counter.

THE CARRY

This is the most functional and practical movement pattern of them all. It is a movement pattern we use all day long, and it is essential for dynamic stability. For that reason, it is one of my favorites.

ROTATION

Rotation is how we transfer power from our lower half, through our core, and out our upper half. It requires head-to-toe stability and teaches our body to work as a single unit rather than as separate halves. Coupling other movements together requires competent rotation.

To access videos demonstrating proper form for the push and pull, squat, hinge or deadlift, lunge, carry, rotation, and more, visit **7WellnessRituals.com**. McLeod Bethel-Thompson, professional football quarterback, will help you with your technique.

DIET AND MUSCLE HEALTH

Gaining and maintaining muscle mass also depends on good nutrition. This includes eating enough nutrient-dense calories to fuel your body. Protein, which helps build and repair muscle, is vital. The amount of protein you need depends on your level of physical activity. Generally, 10% to 35% of your daily calories should come from protein. You also need to consume enough carbohydrates to fuel your muscles. If you're strength training two or more times per week, carbohydrates should make up at least 50% of your daily calories. See Wellness Ritual #2: Consume Healthy Fuel for a more detailed review.

The final tip I have for you is to pay attention to your inner dialogue. When you find yourself thinking negative or angry thoughts about how you look or move, recognize this thought pattern and consciously change the track playing in your head. When you look at yourself in the mirror, say this affirmation out loud:

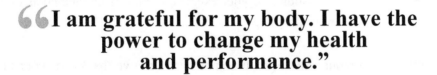

"I am grateful for my body. I have the power to change my health and performance."

Before beginning your workout, express gratitude for your body's ability to carry you through the next twenty minutes. Gratitude releases toxic emotions, eases the nervous system, lowers cortisol, and relaxes tight muscles. Intentionally repeat this track in your mind, even if at first it feels forced. You will find momentum in the practice of self-care and positive encouragement.

There is no changing the past. You are where you are. Your potential lies in the workout you are about to begin. And to answer the earlier question, no, it is not too late.

RITUAL ACTIVATION

RITUAL TARGET

- On the first day of each month, take a good look at yourself in a full-length mirror and ask, "Am I aging well?"

- Consult your healthcare team and ask for their blessing to begin a resistance training program. Go into this appointment armed with the understanding and confidence that it is never too late to start resistance training.

- Hire a personal trainer to help you develop a customized program. Note: Some people enjoy working out with a trainer; others do not. You do not need to spend a lot of money on ongoing training services if money is tight or this isn't your thing, but paying for some clinical guidance to ensure you get off on the right foot is wise.

- Each week, incorporate two to three resistance training workouts of fifteen- to twenty-minutes in duration into your exercise routine. This time counts toward your 150-minute movement target.

- Start each workout with a gratitude practice and give thanks for your body's ability to move, heal, and adapt.

- Keep your focus exclusively on your movement quality for the duration of the workout.

- Vary your training program every six to eight weeks to maintain improvement.

- Prioritize recovery. Your muscles need time to repair and adapt after a workout. Allow for twenty-four to forty-eight hours between workouts.

IN SUMMARY

The goal of Wellness Ritual #5 is to increase your lean muscle mass and make your body stronger. To achieve this outcome, you must incorporate resistance training into your formula and look for opportunities to make your muscles work. Strength training can be done with body weight, resistance bands, free weights, or weight-lifting equipment. A well-rounded program works all major muscle groups twice a week: legs, hips, back, abdomen, chest, shoulders, and arms. Start with a dynamic warm up; aim for one or two sets of eight to twelve repetitions of each exercise using a weight or resistance that is challenging but manageable. The health advantages of maintaining a physically strong body include improved bone, cardiovascular, and metabolic health; increased energy, flexibility, and mobility; and elevated mood, body image, and brain health.

Wired as an extrovert, the role played to Randy's character strengths and preferences. However, **the pace** he was trying to maintain was not sustainable. If he wasn't careful, the **rock star lifestyles** of the talent he was discovering and promoting at Universal would prevent him from becoming the leader **he aspired to become.**

MENTOR PROFILES

RANDY LENNOX

ALISON DANTAS

DR. ROBYNE HANLEY-DAFOE

RANDY LENNOX

Former CEO of Bell Media and Universal Music Canada

Google the best rock frontmen of all time, and you will find Mick Jagger, Freddie Mercury, Robert Plant, Steven Tyler, and Bruce Springsteen at the top of most lists. In addition to their vocal chops, frontmen are known for their charismatic presence, creativity, and big personalities. Their "it factor" lifts their music even higher.

Randy Lennox is a center-stage frontman too. However, his stage is not a 20,000-seat arena. It is the media and entertainment industry. As former CEO of Bell Media and Universal Music Canada, the ripple effect of Randy's talent on Canadian culture is extraordinary. While at the helm of Universal, he signed or elevated the careers of some of Canada's biggest recording artists, including Shawn Mendes, Drake, Justin Bieber, Shania Twain, The Tragically Hip, The Weeknd, Hedley, Alessia Cara, and others. To global superstars, he is known as the "rain maker" or the "make-it-happen captain."

At the 2017 Juno Awards, Randy won the Walt Grealis Special Achievement Award, presented by the Canadian Academy of Recording Arts and Sciences. The prestigious award recognizes the recipient's contribution to the growth and development of the Canadian music industry. U2's Bono kicked the tributes off,[1] calling Randy a "music maven turned telecommunications mogul." Peter Gabriel, a clear admirer of Randy, shared, "I've signed with other labels around the world, but in Canada, I just wanted to be where Randy was." Gene Simmons of Kiss credited Randy for helping to shape the American and Canadian music industry into what it is today. When asked about Randy's influence, Gord Downie from the Tragically Hip cut right to the point with his quirky grin and skilled prose: "Hey Rand, I just want to say, I love you. You only brought a smile and made smiles. You are a gentleman — a beautiful man. Happy days."

In making a move from Universal Music Canada to Bell Media, Randy brought his love for creative content and value creation to Canada's largest media company. While in his role as president and CEO, he set his sights on overhauling and growing Bell Media's streaming operations, signing content deals with U.S. partners, reinvigorating its radio business, and developing new lines of business and content pipelines.[2]

Having already reached the summit twice in his career as a high-profile president and CEO, studying Randy's process is particularly interesting. When we sat down to discuss this book, he had finished his last day at Bell Media only six weeks earlier. January 4, 2021 marked the end of his second act as a leading frontman. Frontmen can find the silence between big performances uncomfortable. Ironically, despite Randy's talent for being at center stage, it was his ability to seek out and embrace times of uncomfortable silence that drove his success. Silence turned out to be the key to unlocking Randy's formula.

SELF-CARE REFLECTION #32

Randy draws strength from times of quietude. If you find it challenging to find moments to yourself or have difficulty turning off the busy-ness in your brain, start with scheduling a ten-minute solitude break into your calendar for some time tomorrow. Honor this appointment when it arrives. Set a timer for ten minutes and switch all devices to airplane mode. Sit quietly, drawing your attention to the rhythm of your breath for the full ten minutes. If your mind wanders (and it will), kindly bring it back to your breath. When the timer goes off, make note of the direction of your thoughts. Recognizing recurrent thoughts often helps identify your leading stressors.

RANDY'S FORMULA FOR HEALTH, STRENGTH & HOPE

Randy is an easy guy to like. He is fun, thoughtful, authentic, wise, and eager to share. After an hour with him, he felt like a good friend. If I were Peter Gabriel, I too would want to sign wherever Randy was. Passionate about the purpose of this book, he offered a transparent look at his process. I assured him that the other mentors profiled in the book were not masters of clean living, and what I was looking for first and foremost were Canadian leaders with clarity and discipline in the practice of their formula. He confirmed he had a solid grip on that, and we jumped into a spirited conversation of leadership, motivation, passion, adversity, pace, reflection, triumphs, failures, growth, and happiness. It was a conversation worthy of its own mini-series.

Randy's formula for success includes all 7 Wellness Rituals, although he leans most heavily on Nurture Mental Fitness. In telling me his story, four key life events stand out, with each playing a significant role in helping Randy develop the way he approaches life with all of its challenges and successes.

LIFE LESSON #1: IGNORING SELF-CARE CAN KILL A DREAM

He would learn the first lesson as a young CEO. Randy worked his way, literally, from the mailroom all the way to the top job at Universal Music Canada. At age thirty-six, he found himself in the position of his dreams and tore into the role, setting both ends of the candle ablaze. Wired as an extrovert, the role played to Randy's character strengths and preferences. However, the pace he was trying to maintain was not sustainable. If he wasn't careful, the rock star lifestyles of the talent he was discovering and promoting at Universal would prevent him from becoming the leader he aspired to become. Falling into this trap was "a challenge I gave myself unknowingly," he shared. Until he learned to get out of his own way, his actions prematurely capped his potential.

> **I don't want to deliver at an 8.5 on a job that I had spent my entire life dreaming about."**

He remembers a specific period in 1998 when he felt the weight of the industry's gaze on his every move. So much so that it stopped him in his tracks, and he thought, "Randy, don't you dare screw this up. You really had an aspiration to be in this chair." Most leaders learn the hard lesson that an unrelenting pace is unsustainable at some point in their careers. It hit Randy early and hard. We spent some time discussing this period in his life. I asked whether his realization that he needed to make some changes was based in fear or pride. He paused and said, "I remember the thought process was exactly this: I don't want to deliver at an 8.5 on a job that I had spent my entire life dreaming about."

Randy loves music. He spent a good part of his youth in and out of various rock bands. I am not sure if he can still carry a tune, but he does play a mean guitar. Knowing that he would not have a career as a musician gave his leadership role with Universal extra meaning. It put him right in the middle of the action with big talent. The job was a thrill and a privilege. To survive the ride, Randy went all in, placing his trust in his natural abilities as a leading frontman. His default setting is to be on. He can entertain and work a room like no one else. Finding himself at the pinnacle of the music industry in Canada, as a young man still learning how to lead effectively, he was eager to leave his mark. So eager, in fact, that his health and well-being were not getting the attention they demanded. Noticing a few critics in the wings that were hoping to see him fail and resenting his quick ascent, he realized he needed to double-down on his effort. Randy's first step in discovering his formula was to ensure he had a clear mind and a healthy body. He exercised great discipline to dial back the late nights and turn away from alcohol. He began to take better care of himself.

LIFE LESSON #2: GET TO KNOW YOURSELF

Blessed with an ability to block distraction and collateral noise, Randy tapped into his laser-sharp talent to concentrate and began to study the habits of other leaders. "Left undisturbed, I can absorb and drink a book very quickly," he shared. One night on business in Montreal, alone in his hotel room, he stumbled across a personality profile test online. The test results would end up having an enormous impact on the course of Randy's life.

Lesson one taught him the risks of pushing all out, all the time. The dangers of continuing to do so held his attention as a leader. Randy needed more balance in his life. Okay, fair enough — but how? He could feel his performance slipping down his ten-point scale. The idea of falling short of his high standard, which was set closer to an eleven, was not acceptable to him. This motivated a search for answers. He realized he was trying to sprint a marathon but did not know how to slow down and still deliver the same impact in an industry that rewards speed.

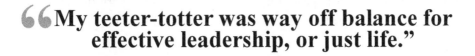
"My teeter-totter was way off balance for effective leadership, or just life."

Taking the profile test, Randy expected the results to confirm what he believed to his core was true — he was an extreme extrovert. Had anyone asked, he would have told them, "I am a 90/10, extrovert/introvert split." It turns out he was wrong. He is actually a 68/32 split. This insight changed everything for him.

Randy's second step toward discovering his formula was to engage therapy and coaching. He was overplaying his extrovert tendencies and choking out his introvert needs. "My teeter-totter was way off balance for effective leadership, or just life."

Lesson two learned. Mixed into the demands he was facing at work, he was also trying to raise a family with his wife. As he entered his forties, his focus and discipline provided an off-ramp yet again — this time creating space for him to make a deliberate effort to express his inner introvert. He set a goal of finding a balance that would increase his introvert tendencies to his 32% target.

LIFE LESSON #3: YOUR MIND IS THE KEY TO NEXT-LEVEL PERFORMANCE

Sharing your process with someone else with the intention and hope that it will perhaps help them on their journey is an intimate experience. At this point in our conversation, the depth of Randy's authenticity and altruistic character was revealed. We had reached the tipping point in the story of his evolution as a leader. As he described the significance of this moment in his life, it felt as though he literally reached through our Zoom call, grabbed hold of my shoulders, looked me directly in the eye, and held my gaze long enough to be sure I did not miss the importance of the point he was making. He said, "Dwight, the best thing I have ever done for my leadership is to give my mind the permission to have that 32%."

I cannot help but wonder if he was taking the opportunity to remind himself of the vital importance of lesson two, as well. I asked him if he had landed at a spot where he was starting to crave solitude. He said, "To get my introvert expression up from 10% to 32% took me ten years. Ten! It was a forcible entry. I am not naturally a quiet guy. If you lined up 100 people that knew me, none of them would say I was quiet. Not a one." I interpreted this response to mean no. It appeared that the silence between performances was still uncomfortable. He valued solitude but was not drawn to it, at least not yet.

Despite the decade-long battle, Randy persisted, and it paid off. The third step in Randy's formula is to never miss his daily practice of solitude and reflection. This practice took Randy's game to the next level in a big way. He discovered silence was not empty. In fact, it offered him a therapeutic detoxification. From a performance standpoint, he felt an immediate improvement in his mental acuity, creativity, memory, and ability to absorb new information. It was like someone had flipped a switch giving him access to a whole new area of his brain. "My 32% is my learning time." He became a voracious reader, constantly learning. Of course, his 68% extrovert got a meaningful bump in performance from the solitude as well. He found his performance for an audience also became sharper and more effective. Physically, he felt stronger and looked healthier, and this only bolstered his extrovert confidence.

The world seemed to notice the changes Randy was making as well. Universal North American Board came calling, as did others for entertainment jobs in LA. Randy noticed the distinct tethering between what he was putting out into the world and the response he was getting from it. Less frenetic, he had figured out how to run at a slower pace and have an even bigger impact.

Twenty years later, Randy still must remind himself daily of the power and importance of lesson two. The extrovert in him stands at the ready 24/7. It requires zero effort, prep, or thought. "I wake up, and I'm there in my 68%. That is just the way I am wired." Finding quiet times off-stage, out of the limelight to give a voice to his introvert tendencies still takes effort. He finds solitude in practicing yoga, reading, playing the guitar, and walking. Walking, always in silence, is his favorite. "My wife and I go for shorter walks together, but I also make sure I have time for my solo 'Randy-park-bench walks,' alone, along the lake."

Lesson three was that he was in good company with introverts. The time spent studying leadership helped him realize that many successful leaders tip toward introversion on the personality scale, including Bill Gates and Warren Buffett. From here, Randy stopped overplaying his hand as frontman. This created space for him to express his empathic nature.

As a huge believer in remembering where you came from, he never allowed himself to stray too far from the guy he was back in his days working in the mailroom. No longer needing to be center stage all the time, he would seek out opportunities down paths less traveled by high-profile CEOs. On his first day at Bell Media, he made a point of introducing himself to the café and building security staff. In short order, he was on a first-name basis with most of them, not because it was strategic but because the mailroom guy is still in him. He also legitimately enjoys the company of people and is not influenced by titles.

LIFE LESSON #4: CARE FOR OTHERS, AND THEY WILL CARE FOR YOU

Randy credits his wife for teaching him the fourth lesson, which was anchored in humility and the importance of trusting your formula. Randy is friends with some of the most talented musicians in the world. He is also surrounded by a wonderful group of close personal friends and his immediate family's love. Despite his success and big life, there is no escaping human nature. Doubt and uncertainty are astute foes.

Following his last day at Bell Media, Randy shared that he had an anxiety attack. "I'll tell you what it was: I didn't know if my phone would ring the next day. I didn't know if Mr. Hot Shot Universal or Mr. Hot Shot Bell Media, who was no longer a hotshot, would get another call."

With plenty of purpose, drive, and energy, he had no interest in going from 100 to zero and retiring. Uncertainty about his next move sparked fear, anxiety, and an innate desire to return to his 90/10 ways, but this is where Randy's inner circle of social support kicked in. Randy's fourth step in crafting his formula was to embrace the love, kindness, and advice of his loving wife, his friends, and the musicians he calls family. Randy Lennox was still a brand the world was interested in. Having treated people with honesty and respect his whole career, with a proven legacy of innovation and a finely crafted formula for success, they assured him that his phone would ring, and ring, and ring — and it has.

A THIRD ACT — NEVER IN DOUBT!

The sparkle in his eye on the day of our interview revealed that Randy will have a third act. Friends and family are calling on him to extend the period of silence between performances and stretch his 32% to 42% before jumping back in. One friend told him, "For God's sake, you had a paper route at age nine, and January 5, 2021, was your first day off. Slow down!" I suspect he will for a while, but not long. Frontmen like the stage, and he is now armed with a formula for success that is locked and loaded. The tickets to his next show will sell out fast.

SELF-CARE REFLECTION #33

Randy was able to identify four life lessons he learned in his personal life and professional career that catapulted major steps forward for success. Are there life lessons you can identify that have had a positive influence on your well-being, even if the lessons were unpleasant and demanded you deal with serious issues? While life events can present themselves unexpectedly and potentially put hardships in our way, consider your life lessons and how you might be better prepared than you think to deal with challenge.

ALISON DANTAS

Senior Executive & Executive Coach, Potential Actualized

When Alison was eleven years old, her family emigrated from Kenya to Canada. The move was full of promise and presented the family with a life-altering opportunity. Unencumbered by the ways of the world, Alison has always dreamed of a big life. From an early age, she remembers a distinct feeling calling her toward leadership, as her profile will reveal.

Growing up in a tight-knit South Asian community, she drew strength from family, friends, neighbors, and her Catholic faith. There was a comfort and confidence provided by these pillars that encouraged her to follow her dreams. Her inner circle knew she was at her best at the front of the room, leading the way.

Alison drove herself hard and enjoyed career success. Her commitment to excellence, consistency, and compassion underpinned every task and challenge she undertook. But as she was to find out, her drive created a blind spot concerning her health and physical limits.

SELF-CARE REFLECTION #34

Are your blind spots known to you? Ask a trusted person in your inner circle for feedback on where your blind spots lie. Does the feedback you receive come as a surprise?

Alison's talent was recognized at a young age and resulted in her appointment to the role of executive director of the Sexual Assault/Rape Crisis Centre of Peel in Mississauga, Ontario, at age twenty-seven. At thirty-six, she was executive director of the Association of Ontario Midwives. By the age of forty-two, she took on the role of CEO of the Ontario Association of Naturopathic Doctors, and by forty-eight, she was named CEO of the Canadian Chiropractic Association (CCA) where she served for over ten years. Alison continues to be widely known and respected for her established brand. After stepping away from the CCA, she turned her attention to her executive coaching practice, Potential Actualized. As a leader, she can be tough, demanding even, but always fair and compassionate. Colleagues and executives attest to her ability to help them stretch, elevate, and adapt. The inner voice that spoke to her as a young girl has become a valued adviser. She calls it her intuition, and it offers clarity and the ability to see windows where others see walls.

Love, it seems, slipped past her intuition quite unexpectedly. Alison met her soulmate, Zahir Ismail, at the University of Waterloo in Ontario. Zahir was completing his PhD in the Faculty of Environmental Sciences and Alison her undergraduate degree. Their chemistry was undeniable, and they were married shortly after. Alison's deep love and admiration are evident in the way she remembers him: "Zahir was so integral to my growth as a human. He was worldly compared to what I was. There was a lot of stretching of my thinking in those first years of our marriage. He was completely intertwined into how I saw the world, how I lived, how I led." Their love story contains all of the ingredients of a Shakespearean masterpiece, reminding us that the course of true love seldom runs smoothly.

With the birth of their daughter, Alison slammed into parenthood at a full sprint. Caring for the needs of a newborn was disorienting for her. She sensed the walls of her life closing in and could not see a window for, perhaps, the first time. Lessons of unconditional, selfless love came quickly as her maternal instincts kicked in; however, so did the punishment of fatigue. She recalls the stark difference in her professional pace, pre- and post-delivery. Before her daughter's arrival, with her husband encouraging her growth, she was accountable to only her ambition. She observes, "At this stage of my life, I was not only performing. I was elevating my game." She noticed a gap that existed between her drive and that of the rest of the pack. Doubling down on effort, drawing on her deep reserves, she widened this advantage. She could operate faster than most and admits to wondering why others struggled to keep pace. Her daughter answered that question.

Maintaining her brand of high-octane performance under the physical limitations of fatigue and stress that come with parenthood tested Alison. But she stuck to her mantra: "Parenting is selfless." The first six to twelve months were chaotic. On a good night, she would piece together five hours of interrupted sleep. Alison and Zahir would try to relieve each other by coordinating schedules and prioritizing work and their daughter's needs above their personal health and lifestyle practices. "As a type-A executive and avid planner, I can't cope with chaos. We were both in survival mode." Compartmentalizing her family's needs and the demands at work, Alison dug deep to find the energy she needed to be what her world had come to rely on.

SELF-CARE REFLECTION #35
In your journal, please reflect on and answer the following:
1. What three titles or labels would best describe your life and priorities?
   To give you an idea, mine are: 1) Husband, 2) Father, and 3) Clinician.
2. List three immediate steps you can take to bring your blind spots out of the dark and align your actions with the priorities you listed above.

Her first indication that her reserves were running low and she was not at her best appeared when food became a comfort rather than fuel. Motherhood and her new eating habits changed her body entirely. Without time for exercise, it was not long before she started to feel back pain. "My modus operandi was sit and stress, driven by high levels of adrenaline and cortisol," she says. She was aware of her declining physical health and the toxic effects of chronic stress but could not break free from it. And then tragedy struck.

Shortly after purchasing their first family home, Zahir was diagnosed with a terminal illness. In the blink of an eye, Alison's life went from stressed and chaotic to unpredictably volatile.

> **❝I found myself with a three-year-old, a new mortgage, in a challenging new executive role, with my soulmate dying, and to cope, I was stress-eating.❞**

Alison was taught to believe that good things happen to good people, hard work is rewarded, and putting your nose to the grindstone pays off. Such beliefs steady young parents trying to build careers. Alison tested the truth of each of these promises. Her instincts to care for, provide for, and protect her family kicked into auto-pilot. Her brand now extended to her family. She said, "There was no doubt in my mind that I was shortening my life at some level." By pushing her daily performance well past her peak, she continued to stray further from the formula she had developed as a young executive, leaving little, if any, time for self-care. Over the subsequent months, there would be countless hospitalizations as her husband's health declined. It was a horrible time in her life. Alison's parents were a huge support, caring for her daughter whenever needed. Neighbors also jumped in to help and would come over in the middle of the night if Alison needed to rush her husband to the hospital. Leaning into her family's strong community bond and foundational faith helped her keep her head above water as her confidence to face adversity continued to grow.

> **"What I realized about myself is that, no matter what the challenge was, I can compartmentalize and overcome anything. And I really mean that because I lived it."**

At her core, she believed that there was a purpose to her life, and there was no problem that she could not solve — this included Zahir's medical condition. For the better part of five years, it was a fight every day. Pouring herself into the challenges at work, parenting a toddler, and nurturing her ill husband, Alison gave all she had to give.

In the end, it was not enough. Zahir could not be saved and passed away at the age of fifty-two. Alison was thirty-nine and now a single mom.

On her husband's death, Alison felt utterly abandoned. "Any construct I had of faith, of believing good things happen to good people, was blown up. Grief brings you to ground zero." For a time after his passing, she even struggled to find tolerance for the language of recovery. "I heard the language used to help people in grief, encouraging me to move on, and it made me angry. Really angry. Move on? If I moved on, I left behind." With each day, the conflict and weight of her burden grew, and her intuition fell silent.

Staying put would ensure the torture of her grief continued. Moving on presented the risk of leaving his memory behind and letting go of the life she had come to know and love. Grief and stress presented an onerous intersection. It left her senses dull, except for the feeling of immense pressure on her heart. Described as anvil on her chest, this pressure intensified, and her grief deepened as she struggled to find relief. She described the grief like an explosion that literally flattened the life she knew and all the beliefs and experiences that had played a role in creating it.

For five years, Alison walked in this void, her interactions shallow and without meaning. She says, "I was still functioning. No one knew what a terrible place I was in. I was still a mom and an executive, trying to be everything to everyone else with literally nothing alive on the inside. Nothing." Her old construct of family and faith attempted to provide support and encouragement. Grief counseling was helpful in a group setting, but Alison quickly found herself trying to pick up the rest of the room. This process was not going to be her process. She did not have the energy to fight her instincts to be the strong one. Her path would have to be a different one. Deep down, she knew that she could not be convinced to heal from the outside. If Alison was to move forward, she needed to integrate new ways of looking at her life.

This realization sparked her recovery and gave volume to her intuition. If she listened closely enough, she could hear her voice was telling her, "You can handle this." Louder by the day, its call for action somehow seemed less offensive as time passed. Arriving at a place where she could finally welcome the experience of her husband's death into her awareness, she could hear her husband saying, "Your life did not end. You were always supposed to go out and leave a mark on the world, so go do it." On reflection, she suspects her intuition never stopped calling for her attention; the grief simply smothered it. Mustering the courage to listen was a defining moment in her life.

The strength required to move forward was drawn from her immigration experience as a young girl. Her family arrived in Canada from Mombasa, Kenya, on a Friday. School started in Scarborough, Ontario, on the following Tuesday. She was welcomed in the playground by every derogatory name in the book. It was both shocking and hurtful. Alison recalls, "In Mombasa, racism is not something I had personally experienced. We grew up white, Black, Chinese, Indian, all side-by-side. Our parents were merciless on acceptance. If you went to someone else's house, you practiced their rituals with respect and did not ask any questions. And when you came home with a friend, the same was reciprocated. There was never a notion of someone being different because of the color of their skin. I knew I was brown. I didn't know that I was perceived as less than."

The determination to be seen as an equal and fight back against a force unfairly skewed had helped her find a voice as a new immigrant to Canada. Calling on this strength once again would also help her defeat grief.

Studying traditional Buddhist writing and meditation also helped. Alison read Deepak Chopra and Pema Chodron's work, and found comfort in the belief that you never own another soul. She realized that she could love deeply but needed to love in detachment. "A part of me died when *my husband* passed away." By releasing her attachment to the love they shared, the pace of her recovery hastened. "It would have killed me if I didn't choose to move through my grief and restore my health. It was a choice I consciously needed to make. I chose to live."

Having lived the better part of her adult life in crisis, caring for the ones most dear to her, she was deprived of the opportunity to develop self-care skills along the way. Wired to help others first, Alison's instincts trumped her personal needs. Prioritizing her health, thus, felt both unfamiliar and uncomfortable. Every day triggered a daily reconsideration of the choice to put her needs first. It would have been much easier to go back to her old habits. Grief wanted her attention back.

SELF-CARE REFLECTION #36

Adversity is a part of the human experience. There is no avoiding it. As you continue reading Alison's story, you will discover how she learned to accept her grief and regain control of her life. Her journey reminds us of the conscious choice we have when we get knocked down. Do you get up and embrace the opportunity to grow or do you stay down? I encourage you to have the courage to ask for help if you find yourself in a dark space. In your journal, list three people you could call on in a crisis, and then let them know they are on your "in-case-of-an-emergency" call list.

ALISON'S FORMULA FOR HEALTH, STRENGTH & HOPE

To restore health, Alison began by repairing her sleep ritual. She had to normalize her sleep patterns and activate the rejuvenating powers of recovery discussed in Wellness Ritual #1: Prioritize Sleep, Rest, and Recovery before making any other adjustments to her lifestyle. The target was seven to nine hours of sleep a night, but after only four to five hours for the better part of the last decade, her healthcare team set a goal of six hours a night to start. When this pattern was established, they moved the bar to seven. At seven, she had the reserves to begin focusing on nutrition and exercise.

Raised in a South Asian family, mealtime was always an important shared experience. Meals were prepared fresh. Nothing was processed, and takeout was unknown. The kitchen was the place to be in her home. A focus on nutrition was as much about healthy eating as it was about stress reduction, cultural expression, building community, and conveying love. Returning a keen eye to her nutritional choices had the desired effect on her weight, but it also strengthened her recovery as she took another step toward community and away from the isolation of her grief. With a genuine interest and enjoyment in cooking and the knowledge of how to properly fuel her body, her nutritional rituals were now lifting her up, not slowing her down.

As her energy reserves continued to replenish, Alison found joy in life again. In celebration, she began planning a trip for her upcoming fiftieth birthday. However, once again, her life would not follow a standard script. Instead of taking the trip she had planned, she spent her birthday coaching her sixteen-year-old pregnant daughter through labor and delivery. The teen pregnancy was an unexpected curveball that opened the door of chaos once again. Regardless, her grandson was welcomed into their loving family, and she threw out any idea of her fifties holding a predictable path. Alison's commitment to her health would be tested again, this time by the needs of a grandchild and her teenage daughter.

She said, "I keep praying for a little normalcy. Boring and predictable for even two weeks would be really nice." From the outside looking in, the benchmarks of life seem scrambled and out of sequence for Alison. When asked whether she saw her life that way, she said she sees life playing out as a series of waves: "For some, waves come crashing in, more powerful and closer together than desired or expected. For others, they play out as calm, gentle ripples. I haven't figured out why the journey is so different for everyone, but I do still sometimes hold onto resentment on the disparity." She keeps this resentment in check and is able to express gratitude for her journey through the practice of meditation.

Meditation anchors her formula. She now wakes between 6 or 6:30 a.m. and practices the twenty-twenty-twenty morning routine developed by leadership expert Robin Sharma. Every day starts with twenty minutes of movement, twenty minutes of reflection, and twenty minutes of learning. This practice has brought structure to Alison's life. It provides an opportunity to feed her soul and nurture her mind and body at the beginning of every day. By prioritizing her personal well-being, she became a more resilient leader, mother, and grandmother.

SELF-CARE REFLECTION #37

A healthy morning routine can set the tone for your entire day. How do you spend the first thirty minutes of your day? Is your first action directed toward self-care or serving the needs of others?

It took time for Alison to learn how destructive her autopilot default was, but she got there. With chronic back pain and three bouts of pneumonia following her grandson's birth, she briefly caught a glimpse of the despair she had known all too well during her years of mourning. Sensing her struggle, a good friend offered the following advice: "Alison, the only thing that has changed is that you are not listening again." Good friends have a way of cutting through the smoke. This was the same friend who, on returning home from the cemetery after Alison buried her husband, told her she would need to choose whether she wanted to live or die. The truth struck a chord and Alison flipped a switch, bringing her executive A-game to her health. By making this decision, she took firm control of her script.

The uncertainty of what lies around the next corner yields zero power over her. Her recovery taught her how to master uncertainty. "I am fearless. I don't fear death. I don't fear conflict. I don't fear the unknown. I don't fear any of it." She has reconciled with who she is and what she stands for. Alison found her place in the world and honors her husband's memory by living her truth and stepping into courage every day.

She now holds tremendous respect for her body. It carried her through her grief with tremendous patience, for which she is extremely grateful. She recognizes that this journey came at a cost, and she must now integrate all 7 Wellness Rituals if she is to live a full life and reach her potential. The legacy she strives for is to change the world one experience at a time. In everything she does, she asks what she can bring to the table to elevate the experience. "For me, tiny changes are the most momentous kind of change we can make because tiny changes are more accepted by others, and incremental changes on that scale become contagious."

Former CCA Board Chair, Dr. Debbie Wright, shared, "Working with Alison has been akin to having a front row seat in a Master Class on change management. Her bold and courageous style of leadership has been an inspiration to me and to all that have had a chance to serve alongside her."

DR. ROBYNE HANLEY-DAFOE

Author, Psychology and Education Instructor, Stress Resiliency Expert

At sixteen years old, Robyne found herself drowning in icy water in the dead of winter. Her car had crashed off a rural road into the Otonabee River. After escaping through the driver's window into total darkness, it took a moment for her to figure out which way was up. With a sudden searing pain striking the side of Robyne's face, she realized she had finally reached the surface but was trapped under the ice. Weighed down by her winter coat and boots, searching desperately for open water and air, she reflected on her mother's words: "Robyne, you can do hard things."

The current had pushed her downstream from where her car plunged through the ice. She went with the current, kicking her legs, and then the ice sheet gave way to open water. Gasping for air, she struggled to hold onto the edge of the breaking ice. Robyne recounted that during this season of her life, she felt anger toward the professionals who predicted she would not survive her teenage years — they believed she was too far gone. She feared that they might be right despite her family's best efforts to get her help. The idea that her death would separate her from her mother was agonizing. If freezing to death was the end, so be it, though knowing how her parents would suffer kept her in the fight of her life.

Thankfully, Robyne's miracle was already in motion. A thirty-year-old man heading home from his evening shift happened to see her car tracks veer off the road and stopped his truck to look for anyone who might need help. Making an "X" with lumber in the back of his pickup, he headed out onto the ice with a chain in hand, hearing it crack under his feet. He saw Robyne, got down on his belly, and slowly crawled toward her. She was able to grab the chain and he pulled her to safety. Her hero would later receive the Governor General's Award for the bravery he exhibited on this night.

Robyne holds a special place in her heart for her hero but credits her mom for her survival. "I survived because of my mother's faith in me and her faith in the world. She told me my whole life that I could do hard things. Even in the most difficult circumstances, she would say, 'I don't know how to fix this, but you don't have to walk it alone.' She has always been in my corner."

EARLY TRIALS AND AFFLICTIONS

Robyne's family had moved from a larger city to a rural area to give her a fresh start. By this time, she had already dropped out of school, been hospitalized for mental health treatment, and was struggling with aggressive addictions and self-harm behavior.

Robyne got clean before her seventeenth birthday, but an eating disorder manifested as she tried to regain control of her life. "When you start losing weight and appear fit, society rewards you. People tell you you look great and that you look healthy. I was all of that, but I was still in a very dark season, which most people didn't realize." The eating disorder stemmed from her unresolved trauma response. With determination, love from her family, and the skilled clinical guidance of a team of health professionals, Robyne eventually repaired the fractured relationship she had with herself and got her life back on track.

She spoke to me about what it meant to be a mother for the first time: "The birth of our first son helped me get on the other side of my issues in a very significant way. I realized it's not about me anymore — there's somebody else counting on me, and that was that. I got back into that place of perspective-taking and being able to live within my values. I did the work so I could make sure that I was able and ready to look after our children."

TRANSFORMED AND TRANSFORMATIVE

Now forty-two, Robyne is focused on wellness by helping people cope with stress and change, improve their personal well-being, and be strong and adaptable. At the time of our first interview, her book, *Calm Within the Storm: A Pathway to Everyday Resiliency*, was entering its third printing. Robyne is passionate about her work and offers kind, research-informed, and achievable personal development practices for everyday resiliency. She has an extraordinary sensitivity to emotion and is described as tender and fiercely loyal.

Woven into Robyne's formula are techniques to help her manage her Attention Deficit Hyperactive Disorder (ADHD). "I was much older in my life when I was diagnosed and treated for my ADHD, and of course, when you look back, it's easy to see how it contributed to a number of my issues." Her ADHD holds an element of distractibility, but it has more to do with impulsive thinking, time blindness, and relentlessness. She can stay on task but will sometimes miss things because of her ability to become hyper-focused. "Having schedules, routines, checkpoints, and a disciplined self-care routine help me organize my thinking and find adaptive ways of working with my ADHD."

---

66 I'm not worried about every single night. I think about my sleep and energy in seventy-two-hour windows."

Robyne's sweet spot to enter the day is 6 a.m., and days where this is not the case are rare. This ritual stands independent of the day of the week, holidays, or birthdays and appears to be locked in 365 days a year. Waking any earlier leaves her feeling sluggish and any later cuts into her morning self-care routine.

By framing her rest and recovery behavior in three-day windows and playing to averages, Robyne keeps a keen eye on her sleep. She listens to her body and builds buffer zones for each rule she sets, placing a high value on knowing the limits of her physiology and the flexibility of her formula. "I'm not worried about every single night. I think about my sleep and energy in seventy-two-hour windows."

When it comes to bedtime, she operates within a wider margin. Most nights, Robyne aims to have her head on the pillow by 10 p.m., but this is not a hard target, unlike her wake-up time. "One of the things I often talk about in my research is the importance of flexibility. When we subscribe to rigid practices, like 'I have to be in bed every night by 10 p.m. if I'm going to get up at six and still get eight hours of sleep,' we can create some unnecessary anxiety when things don't go as planned." If she gets pulled off track, she is cognizant of getting to bed earlier the next night or the night after that. Managing sleep in three-day chunks keeps her from forcing rest, which can boost her stress. It also holds her accountable to her desired eight hours a night average. Through trial and error, she has found forecasting beyond three days unproductive and unrealistic.

Robyne brings mindfulness to rest and recovery by taking deliberate steps to quiet her mental chatter as she enters the final few hours of a day. "We pick up energy, thoughts, and emotions all day. It is not realistic to expect to turn these off and enjoy a restful sleep on demand. One of the goals that I have before I go to bed is to find a way to wind down and hold peace. I need to find a sense of stillness before I sleep." It is in this state that Robyne appears to have discovered a way to elevate her recuperative powers.

Sometime before dinner, she begins her unwinding ritual by emptying her short-term memory and placing tomorrow's to-do list on post-it notes. With these priorities accounted for, they lose their authority and no longer distract her thinking or spark rumination. She will then deliberately begin to redirect her thoughts toward recovery. The weight of a busy day or anticipation of a future big event immediately feels lighter by shifting her mental focus. This process grounds her.

> 66 **You can't do this decompression mind work in the last ten minutes of a day... it's not like I'm meditating or isolating, disconnected from the world in a quiet darkroom. It's literally just knowing that I need to start winding down to balance the pace that I push at each day."**

As Robyne prepares for bed, she will limit her screen time, ensure the temperature in their bedroom is cool, and complete a meditation. She enjoys listening to sleep-cast stories on the Headspace App with a daily goal of drifting off to sleep with peace in her head and heart. "Before bed, I look to land in a place of positive energy, find a sense of calm and a knowing that, yes, there's still work to be done, but mental loose ends are tied up, and everything is in its place." There is a sense of mental, physical, emotional, and spiritual order in this state for her.

ROBYNE'S "TELLS"

If Robyne finds herself stuck in a "go" mindset and cannot find quietude, it is usually because she has fallen into a feeling of scarcity. She knows that holding this position on her stress curve invites trouble. "If I cross that threshold where stress is no longer serving me, and it starts to pool up in my nervous system, I have 'tells.'" Becoming proficient at recognizing these helps her course-correct. She describes this slide as a *cognitive confusion*. At first, her time on task increases, she gets a little clumsy and is more indecisive. She may start mixing up her children's names, notice a hint of uncertainty, or experience a falloff in her energy at top-speed in the early stages of this slide. "Physically, emotionally, and energetically, I notice a low but recognizable erosion if I push past this point."

> " I go over the basics in my mind, starting with what I'm grateful for, and use gratitude reflections as a way to knock myself out of a toxic hustle mode."

Another "tell" is when her inner voice starts complaining and calling out for "more" — more time, more energy, and more effort. Experience has taught her the best way to silence this voice and move out of a scarcity mindset is not to push harder or extend a day. Instead, she must move toward a "sufficiency mindset" through gratitude. From here, she taps into a rich energy and feels fulfillment, safety, and love. "I go over the basics in my mind, starting with what I'm grateful for, and use gratitude reflections as a way to knock myself out of a toxic hustle mode."

Robyne's family is her gratitude anchor.

FAMILY HUDDLES

Family huddles help Robyne and her husband stay present throughout their teens' busy lives. Mornings seem to offer the most impactful exchanges. Huddles are kept short and do not spill over into long lectures. Together they share stressors, lean on each other for help, and align next steps. Robyne will ask her husband and kids who needs her on her A-game today? The kids might express some nervousness about an upcoming try-out or exam, allowing the family to rally support in their direction. "The key message is that they have a Home Team, and the Home Team is always on their side. I find that two or three times a week, our huddles create a family culture that makes it so we can have difficult conversations if needed." When it comes to resiliency, they encourage their children not to waste a mistake and to embrace stumbles as an opportunity to discover a blind spot. Having a mom as a resiliency expert has its perks.

The family huddles also present Robyne with an opportunity to ask for help. "Heading into a demanding stretch, I'll let my family know that I'm probably going to be operating at about 20% on the home front, so that means 80% of what I usually do is going to have to get picked up elsewhere, or we need to find a workaround. Teenagers understand this concept, and my husband is brilliant at stepping up."

SELF-CARE REFLECTION #38

As you read about Robyne's "tells," are you thinking about your own "tells" — those signals you get from your body that something is off, that something is not quite right. In Robyne's case, she knows she has to shift to a sufficiency mindset and tap into sources of safety and love when her tells appear. What is your version of Robyne's "sufficiency mindset"? Can you grow that mindset? Make notes in your journal.

ROBYNE'S FORMULA FOR HEALTH, STRENGTH & HOPE

GET MOVING FIRST THING

Robyne works with people experiencing the worst seasons of their lives. To bring the best version of herself into each day and protect herself from the stress of her work, she pre-loads her self-care and looks to win her morning. "I'm able to show up and be of service to others, run my company, still do my research and my teaching because I have dialed in a morning routine of self-care that I practice before opening myself up to the world."

Regardless of the weather, once up, she is out the door with the family dog for a thirty-minute walk in nature. This time in nature, or, as Robyne calls it, her dose of "vitamin N," is how she starts every day. Returning to the house, she enjoys a cup of coffee and then moves to thirty minutes of more vigorous exercise. Some days, this is a cardio HIIT; other days, it's resistance training or a gentle yoga practice.

"I have had a very fractured relationship with food and exercise, and I'm now in a place where I move and eat to feel well. I tried to 'hate myself healthy,' and that didn't work. I tried to punish myself into perfection, and that didn't go very well either. So for me, I exercise in the morning because it breaks me through the fog. It breaks that autopilot-sleepwalking feeling and really helps me get in tune with my body.

> **" Prioritizing this time alone for reflection and exercise keeps me at my best. It is not selfish — it is science."**

Robyne also integrates movement with short stretch breaks, a few minutes of jumping rope, or a couple of reps of light resistance training with exercise bands periodically throughout her day. "I'm a big advocate of really working with my energy, so if I've been on Zoom calls, I'll find different ways to move and get my heart rate up." She is not breaking into a sweat here, just changing her physical pace and posture to boost her energy instead of reaching for an afternoon coffee. Her proactive efforts to sustain high energy levels throughout the day with these simple techniques have significantly improved her productivity.

She also has a team of clinicians that she leans on to keep her body in peak shape. "If I have a big deadline or I know I'm coming into a busy period, I'll preemptively go ahead and book appointments with my chiropractor and massage therapist, knowing that my future self will thank me." Robyne has connected the importance of her movement quality with her physical performance.

SELF-CARE REFLECTION #39

Robyne prioritizes movement early in the day to wake up her mind and body and to get energy flowing. Many mentors do the same. Consider carving time out every morning for ten to fifteen minutes of movement before checking your inbox. Paying yourself first with this physical investment will boost your mental fitness.

NUTRITION AND RESILIENCY

When it comes to nutrition, she brings mindfulness to healthy eating and speaks passionately about intuitive eating and breaking through the challenges of diet culture. Nothing is off-limits. "I do not want our children falling into the diet culture practices of good versus bad or clean versus not clean. Food is food, and we encourage the importance of listening to the needs of our body." Careful not to fall into a three-meal crescendo eating pattern of light, light, and then heavy, she avoids heavy calorie loads toward the end of the day.

Given her personal experiences and professional expertise, Robyne brings a unique perspective to the impact diet has on resiliency. "It is essential to make nutritional choices that honor our relationship with our bodies, especially for women. Diet culture has just ravaged our confidence with food and established a set of rules and pressure points that block many from developing a good relationship with food. We are intellectual beings, but we're also emotional beings that possess an intuitive knowledge of what our bodies need. If we only think about trying to make our bodies smaller so they take up less space, that's not going to bring enrichment or a sense of peace into our lives." She encourages her clients to be mindful of who they follow on social media; keep healthy, realistic role models close, and disregard the rest. "We will never be satisfied with external measures; finding that place of inner attunement instead of outer attainment is vitally important."

FAITH AND RESILIENCY

Robyne's inner attunement is derived from her faith. She explained, "It always comes back to living within my values. The greatest gift my mother gave me was my faith to trust." As a scholar studying resiliency, defining the role of faith, spirituality, and religion can be a challenge. Her research shows that when people are in the darkest hours of the worst of experiences, faith provides hope that improves how humans cope during difficult times. "Trusting in the goodness of the world makes a real difference in our resiliency. For me, this goodness is God."

Standing firmly rooted in her values helps Robyne make difficult decisions with confidence. She places a high value on her social support network of family and close friends but will also regularly check in with mental health professionals for a mental tune-up to keep her A-game in play. "I often let folks know that at least once a year, it is a good idea to talk to someone outside of your inner circle and speak to a professional. Things that are tucked away have a tendency of finding their way to the surface. Healthy people that are living the good life demonstrate a consistent practice of radical honesty with a trusted person." Seeking professional help to identify undesirable patterns of behavior and implementing intentional actions to address them at an early stage is one of her resiliency secrets.

PLAY AND RESILIENCY

Unstructured play is another. "Lighthearted play brings merriment to our lives that keeps us in a place of active discovery and inquiry, which is essential to mental health." She looks for opportunities to break away from the calendar or clock to be curious and wonder or sometimes just to be bored. When Robyne plays with purpose, she feels free from obligation and experiences a sense of spaciousness that fuels her creativity and opens her mind to discovery.

Even during heavy lifting, integrating play helps her juggle her many responsibilities and keeps her mind on task and her attitude positive. Her playfulness is instantly recognizable in her smile, the stories she shares, and even in how she actively listens. Robyne will intentionally set her mood heading into a task, using external cues and routines. "I use things like music, color, movement, even different smells to stimulate my senses and get integrated into my day." By having smaller check-in points and mindful moments of renewal built into her day, she uses play to elevate her performance.

A FINAL BIT OF ADVICE

"One of the big misconceptions in our culture is that we allow ourselves to get depleted before we practice self-care. My message and my research are that we can pre-load self-care. We don't have to wait until we're burned out or exhausted to start looking after ourselves. If we go in game-ready, use that energy throughout the day, and then do more passive recovery in the evening that doesn't take a lot of energy or effort, we can perform with consistency and avoid a lot of trouble."

Life is unpredictable and, at our darkest moments, we can feel trapped under ice and desperate to find open water. Having the discipline to hold onto her faith, come what may, and trust that things are going to be alright is how Robyne stays game-ready.

No one needs to tell you that **you are loved no matter what**; you just know it. Possessing a high level of mental fitness feels much the same way.

WELLNESS RITUAL #6

NURTURE MENTAL FITNESS

7 WELLNESS RITUALS
FOR HEALTH, STRENGTH & HOPE

WELLNESS RITUAL #6: THE SCIENCE

The wave of mental illness accompanying the pandemic is alarming. Sadly, high levels of stress and anxiety have become the norm for many people. When left untreated, mental illness can cause severe emotional, behavioral, and physical health problems. Evidence shows that chronic stress levels can shrink parts of the brain that handle higher-order tasks while increasing activity in primitive parts of the brain focused on survival, making us even more receptive to stress. Techniques to develop your mental fitness are essential to protecting and supporting your mental health in today's society.

*M*ental fitness is a state of emotional, psychological, and social well-being. To have it is to live with your A-game accessible on demand. The experience is much like the feeling of unconditional love. Such love, whether from a partner, parent, sibling, friend, or dog, provides an emotional safety net that inspires confidence, sets a purpose, and offers great comfort.

No one needs to tell you that you are loved no matter what; you just know it. Possessing a high level of mental fitness feels much the same way. It too provides confidence and inspires action, but it also gives you the power to push through a challenge and have the presence of mind to recognize when it is time to pull back into recovery. It is what helps Dr. Robyne Hanley-Dafoe know in her heart that she can do hard things.

OUR PRE-PANDEMIC PACE

Pre-COVID-19, by the time Canadians reached age forty, one in two had experienced a mental illness.[1] Contributing to our alarming levels of daily stress was the extension of our workweek. In the early 2000s, the forty-hour Monday to Friday gig was on its way out. By the 2010s, a sixty-hour workweek, once a reliable, well-worn path to career advancement, appeared light, as a trend recognized as "extreme work" emerged. Individuals worked harder, faster, and longer to keep a shot at the middle class within reach while businesses prioritized efficiency and the bottom line.

A 2006 study by the *Harvard Business Review* revealed that 62% of high-earning individuals worked more than fifty hours a week, 35% worked more than sixty hours a week, and 10% more than eighty hours a week.[2] At the time, there wasn't much discussion about the sustainability of this pace or the preservation of mental fitness. When making kids' lunches, overseeing homework, driving to and from extracurricular activities, completing household chores, caring for elder parents, and grinding out a commute to and from work get packed into the margins of a sixty-hour workweek, there isn't much time for anything else besides sleep. This script had people leaving their homes by 6 a.m. and returning by 8 p.m., Monday to Friday, with additional work often bleeding into the evenings and weekends. Is it any wonder that our mental health suffered?

As competition intensified, vacations and dedicated downtime also started to shrink. Among the extreme-job crowd, 42% averaged ten or fewer vacation days per year.[2] Work pressure to perform at peak was seen across the economy as people pushed their limits to stay in the fast lane. The day-to-day survival for many was like an episode from the hit Netflix series *Squid Game*, where individuals risk their lives playing a series of deadly games in hopes of financial reward. Think of musical chairs with fatal consequences for the person left standing.

THE PANDEMIC DISRUPTION

By the time COVID-19 revealed itself, many of us were already living with toxic levels of chronic stress; the additional burden of the pandemic added a breaking point accelerant. In March 2022, the World Health Organization warned that COVID-19 had triggered a 25% increase in anxiety and depression worldwide.[3] Statistics Canada released a survey in June 2022 that showed 95% of healthcare workers felt that the pandemic had negatively impacted their mental health and added considerable stress to their work-life balance.[4] One in four nurses surveyed said they planned to quit within the next three years.[4]

Experts agree that a mental illness tsunami fueled by the pandemic's ripple effect on our pre-pandemic, fragile mental state has set the stage for a health crisis unlike anything we have ever seen.

From the ashes of extreme work, two new trends have started to emerge — "The Great Resignation" and "Ergophobia." By 2021, record numbers of employees had quit their jobs. Workers began retiring in greater numbers, reevaluating their work-life balance, and switching industries.[5] Heading into the fall of 2022, the preference to work from home had become entrenched. Ergophobia, a morbid fear or hatred of work, leading to panic attacks, burnout, and depression disorders, made returning to the office even more difficult for some.[6]

Businesses that flourished during the pandemic operated on thin ice as essential staff pushed to keep up with demand and inevitably burnt out. Manufacturers of masks, hand sanitizer, and cleaning wipes tried but couldn't. When the run on toilet paper and baby formula hit, the vulnerability of the supply chain that we have all come to rely on was exposed, and our collective stress grew.

Burnout hit frontline workers, parents, caregivers, and organizational leaders particularly hard, with working women shouldering the brunt of the load. A 2021 *Women in the Workplace* report published by McKinsey and Company highlighted that one in three women were considering leaving the workforce, switching jobs, or cutting work hours as care obligations fell disproportionately to their watch.[7]

An article published in *The Globe and Mail* in June 2022, titled "Taking a 'momcation' — a holiday without my husband and kids saved my sanity," revealed that working mothers were on the verge of collapse.[8] Carrying the load of the day-to-day decision-making and the responsibility for their family's mental and physical health left nearly half of the mothers surveyed in a national poll at their breaking point by April 2022.[9] Three in five mothers wished they could make their mental health more of a priority but were unable to find time for self-care.[9] Mothers held the line, but now they need relief.

Businesses of all sizes attempted to adapt, but managers and HR staff were embattled by frustration, disagreement, and confusion surrounding the vaccination statuses of their employees and the criteria for a "return-to-normal," resulting in staffing shortages and declining customer service. The acute focus on delivering essential products and services meant that opportunities for specialized training and professional development, mentorship, and client and colleague interactions were no longer part of the work experience. The threat to employee engagement and a healthy workplace hidden in sustained work without reward was now out in the open.

Outside of the workplace, the mental health of seniors also suffered. Isolation from family and friends and disruption in daily routines had unintended, harmful consequences in the older adult population despite its benefit of slowing viral transmission.[10] Anxiety, anger, and emotional instability accompany loneliness. Isolation calls on the sympathetic nervous system and promotes hypertension, inflammation, and elevated stress hormone levels, which, over the long term, can be dangerous. While younger generations reported higher rates of anxiety and depression during the pandemic than older adults, some seniors felt their lives were expendable.[11]

MILLENNIALS ARE LEADING THE CHARGE FOR CHANGE

Recognizing the vital importance of mental health and leading the charge for change are Millennials. Born between 1981 and 1996, Millennials are beginning to exert their influence on workplace cultures and hiring practices. They want a flexible work environment that provides authentic feedback and positive encouragement. They want to feel connected to their purpose at work and be recognized for their efforts. Five o'clock TGIT — Thank Goodness It's Thursday — parties, whether in-person or virtual, hold greater appeal and retention power than the allure of a bigger wage or corner office. They value their mental health and possess a self-awareness that previous generations have taken much longer to develop.

Thanks to this Millennial nudge and the pandemic-induced timeout, we appear to have landed at a spot where work and what people are willing to sacrifice to make a living are changing. People have had enough and are emerging from their time in the corner wanting to work smarter — not longer or harder. Companies are responding with increased wages, corporate wellness programs, and benefit packages that include paid time off, childcare support, flex hours, and health spending accounts, understanding that as job satisfaction decreases, stress and turnover skyrocket.

The disruption caused by the pandemic has sparked a health awakening, which is likely one of the trends that triggered your interest in this book. There is a transformational shift occurring that is changing how we live and work and the priority we place on our health and well-being. For those inclined to look for the silver lining of the last two years, this may be it. If you listen closely enough to your inner voice, you will hear it call for a healthier experience. Many patients tell me this voice is no longer a whisper.

The mentors' stories show us that, to realize our potential, we must learn how to leverage our stress response, respect our biological limits, and embrace adversity. To experience your full biological potential requires a solid mental game. Welcome to Wellness Ritual #6: Nurture Your Mental Fitness, where we will explore how mental fitness leads to increased cognitive function and capacity, an improved mood, and a boost in positive emotions, confidence, concentration, and memory. By incorporating this ritual into your formula, your resiliency will expand, your energy reserve will begin to replenish, and you will discover a healthier relationship with yourself and, subsequently, with others.

IF YOU ARE A HEADACHE SUFFERER...

Just because headaches are common does not make them normal. If your current strategy to combat a stress-induced tension headache is to keep your head down, throw back another cup of coffee with a few analgesics, and grind through the day, your headaches will likely continue. This remedy may even make your headaches worse. When dehydrated, your brain and other soft tissues shrink. Think of a shriveled-up grape left in the bottom of the fruit basket for too long. Dehydration, even at mild levels, can cause headaches.[14] Reaching for an over-the-counter pain reliever, like acetaminophen, aspirin, or ibuprofen, can help relieve a headache. However, overuse of these medications or failing to follow the instructions on the bottle can actually increase your headaches, triggering what are called "rebound headaches."[15] Daily caffeine loads from coffee, soda, and pain relievers can accelerate both dehydration and medication overuse headaches.[15] As a side note, the best approach to alleviating tension headaches is to keep them from happening in the first place. Move, drink water, stretch, get enough sleep, learn how to maintain a neutral spine, practice healthy ergonomics, and clean up your diet, and your body will turn off the check engine headache light.

The previous five Wellness Rituals are dedicated to achieving peak physical health and fitness. This one is all about the health of the mind, and it should come as no surprise that its required upkeep and maintenance are just as essential. Learning how to recognize your stressors and acknowledge the signs and symptoms of stress is where this journey must begin.

DO A MENTAL STATUS CHECK

Think about the last time you held a sustained peak effort. Were you aware of when you reached your peak, or did you blow right past it? When at your peak, how did you feel? Were you energized or exhausted? Did you feel confidence or doubt? As the event passed or you had a minute to finally catch your breath, how did your symptoms change?

THE PERKS OF STRESS

We all have a baseline operating level that is a function of our age, genetics, and the quality of our practice of the Wellness Rituals discussed in this book. When faced with a challenge, our body's ability to mobilize its resources and elevate its performance from this baseline to our best effort is extraordinary. This is a normal response and no more of a threat to our health than breathing. Stress is a part of life. It is necessary and, in healthy doses, can be very positive.

Research has shown that how we view our stress matters. Individuals who see stress as debilitating tend to either over- or under-react when feeling pressure. In contrast, those with a "stress-is-enhancing" mindset tend to demonstrate greater control over their response to it. This positive shift in perspective leads to a lighter physiological burden and greater capacity for stress, thanks to a more moderate cortisol release.[12] The "stress-is-enhancing" group also tend to be more willing to seek out and receive feedback during times of stress.[12] Perspective, feedback, and a hopeful outlook are all significant players when it comes to developing mental fitness.

While heightened stress can feel overwhelming, moderate levels can enhance our motivation and help us push to a deadline with greater focus and attention. The stress that accompanies our life experiences helps us develop problem-solving skills and gain confidence in our ability to deliver. From these experiences, our resiliency begins to take shape. Times of struggle and adversity are often the experiences we feel most proud of and hold the greatest meaning in our lives. *The problem isn't stress — it is our unrelenting, chronic exposure to it.*

SYMPTOMS OF STRESS TO WATCH OUT FOR:

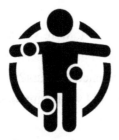 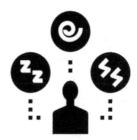

PHYSICAL	EMOTIONAL
LOWER LIBIDO	AVOIDANCE OF OTHERS
DIZZINESS OR LIGHTHEADEDNESS	STRESS EATING
DIGESTIVE TROUBLE	LONELINESS
HIGH BLOOD PRESSURE	LOW SELF-ESTEEM
HEADACHE	IRRITABILITY AND MOOD SWINGS
FATIGUE AND TROUBLE SLEEPING	ANXIETY AND DEPRESSION
BACK, SHOULDER OR NECK PAIN	FEELING OVERWHELMED
MUSCLE TENSION OR JAW CLENCHING	DIFFICULTY QUIETING MIND OR RELAXING

COMMON SYMPTOMS OF STRESS

The body is brilliant at letting us know it is running on fumes. We are just not very good at listening to it. If you are feeling worn thin, here is a list of common physical symptoms of stress to keep an eye on. Acknowledging these early warning signs is not a sign of weakness. Greater self-awareness provides an off-ramp and the opportunity to course-correct, recover, and prepare for a subsequent push while avoiding the toxicity of chronic stress exposure.

The well-established relationship between stress and disease was not always recognized. It was Dr. Hans Selye (1907–1982), a pioneering Hungarian-Canadian endocrinologist, who first linked stress to disease.13 Considered the "father of stress research," Dr. Selye's work remains the basis of all modern discussions of biological stress. In the field of stress resiliency, he is a legend.

When signs and symptoms of stress start to show up in your life on the regular, it is your body's way of calling attention to your pace and load. Think of it as your "check engine" warning light. Ignoring the light will undoubtedly land you in the mechanic's shop with a bigger problem and more expensive repairs. Dr. Selye defined this recklessness and our body's response to chronic stress as "that which accelerates the rate of aging through wear and tear of daily living." He made a point of highlighting the influence daily choices have over our rate of decline.

WHAT STRESSES YOU OUT?

Knowing your stressors will help you understand how, when, and why you respond to stress the way you do and what is fueling the familiar symptoms listed above. Flying off the handle when someone cuts you off on the highway seems like a wasteful use of energy in the face of all the other stressors currently fighting for our attention. Frustrating? Yes. Inconsiderate? Sure. But is it worth the rage? No. Acknowledging the frustration and choosing not to react is powerful. Maybe the other driver was rushing home to a sick kid, or maybe he is just a jerk. Regardless, you have zero control over his behavior, and his influence on your life is insignificant. Investing your emotional energy and thoughts wisely, even selfishly, saves your energy for a greater purpose. This practice creates a buffer from distractions and annoyances and allows you to clearly identify challenges worth investing in. Choosing not to respond is rewarded down the road as you discover additional fuel in the tank when you do decide to jump in and engage.

This skill takes time to develop. Until you are capable of pausing long enough to make a conscious choice to respond or not in real-time, you may be well into a full offensive attack before you even realize you have been triggered. This biological phenomenon is called your stress response, and evolution has favored its speed and scope. Buckle up. It is a fast ride.

THE STRESS RESPONSE: FIGHT OR FLIGHT

A "giddy-up-and-go" event that triggers an emotional response releases a biological storm that lifts your performance from baseline to a level otherwise inaccessible. This kind of stimulus opens the door to an awesome cascade of biochemical reactions, some of which occur in fractions of a second. Neurotransmitters are activated, hormones are released, and nutrients are metabolized in a coordinated sequence that rivals the end-of-day firework show at Disney's Magic Kingdom. Some body systems (e.g., the cardiovascular system) accelerate their function, and others (e.g., the gastrointestinal system) slow down their operation in a top-down call to shunt all resources to the task at hand. This action prepares our body for a physical response regardless of the nature of the challenge.

Evolutionarily speaking, this mechanism has served us well. However, in modern times, most human stress is psychosocial, so our need to respond physically in most cases is unnecessary. When confronted with stress — physical or emotional, real or imagined — a center in our brain called the amygdala causes the nervous system to release hormones (specifically epinephrine and norepinephrine, which are also known as adrenaline and noradrenaline), which propel us into a state of arousal.

Here is how I explained this to my fourteen-year-old son, anxious about facing his first set of in-person high school exams. After praising him for recognizing and acknowledging that he was feeling some anxiety, I told him that his body was revving up its engine to help him be at his best. Adrenaline and dopamine were flooding his brain and body with blood and oxygen to increase his energy, heighten his alertness, and narrow his focus. I encouraged him not to shy away from his nervousness but embrace it by connecting with the clear and present changes he was experiencing in his body. He described the butterflies in his stomach, the nervous anticipation, the sweaty palms, the beating heart, and the overactive GI tract and questioned exactly how any of those changes would help him with the Pythagorean theorem. Fair point. Pivoting to more friendly ground, I told him that he could unlock a superhero version of himself by embracing his excited state.

At breakfast the morning of his math exam, his fight or flight response was in full go-mode; his metabolism, heart rate, blood pressure, breathing rate, and muscle tension were all on the rise. Even at fourteen, he could tell something significant was happening. He could feel his body preparing for a physical challenge and shared that if the exam included a Tough Mudder obstacle course, he'd be ready. I suggested that he think of his elevated state as an avatar that possessed superhuman strength and a creative, fast, and intelligent mind. He had put the work in; now, he needed to learn to trust his body to perform in its excited state. He went off to school with the mindset of an exam-conquering avatar, ready for whatever the teacher decided to throw his way — including a mud pit.

In this state of arousal, your avatar stays "alert" until your mind tells you the situation requiring your best effort has passed. In the safety of retreat, your brain signals an "all clear," the amygdala chills out, and your body gradually returns to normal. Toggling between our baseline and peak performance is not like a light switch that can be flipped on and off. It takes time for our biochemistry to normalize. Suppose another stressor is introduced while you are still within your original recovery window. In that case, the second stress response builds off the first, and an even longer recovery period will be required before you return to your baseline. In this regard, stress is biochemically cumulative, and our health can really suffer from it, as I explain below.

HOW STRESS AFFECTS PERFORMANCE: THE YERKES-DODSON LAW

The Yerkes-Dodson law models the relationship between stress, arousal, and task performance.[16] It dictates that our performance increases in response to a physical or mental challenge, but only to a point. Too little or too much arousal results in poor performance. Attempting to operate in your avatar for prolonged periods without allowing for proper recovery is where our health starts to suffer. See Figure 1 below. The right side of this bell curve is the danger zone. Unfortunately, this is where many lived pre-pandemic. It is an existence that features insomnia, errors in judgment, declining concentration, mood swings, heart disease, ulcers, and anxiety. There is no back door access to the peak from the right side of the curve.

YERKES DODSON
STRESS PERFORMANCE CURVE

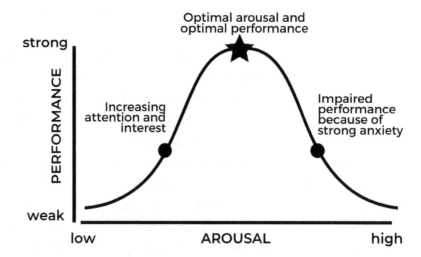

Figure 6.1: The Yerkes-Dodson Law

Source: Robert M. Yerkes and John Dodson, https://www.healthline.com/health/yerkes-dodson-law

If you attempt to make the star at the apex of your stress response curve your new baseline, it will be equivalent to driving at top speed, hoping to cover an additional 200 km when the fuel gauge reads EMPTY. When you inevitably end up at the side of the road, well short of your destination and a long walk to the closest gas station, it is hard not to see the severe error in judgment. Evidence shows that exposure to chronic stress can shrink parts of the brain that handle high-order tasks while increasing activity in primitive parts of the brain focused on survival, making us even more reactive to the fight or flight trigger.[17] In other words, by keeping your amygdala on high alert, you are willfully sprinting to your breaking point and training your mind to be on the lookout for threats.

By anticipating and planning for a recovery period, you can break free from this cycle and learn how to intentionally bring yourself toward your peak as you head into an important meeting or enter a challenging conversation. Playing on the left side of your curve offers access to your best effort and long-term health. Mentors maintain an appreciation for where they are on their curve relative to their baseline and peak at all times and will proactively schedule their recovery time to keep their peak within reach. Dr. Greg Wells and Silken Laumann do this exceptionally well.

OBSERVE AND CHALLENGE YOUR THINKING

To help craft a practical, proactive approach to mental fitness, I turned to Dr. Ian Dawe, a patient-centered practicing psychiatrist, associate professor of Psychiatry at the University of Toronto, and former Chief and Medical Director of Mental Health at Trillium Health Partners. Dr. Dawe knows the inner workings of the human mind better than most and is widely respected for his clinical passion for mental health. "Leaving people who are most in distress to manage their care can't be the way it continues to happen," Dr. Dawe says. "That is unconscionable."[18] When I asked him about mental fitness, he shared that "there is an identifiable connection between our thoughts, feelings, and performance. To be mentally fit is to understand this connection, and that discovery begins with learning how to recognize and modify negative thoughts. If you learn to control your thoughts, you can begin to alter your feelings and behaviors."

To drive this point home, he offered the following scenario: "Imagine that you hear a loud noise in another room while at home alone in the middle of the night. If your first thought is, 'There is a burglar in the house,' you are likely going to feel anxious and take action that will minimize the perceived danger, like hiding or phoning 911. However, if your first thought was, 'It is windy outside. I left the window open in the other bedroom, and the wind has likely blown a picture frame over again,' your behavior will look quite different. You might calmly get up, close the window, pick up the frame off the floor, and go back to bed."

Pausing to challenge automatic thoughts verbally can help us gain some control over our stress response and modify our behavior. Dr. Dawe suggests that when faced with a stressful situation that triggers doubt or negative thoughts, you recognize the audio track playing in your mind and ask yourself the following questions:

- What evidence do I have for this thought?
- How would someone else feel about this situation?
- Are my judgments based on how I feel rather than what I did?
- Am I setting an unrealistic or unobtainable standard?
- Am I forgetting relevant facts or over-focusing on irrelevant facts?
- Am I thinking in all or nothing terms?
- Am I overestimating how much control I have over the way things worked out?

- What if "it" happens? What would be so bad about that?
- How will things be in x months/years down the road?
- Am I overestimating how likely an event is or under-estimating what I can do to deal with the situation?

WAYS TO COPE WITH STRESS

There is no one "correct" way to cope with stress. Dr. Andy Smith walks his "stress-monster" into submission. Michael Grange hits the gym. Alison Dantas meditates and practices yoga. Jim Leech walks his dog. Regular movement increases self-confidence, improves mood, aids relaxation, and lowers symptoms of depression and anxiety. But what else can you do? Dr. Dawe recommends the following strategies to individuals who come to him feeling overwhelmed.

Identify your key stressors: What is keeping you up at night? Are you happy at work? Are you struggling with a challenging relationship? Is your health troubling you? Do you have financial worries? Are trivial concerns masking a deeper issue? Identify your key stressors, and you can begin to do something about them.

Craft a solution: Having a plan helps. What can you do to change your current situation? What will be the consequences of taking this action? Should you be looking for a less stressful job? Do you need marriage counseling? Do you need to review your care plan with your doctor? Would a second opinion help? Should you talk to a financial expert about money management? What will happen if you do nothing?

Share the load: You may find it helpful to talk about your stress. Friends and family members may not realize you are having a hard time. The simple action of venting to a trusted person can significantly reduce stress levels, and they may think of a solution you haven't considered. If you prefer to speak with someone outside your circle of friends and relatives, approach your family doctor and ask for a referral to a mental health counselor.

Invest in your stress resiliency: Time spent in the company of an experienced business coach or counselor specializing in stress management can provide a fresh perspective and an opportunity to reset.

Take a mental holiday: You may be able to get rid of stressful feelings temporarily by shifting gears and carving time out to enjoy the outdoors, gather with friends, or decompress in a hobby. The practice of a simple ten-minute, end-of-day meditation can also provide a nice reset.

DR. ROBYNE'S PILLARS OF STRESS RESILIENCY

Mentor and stress resiliency expert Dr. Robyne Hanley-Dafoe's book, *Calm Within the Storm: A Pathway to Every Day Resiliency*, is a must-read if you want a deeper dive into building resiliency. She provides readers with an easy-to-follow roadmap to redefine resiliency for everyday life. She writes, "Resiliency is not simply the ability to bounce back from adversity; but it is also the steadfast belief that we can and will navigate the hard parts of our lives, no matter what." When I spoke with her about Wellness Ritual #6, she said, "Resiliency is not something that we either have or don't. It is a life skill we can learn to develop with effort."

Dedicating her research to what resilient people do differently and where they draw their strength and focus from has led her to develop a resiliency model based on five interconnected pillars that establish our baseline for coping with life's challenges. These pillars are Belonging, Perspective, Acceptance, Hope, and Humor. Here is an overview of her model.

Dr. Robyne's Resiliency Pillar: Belonging

Dr. Robyne shares, "At no other point in history have we been so connected yet so isolated and lonely. Connection has become competitive. How many likes, followers, and retweets one can get have become markers of popularity. People are hurting. We feel alone. We are thirsting for true connection and meaning in our relationships, but we are filled with feelings of lack and inauthenticity."

To connect with a sense of *Belonging*, she believes we must foster a connection with ourselves by spending time in reflection to cultivate a "caring companion champion" — someone who will have our back and defend us, even from ourselves, if or when necessary. Our resiliency grows by getting out of our way and seeing ourselves as part of something bigger.

Dr. Robyne's Resiliency Pillar: Perspective

With the second pillar, *Perspective*, Dr. Robyne emphasizes the importance of how you frame your circumstances and align your feelings. She calls on the importance of developing nimble and flexible thinking. When you view yourself as capable of handling and even learning and growing from the stress in your life and accept stress as an energy that everyone must deal with, its grip on us changes. You can sharpen your perspective by connecting with what matters to you the most.

Dr. Robyne's Resiliency Pillar: Acceptance

The third pillar, *Acceptance*, is achieved with time and life experience. At its core is the practice of living an examined life. Dr. Robyne writes, "We can't practice acceptance when we are not mindful. We need to tune into feelings, thoughts, and behaviors, as well as their respective

AM I BURNT OUT, OR DO I HAVE A MENTAL ILLNESS?

Extreme commitments that leave you neglecting your self-care will result in exhaustion, but does this mean you just need rest, or are you at risk of developing a mental illness?

Emotional, mental, and physical exhaustion from long-term exposure to emotionally charged situations, overworking, and poor self-care practices increase your risk of experiencing burnout.[19] The emotional exhaustion at the core of burnout reflects a combination of a low mood and fatigue or loss of energy which correlates very highly with other depressive symptoms.[20] Both career and parental burnout are on the rise, but this does not mean that you are clinically depressed.[21, 22] If this question has crossed your mind, take action. Approach your family doctor and discuss your mental well-being.

impacts." It takes patience and discipline to choose to pause, observe, and reflect. When we make a choice to push back against life, we run the risk of getting stuck."

Marsha Linehan, American psychologist, author, and creator of dialectical behavior therapy (DBT), a type of psychotherapy that combines behavioral science with concepts like acceptance and mindfulness, talks about "radical acceptance" in a similar way. Radical acceptance is when you stop fighting reality, stop responding with impulsive or destructive behaviors when things aren't going the way you want them to, and let go of bitterness that may be keeping you trapped in a cycle of suffering.[24] Linehan encourages us to allow for disappointment, sadness, or grief, and acknowledge that life can be worth living even when there is pain.[24]

Dr. Robyne's Resiliency Pillar: Hope

After reading Dr. Robyne's profile, you will understand why she is particularly passionate about the fourth resiliency pillar, *Hope*. She calls hope the heart of resiliency and leans on the importance of believing and living a hope-filled life. Much like *Acceptance, Hope* is a choice. "When we feel as though hope has escaped from our lives, whether because of disappointment, setbacks, loss, grief, or any other form of injustice, or perhaps even for no reason whatsoever, it is nearly impossible to trust that we will bounce back."

To nurture our hope, she echoes Dr. Dawe and believes that we must first acknowledge our inner dialogue and change our thinking. "Hope is more than optimism, it is the motivation that gives us the capacity to believe that we can experience positive outcomes by working toward a goal."

Dr. Robyne's Resiliency Pillar: Humor

The final pillar, *Humor*, focuses on setting a goal of lifting the weight off your shoulders and softening your heart by looking for wonder in the everyday. "In times of stress, change, challenge, and uncertainty, humor is often the first thing to go, but interestingly, it is in those tense times when we need it the most. By taking a step back and being willing to be humble, you can find surprises that provide relief and lighten the load."

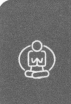

Children laugh approximately six times more than adults do in a day.[27] Even if smiling feels a little forced, the simple act has been shown to activate mood boosters and improve your state of mind. Tap into your inner child and have some fun.

CHAPIN CLINICAL CORNER

SELF-CARE REFLECTION #40

If I were to ask you to list the stressors that make your life extreme, you could likely do so very quickly. It is natural to keep this list top of mind. Dr. Dawe highlighted the importance of knowing your stressors. However, knowing them and letting them run the show are entirely different. Take a moment to consider the three stressors that currently sit at the top of your list. Write down a single word to represent each one in the spaces below. Label them with whatever word you want. Profanity and sarcasm are encouraged, especially if it brings a smile to your face.

1. _____

2. _____

3. _____

Identify the stressor that troubles you the most. We will consider this the kingpin. Neuroscientist Matt Lieberman has shown that purposefully acknowledging and labeling your stress lets you pause the visceral amygdala reaction and allows you to choose a more enhancing, deliberate response.[12]

Renowned clinical psychologist Dr. Richard Earle helps high performers disarm their kingpin with a single question. As Dr. Selye's last post-doctoral student, Dr. Earle worked hand-in-hand with the father of stress research. As such, he shares his curiosity and is quick to get to the root source of burnout. As the managing director of the Canadian National Institute of Stress and the Hans Selye Foundation, he continues to develop the research of his mentor and colleagues. Earle is currently working on a coaching tool that leverages the influence of mirror neurons to enhance self-awareness.

Before asking his kingpin-killing question, Earle presents his clients, weakened by the chronic toxicity of stress, with a gift box.

Handing them the hypothetical gift, he asks them to imagine that within the box is the solution to eradicate their number one stressor. Like a genie who grants a single wish, opening this box can erase your kingpin from existence, thus terminating its influence over you.

After sitting for a minute with this thought, he encourages his clients to experience the emotional response it triggers, and then he asks his question. Assuming you opened the box, applied the solution, and as a result, things were in fact better for you, *what does better look like*?

Earle shares that when a top performer's personal or professional return on investment is unclear or fragile, or they become blinded by their kingpin, their potential for health and well-being becomes unnecessarily capped. In an overwhelmed state, we can become so consumed by the stressors that make our lives feel extreme that it can be difficult to answer the simple question above.

To understand what your better would look like, you need to explore your kingpin mindset and inner dialogue. How would it make you feel if your kingpin was no longer in your life? What emotions would be triggered? Is it a feeling of happiness and gratitude, or is it simply relief? How would this state change your actions? How would it change the way you speak to yourself and others? What influence would it have on your outlook and attitude?

SMILING IS CONTAGIOUS.

Have you ever noticed that when you see someone yawn, it triggers you to yawn as well? This is thanks to "mirror neurons." Important in early human development, these neurons allow babies to mimic facial and emotional reactions in response to sensory input. Smiling and laughter activate mirror neurons in the same way. Bringing more laughter to your day will lift your mood as well as the moods of those around you.[25]

"The most radical act anyone can commit is to be happy."
– Patch Adams

The point of this exercise is to highlight the powerful downstream effect our thoughts have on our emotions and behavior. Fixating on our list of stressors or struggling to find a viable solution that may or may not exist can fuel a mindset that prevents any advancement in our mental fitness or enjoyment of life. Accepting, reframing, and choosing hope offers a different experience.

RITUAL ACTIVATION

TAKE THESE STEPS:

- **Schedule more "Me" time.** Devote at least 1% of your day (fourteen minutes and twenty-four seconds) to personal development and stress resiliency. I start my day with my mobility practice and pushups and end it with a short ten-minute meditation. These bookend rituals make me feel physically and mentally strong and reinforce my commitment to take charge of my health. What matters isn't what you choose to do, but that it makes you feel good about yourself. Keep the task of emptying your email inbox off this list.

- **Reward yourself for "me-time" streaks.** Reinforce your commitment to your "me-time" with a reward that triggers your brain to associate the reward's pleasure with your health goal of nurturing your mental fitness. Scale and vary your rewards to stay on budget and incentivized. Dr. Dawe shares, "Acknowledging and celebrating success helps us cement our confidence in building gains, rather than just chalking them up to chance, luck, or the efforts of others. To genuinely say, 'I did this, and it worked,' helps us articulate the confidence to move forward."

- **Play to your strengths.** Research has shown that the following nine personality traits are associated with resiliency: decisiveness, a sense of purpose, strong values, flexibility, self-care discipline, humor, responsibility, social support, and optimism.[26] Think about which traits you possess and begin leaning on them during stressful situations. You will see the most significant growth in your areas of interest and strength.

- **Ask for help.** Drs. Dawe and Hanley-Dafoe insist that developing a trusted social network is essential for mental health. Recognize the early warning signs of excessive stress and take action by speaking up. Do not live life on the right side of your stress response curve.

- **De-stress your diet.** Following Wellness Rituals #2 and #3 will enhance your resiliency. Discuss the appropriate use of vitamins and supplements with your team of healthcare professionals given your medical history.

MIND GAMES: CAN PLAYING BRAIN-TEASER MIND GAMES HELP KEEP YOUR MIND FIT?

There isn't definitive evidence to give us a clear answer to this question. However, experts do agree that keeping your mind active is essential to healthy aging. What the brain needs most is something new every day. With this exposure, it responds more like a muscle than the organ it is. Use it or lose it. Games designed to test your memory can be effective at sharpening certain mental skills, such as reaction time, short-term memory, and decision making. Here is a short list of activities and techniques that will give your mental fitness a further boost:

- Completing crossword or Sudoku puzzles
- Memorizing a shopping list or phone number
- Playing card games, like bridge
- Playing chess
- Driving without using navigation
- Learning a new language or instrument
- Trying a brain game app, like BrainHQ

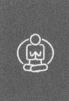

- **Get your 150 minutes of activity every week.** Still struggling with this commitment? Re-read Wellness Rituals #4 and #5.

- **Prepare for success.** Be honest about what you have control over and what you don't. If you have control, take action and plan for a resolution. Identify anything that can be done ahead of time to reduce stress, and then do it. If the task belongs to someone else, let go of it. Practice making the choice not to react. A number of the mentors practice guided imagery to become more familiar with the nerves that precede a big event. Khamica Bingham runs her race in her mind hundreds of times before the gun actually goes off. Using the same mind-body connections that can create tension, insomnia, anxiety, and over-eating in response to stress can be used to develop a sense of calm.

- **Practice Wellness Ritual #1.** Like your life depends on it.

- **Choose hope.** Even when life feels hard.

IN SUMMARY

Take the opportunity afforded by the pandemic's disruption to consider the sustainability of your pace and the priority you are placing on your health. Moving through adversity and learning from life's challenges is easier with a "stress-is-enhancing" mindset and a dedication to mental fitness. The practice of nurturing your mental fitness leads to improved coping skills and greater consistency in delivering a determined, focused, and confident response to a stressful event. It will help you remain in control when under pressure and give you the capacity to change your behavior to realize your goals. A strong self-awareness developed through Dr. Dawe's coping strategies and the regular practice of Dr. Robyne's five pillars of stress resiliency will get you on your way.

HOW DOES FAITH OR SPIRITUALITY IMPACT RESILIENCY?

If belonging to something that is greater than yourself has been shown to enhance resiliency, then you would expect individuals with a strong faith or spirituality to showcase tremendous mental fitness. After twenty-four years of clinical practice, there is no doubt in my mind that faith, spirituality, and resiliency are intimately connected. Growing up in a Christian home, my parents both lived their lives dedicated to the glory of God and modeled an unshakable faith for my sister, brother, and I. As a child, this gave me comfort and created a structure to my world. We learned to "do unto others what you would have them do to you" (Matthew 7:12) and to "love your neighbor" (Mark 12:31, Luke 10:27).

My upbringing allows me to place trust and belief in a higher purpose that cannot be seen or measured, despite my scientific curiosity. As a clinician, I've witnessed healing and recovery that cannot be explained by science, and patients confront tragedy with a faith that provides unfathomable resiliency.

Current medical models of evidence-based practice extend beyond double-blinded, randomized, controlled trials to include clinical experience, and that is what I offer you here. Spirituality and religion are historically linked with tremendous human suffering, but they can also be powerful sources of hope, meaning, peace, comfort, and forgiveness.[23] On the topic of faith, Dr. Robyne writes, "When life is complicated, unforgiving, and relentless, as it often can be, having a rock upon which you can rest and cast your worries is the universal root of belonging and being connected to something greater. Our faith has the capacity to bind us to our past, ground us in our future, and foster hope for tomorrow."

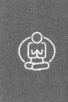

On turning forty, Michael reached **a defining moment in his life.** He recalls waking one day and realizing that he **was at the midway point** of his life and was living on autopilot...he had become complacent and blind to the impact his **day-to-day decisions** were having on his health and performance.

MENTOR PROFILES

MICHAEL RICHARDSON
LYNN LANGROCK
JANN ARDEN

MICHAEL RICHARDSON

CEO and Co-founder of Eclipsys

Michael's son Matt is severely autistic, non-verbal, and lives in a group home with other high-needs residents. At a height of 6'4" and weighing 270 pounds, when Matt wants to move, he is a force difficult to stop.

Intellectually, Michael grasped his son's reality soon after his birth, but emotionally, a parent's journey with a special needs child is mercurial. The pendulum quickly swings from anger and questions of "why me?" to amazement and love. The initial learning curve can be steep for both the parent and the child. One minute, Michael would find confidence in a new communication technique that Matt would appear to respond favorably to, and the next, he would fall back into doubt and frustration. Determined to position Matt for success, Michael continued down a difficult path confronted with challenges beyond his control. Along the way, quite unexpectedly, Matt unlocked Michael's true potential. In a role reversal, the son was the one to teach the father life skills, impacting Michael's life in the most profound way in the process.

Michael admits that he moved through his own youth and early adulthood with relative ease. His childhood had structure and security that established a strong foundation in learning and values. When he encounters a problem, Michael is able to respond quickly, typically with a creative solution. He refers to himself as a "fixer," and he learned to lean on this talent from a young age. "School was not tough for me, and I never found work to be that difficult either. When Matt came into my life, it was like somebody decided, 'Here is your challenge. Here is your thing, and you are not going to be able to fix it.'" Michael was thirty-four when Matt was born.

With the guidance of leading professionals, Michael learned effective strategies to best support Matt. "By speaking directly to him, making eye contact, and using pictures and photographs when communicating, I can connect with him." Matt became agitated when home for dinner recently, and with the source of his frustration unknown, his size and physicality presented a challenge. Michael's ability to de-escalate these encounters is essential to the smooth functioning of their supportive family unit. Michael and his wife, Monica, also have a daughter, Stephanie, a few years younger than Matt. Raised voices, sharp tones, impatience, or physical confrontations do not work when settling Matt down. He does not respond to directions or commands. The best way to hold Matt's attention is to speak softly and engage him with eye-to-eye contact. Michael found success with his son when he realized that "You can't tell him things, provide detailed instructions, or reason with him. To communicate, you have to ask him direct questions. Would you like this or that?" When Michael lands on the correct answer, Matt hits his chest to indicate his preference. Michael and Monica have become a great team in managing and prioritizing Matthew's care and development. His sister, Stephanie, has a deep connection to his well being.

FATHER AND SON

> ❝ I don't have a single memory of playing with my dad as a child. He worked hard, provided for the family, and then retired. And on his retirement, because of some health challenges, he got old in five years. ❞

Learning to be patient, aware, and focused with Matt are life skills complemented by those born in his relationship with his father. His father had a challenging childhood. Leaning on his intelligence and the Richardson work ethic, his dad found success with IBM Canada Ltd., retiring as an executive after a long career with the technology giant. He passed away in 2013 at the age of seventy-nine. Michael loved his father, looked up to him, and had great respect for him as a man. However, his dad seemed to have the time and interest for two passions in life — work and family. He had few hobbies and just a handful of close friends. With a hint of sadness, Michael remembers his dad driving him to soccer, hockey, and lacrosse games, but never did the two of them take advantage of a lazy Saturday afternoon to head down to the park and throw a ball. Once in a while, they played golf.

"I don't have a single memory of playing with my dad as a child. He worked hard, provided for the family, and then retired. And on his retirement, because of some health challenges, he got old in five years." Trouble with an arthritic hip, poor knees, Parkinson's, and eventually dementia would all hasten his dad's rapid decline and leave a lasting impression on what Michael wanted from his own life.

Following in his father's footsteps, Michael joined IBM Canada Ltd. in the early 1980s. He found himself fresh out of school with a history and economics degree, sitting at the table next to talented engineers with cutting-edge expertise. At the time, the organization placed a high value on the engineers' specialized skill set, often leaving Michael feeling like the odd man out. "For the first five years of my career, I felt like the dumbest person in the room." He dug in and worked hard to carve out his role. After several years, it became apparent that career advancement was awarded to those with superior technical abilities. Engineers were recognized as a priority for promotion over those with leadership potential, giving Michael's peers an advantage over him. He would leave in 1998, after fourteen years, deviating from his father's path. By jumping tracks, he created an opportunity to redefine his value and brand by becoming an innovative entrepreneur capable of achieving next-level success.

SELF-CARE REFLECTION #41

In his son and in his father, Michael has learned valuable life lessons about love, patience, kindness, and health. In your journal, write about lessons you have learned from others that have shaped your attitude toward self-care.

COMPLACENCY LEADS TO A WAKE-UP CALL

As a hard driver and hyper-competitive executive, Michael continues to strive for a big life. "I like to win." A self-proclaimed "late bloomer," he now owns three companies. His most prominent role is as CEO and Co-Founder of Eclipsys Solutions, a company that solves problems around enterprise IT requirements, security, and performance. This position draws on Michael's unique problem-solving skills and emotional intelligence. At Eclipsys, he appears to have found his niche.

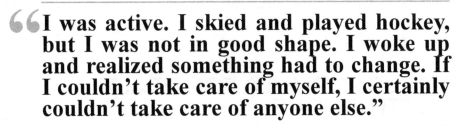

I was active. I skied and played hockey, but I was not in good shape. I woke up and realized something had to change. If I couldn't take care of myself, I certainly couldn't take care of anyone else."

On turning forty, Michael reached a defining moment in his life. He recalls waking one day and realizing that he was at the midway point of his life and was living on autopilot. A personal audit of his lifestyle choices revealed that he had become complacent and blind to the impact his day-to-day decisions were having on his health and performance. He was fifty pounds overweight, unfit, and overworked. "I was active. I skied and played hockey, but I was not in good shape. I woke up and realized something had to change. If I couldn't take care of myself, I certainly couldn't take care of anyone else."

Michael stood at this crossroads and made a decision guided by his love for his family, his father's decline, and the excitement he had tapped into as an entrepreneur. If he was going to realize the vision he had for his life, he needed a new formula and an immediate reason to get into shape.

He would often fantasize about taking a back-country ski trip with one of his closest childhood friends. Armed with a sudden desire for change, Michael called their bluff and challenged the friend, "Are we ever going to do this or just keep talking about it?" By the end of the week, the ski trip was booked, and Michael had the urgency he needed to begin his transformation. The trip would be physically demanding and require respect and preparation if it were to live up to their dreams. Michael started to train aggressively, determined to drop his weight and improve his core and leg strength in advance of their departure. The experience was everything they hoped it would be, but the true gift was the ripple effect it created. Michael came back a different man, more determined than ever to get into the best shape of his life. He reverse-engineered his formula to achieve these fitness goals. He says, "I am now on year nineteen of that ski trip."

Michael began approaching each day with purpose, and his body responded favorably to the winning formula he developed. He continues to embrace all 7 Wellness Rituals and views each one of them as a unique "dial." Adjusting his dials accordingly has allowed him to elevate his performance in all aspects of his life. Here is a look at how his formula plays out.

MICHAEL'S FORMULA FOR HEALTH, STRENGTH & HOPE

Michael places a priority on sleep out of necessity.

> **I can't go to bed at midnight, get up at 6 a.m., and expect to perform. I had to acknowledge that at sixty-one, I needed more sleep than I thought I did — especially in the last ten years."**

As an avid cyclist, regular three-hour bike rides empty his tank quickly. His sleep routine now consistently delivers seven hours a night, and he has developed an impressive self-awareness of his stress versus satisfaction ratio. If he finds his energy falling off or his performance slipping, a twenty-minute power nap usually gives him a meaningful boost. Michael will enjoy quiet moments at home at the end of the day before bed, but otherwise does not seek solitude. He appears to recharge quicker when surrounded by friends and is more inclined to add community and social engagement to his life, not escape from it.

For twenty years, he had never gone longer than three days without getting his heart rate up from exercise. In the early days, motivated to see change quickly, he would work out seven days a week. At the time, Matt was still living in their home, and Michael would do whatever he needed to do to get his workout in regardless of the hour. "Finding time to exercise became stressful. There would be nights where I would be heading down to the basement to jump on the stationary bike at 10:30 p.m." Post-workout, lying in bed, wired from the high-intensity exercise, Michael would often have difficulty falling asleep until sometime after 1:30 a.m. "Up at 6 a.m. to start my day, completely exhausted, with less than five hours of sleep, I realized this probably wasn't sustainable or all that helpful." He abandoned this approach and hired a personal trainer with whom he has worked out ever since.

When in the gym, he pushes his body hard. On off-days, he prioritizes recovery. His trainer emphasizes the importance of both. "I can still routinely maintain an elevated heart rate of 160 beats per minute on long bike rides." He is proud to report that he has never suffered a sports injury while under his trainer's supervision and attributes his improvements in mental acuity and stress resiliency to his commitment to fitness. After years of training, Michael can literally feel his endorphins kick in at the twelve- to fifteen-minute mark of exercise. His body's response to the natural painkiller and mood elevator triggers a euphoria that keeps him coming back for more. There is a rhythm to his training that peaks his interest and allows him to participate in various sports, including skiing, hockey, and cycling, at a high level. Cycling is his favorite activity.

Pouring himself into the world of cycling has given Michael immense joy. Not only has it provided him with a physical outlet to reach his fitness goals, but it has also allowed him to cultivate valuable friendships. Michael is conscious of building a community in his life outside of work that he can access easily. He understands the scientific connection between social support and longevity and has found neighbors who share his passion. He loves the cycling community as much as he does the physical challenge of a long ride. Michael averages 250 km a week between April and October and cycles all year round. A weekday ride into the sunset around 5:30 to 6 p.m. is his happy place.

His cycling friendships provide encouragement and establish accountability beyond the time the group spends together in the saddle. Conversations range from cycling performance metrics, gear, and cycling routes to work issues, family challenges, and aging. It is a community passionate about performance and perceptive about resiliency. There is no place to hide on a 100 km group ride. The group takes good care of each other, and no one is ever left behind. "I am at a stage of life where I can go out for a three-hour ride. We can be forty km in before we really get going. That first hour is spent yakking and catching up with friends as we bike out of the city. After a nice social warm up, we get up into the country, hit it hard for an hour or so, and then return home." The friendships he has made in cycling represent an important dial in his life that he values dearly.

SELF-CARE REFLECTION #42

There is a special social component to Michael's health formula. He is part of a cycling community, people who share a common passion for cycling and for each other. What role does community and a sense of belonging play in your formula? How could you enhance this key ingredient to good health in your life? Are there volunteer or mentorship opportunities available to you? Have you considered joining a community social or sports club?

ON AGING WELL AND MENTAL FITNESS

In addition to Michael's trainer, an executive coach and dietitian hold him accountable to his formula. For the better part of ten years, he has met with his coach over regularly scheduled breakfast meetings at a local restaurant around the corner from his home. "My coach provides me with professional counseling to help me with my business and has been a tremendous sounding board and pillar of support for many years."

While his coach helps him develop his leadership skills, his dietitian helps him confront his sweet tooth. "When I'm riding hard, I can literally eat whatever I want. Calories melt away." Michael's level of exercise masks a few poor dietary habits. However, each winter, as his mileage drops, his snacking habits start catching up with him, and his weight starts to rise. "I put on five to seven pounds each winter." He weighs himself daily and keeps a close eye on his waistline, determined not to let his weight gain pass this mark. Now at 215 pounds, he is curious to see what his cycling performance would look like if he were ten to fifteen pounds lighter. To get there, his dietitian is helping him with portion control, the timing of his meals, and how to incorporate healthy carbs into his diet to fuel longer rides and quicker recoveries.

Movement quality is another dial Michael monitors. Adapting his training intensity and placing a greater focus on his flexibility as he ages is an ongoing discussion he has with his trainer. She has helped him appreciate that a tight muscle is a weak muscle and will vary his workouts to improve his balance and functional range of motion. "When it comes to cycling, I'm fortunate that I can keep up with guys many years younger than me because of my ability to maintain a higher heart rate for my age — some of this is genetic, and some is earned. Where I struggle is my flexibility. My frame is built to be internally rotated. I don't love stretching."

The idea of retiring or escaping work pressures in any capacity carries zero weight in Michael's formula. "I have worked hard to be in the position I am, free from any outside influences. I enjoy my work and see it like another dial in my life." He has found a balance in his approach that fuels his passions for work and play, which are often one in the same for him. Exercise is his release and keeps him mentally fit. The demands of work appear not to trouble him.

"The skills I've developed to help my son I now use in everyday life. They are skills that, quite honestly, Matt has helped me to build." Learning to slow down and step back to allow time and space to be curious, make eye contact, speak quietly, and communicate with intention have helped Michael immeasurably with both his son and his professional life. "Instead of trying to get people to where I want them to be, I've learned to meet them where they are. Over the last twenty-five years, Matt and I have practiced this technique." When Michael started applying these skills in business, he found they worked just as well. He credits his son for helping him develop his emotional intelligence and, in doing so, change the trajectory of his career. "I now have a level of empathy and curiosity that allows me to connect with people in a special way."

Learning to engage with Matt on Matt's terms, drawing motivation from his father's choices, seeking guidance from a team of professionals, implementing their recommendations, and cultivating a love for exercise have all played a huge role in how Michael's formula came together. He has learned to accept the things he cannot change and leverage the courage to adapt and change the things he can with the help of his community. As Michael says, "Everyone gets their bag of hammers. It is up to you what you are going to do with them."

LYNN LANGROCK

VP of People for Bimbo QSR

*L*ynn's husband, Abe, tragically passed away at the age of fifty-five. Complications following surgery to open a blocked coronary artery, coupled with the early detection of esophageal cancer, ended his life unexpectedly. His sudden departure left Lynn and their two sons stunned with unimaginable heartbreak. Walking provided Lynn with a temporary escape from her grief. Well before Abe's health issues were known, Lynn had set a daily goal of walking at least 10,000 steps. By the day of Abe's memorial service, this streak had extended well beyond three years without a single day missed. There would be no skipping this day either. Lynn woke early that morning, laced up her walking shoes, and hit the road, knowing the movement would help steady her mind in preparation for the day ahead. The autopilot feature of a three-year ritual had kicked in, nurturing and guiding her forward, literally one foot in front of the next. She said, "Even in my darkest days, I had this ritual to fall back onto."

Abe's father passed away as a young man too. He was only fifty when he died. "We had a couple of conversations about the 'what if scenario' before Abe's illness was known. He had seen his mother go on to live a long life alone after his dad's death, and he wanted me to promise that if something were to happen to him, I would not follow in his mother's footsteps. He didn't want me to live alone. I flat out told him that we were not having this conversation, and that this was not going to happen."

And then, it did.

For some time following Abe's death, Lynn was angry. Replaying his forewarned concern and the promise she left unanswered would sometimes trigger an argument. Of course, these discussions only had one voice. Not one to pull punches or shy away from a well-placed, emphatic F-bomb, Lynn's response to Abe's request would play out in her mind something like this: "Fuck you, Abe. You are not here anymore, so you don't get a say. You don't get an opinion. I'll be alone if I want to be alone, and there is nothing you can do about it."

Following the memorial service, Lynn and the boys spent December at their family cottage in Nova Scotia. As the calendar turned to the New Year, the boys prepared to return to university, and Lynn realized that she could not mourn while attending to their needs. It had become evident that everyone needed to move forward, as painful as that might be. "I drove them back to university, made sure they were all set up in their apartment, then Googled the warmest spot in Florida in January, booked an Airbnb, and drove straight to the airport."

There are gaps in Lynn's memory as she re-entered her life. "It probably took me a few years to realize that I had crafted my recovery and life after Abe around coping with competence."

Feeling an unfamiliar fragility, Lynn spent a lot of time in her office, avoiding people and "unnecessary" conversations. The energy to show up each day varied in intensity from overwhelming to startling. "Thankfully, I had a buffer. My team was strong. They took on the role of caretaking, and caught anything that slipped past me. I probably didn't let my guard down with my leader for at least six or seven months into my grieving process." Her decision to return to work less than two months after Abe's death was more about her boys. They needed to feel like things were falling back into place, and her well-being and return to work were paramount to their recovery.

The following two years were spent doing: selling Abe's car, their house, and the cottage. "We owned a DIY MacGyver cottage that Abe was the only one who knew how to run." Unintentionally, Lynn began whittling her personal life down to a transactional to-do list. "Doing" kept her on her feet. For every task completed and crossed off the list, two new ones were added. Pouring her remaining attention into the needs of the boys and her work provided stability and a much-needed distraction that played to her strengths. Lynn's true heart is one of a loving caregiver. "There were some days where it was a victory to leave the house and walk around the block." With personal and professional success forged out of hard work, intelligence, empathy, and discipline, Lynn delivered without hesitation and pushed herself to the point of exhaustion. Missing from her formula was a commitment to proactive self-care. In time, avoiding self-care would have capped her potential.

SELF-CARE REFLECTION #43

In your journal, reflect on your own life experiences when events and attending to the needs of others demanded your full attention, leaving less time for self-care. At what point did you begin to recognize the weight of the responsibility you were carrying? How did this realization show up biologically? Were you tired or resentful? Did you cut your sleep short or experience headaches or elevated physical pain? Learning to act on these alarm bells early offers health protection and enhanced resiliency. If you are in a situation now that demands you think and care for others first, what can you do to maintain your health until things change?

A COMMITMENT TO THE LONG GAME

As Lynn worked through her grief, her approach shifted. Forced to become acutely aware of the precious value of a minute, she re-constructed her formula to support the long game. Possessing a heightened sensitivity to her specific individual needs resulted in a boost in performance, which opened doors to exciting new opportunities. Abe will remain a monumental part of Lynn's life story, but the arguments have stopped. Someday, he may even see the promise he asked Lynn to make fulfilled.

As VP of Human Relations and Corporate Affairs for Bimbo Canada, Lynn was recognized by *Report on Business Magazine* in November 2020 as one of Canada's Best Executives for her leadership throughout the COVID-19 pandemic. In March 2021, she was promoted to VP of People for Bimbo QSR. Founded in 1955, Bimbo QSR is a wholesale commercial bakery that supplies restaurant chains with high-quality buns and artisan rolls from forty-seven bakeries in twenty-two countries. With 2,100 employees, they are a global bakery leader. Their leadership team comprises bakery and foodservice industry experts with decades of business-building experience. "Our business is on a growth trajectory. Working for this team is incredibly exciting. Just this week, I was on the phone with our General Managers in Europe and South Africa. Last week it was China. To my core, I believe that you are never too old to learn. The energy you get back from a new opportunity like this one is profound. And I'm loving it."

LYNN'S FORMULA FOR HEALTH, STRENGTH & HOPE

Lynn's formula is now set to support a world-class performance in her global corporate role. Up between 6 and 6:30 a.m. most mornings, her first action is to put on her running shoes.

> 66 **I look for opportunities to exercise throughout the day but prefer to get the bulk of it done in the morning."**

Walking or running first-thing gives her time to intentionally establish her mindset for the day. This time is a gift that offers an even greater reward when experienced in solitude. If the time is shared, it is only with the best of friends. Last year, she averaged 12,000 steps a day. This year, her average has surpassed 15,000 steps a day.

Drawn to the principles of mental fitness, she holds respect for the value of meditation but struggles with putting it into practice. Wired to serve, her attention is easily hijacked by the needs of others. The book *Meditation for the Fidgety Skeptic* by Dan Harris is one of her favorites and has helped her develop resiliency by incorporating a morning meditation buffer.

"Our divisions in Europe, the Middle East, and Asia are already well into their day when I get up at 6 a.m. If I jump into my inbox first thing or book a call to South Africa, it will be 9:30 a.m. before I know it and I haven't yet had my walk, breakfast, or even changed into my 'good' work-from-home Lululemon gear." Barring some critical issue demanding her immediate attention, the first hour of her day is now reserved for her.

Pre-pandemic, the commute to and from work provided another valuable decompression time. "I would take this time to mentally prepare for work heading into the office or for the family when heading home for what I called the second shift."

FOOD, MEDITATION, AND RECOVERY

Grief dulled Lynn's senses for a period of time. "I began mindlessly eating and started gaining weight despite my daily walks. I wasn't making good food choices and actually stopped tasting the food I was eating altogether." She engaged a health and nutrition coach who turned her focus to mindful eating, eventually awakening her taste buds.

Upon returning from her morning walk or run, she will enjoy a decaffeinated coffee and a quick breakfast of steel-cut oats with cinnamon or egg on a piece of Stone Mill Ancient Grain toast. If pressed for time, she will grab a smoothie and go. This meal anchors her morning energy. Skipping it leaves her feeling a step behind all day and sets her up for poor choices later on as her cravings assume control.

Coupling daily meditation with a heightened awareness of portion control, food flavor, strategic meal prep, and quality food selection, Lynn reconnected with what, when, and why she was eating. "With this practice, I noticed a direct boost in my energy, and the afternoon lethargy that called for an afternoon nap fell away." Lynn has never dieted but admits to a track record of cutting corners when it comes to healthy eating. She no longer skips breakfast or works through the day without lunch. Healthy food choices are now an essential component of her revamped formula, and the discipline provides her with the energy to deliver at a consistently high level.

66 If I don't get that 'me time' at the end of the day, I'm just not my best self."

Lynn's bedtime varies. She will be in bed by 11 p.m. and read until she drifts off to sleep on well-balanced days that play close to the script. Bedtime reading helps her wind down and nourishes her mind. "If I don't get that 'me time' at the end of the day, I'm just not my best self."

Too many consecutive nights that extend past 11 p.m. come at a cost to her performance. Back and shoulder pain used to be the only thing that would slow her down and force an earlier bedtime. Lynn is now much more proactive with her visits to her chiropractor and pays close attention to her sleep patterns. "I used to go hard until my body physically hurt. Now I am much wiser and will recalibrate to my needs earlier."

OBLIGATIONS AND MINDSET

In addition to her two boys, who are now in their twenties, Lynn has several family members who rely on her support.

> **❝I've also shifted my mindset when it comes to tackling my list of responsibilities. I am now very grateful to spend time with family and enjoy the opportunity to help them immensely.❞**

Pivoting to serve the needs of loved ones out of appreciation rather than obligation has allowed her to stay present in their company. This time is no longer a task to strike from the list; it is an event that gives back, leaving Lynn feeling fulfilled and balanced.

SELF-CARE REFLECTION #44

Do you view your duty to attend to the needs of loved ones as a necessary evil or as an opportunity to cultivate gratitude? If you need to pivot like Lynn has, what steps can you take to begin that shift of mindset and perspective? What health benefits might arise from doing so? Please journal your thoughts.

SELF-CARE DISCIPLINES

By managing her calendar differently, Lynn has also discovered new pockets of time during the workday that provide an additional reprieve. "I've started blocking my calendar every day from 4 to 6 p.m. Occasionally, I'll need to schedule something critical in that window, but otherwise, I'll use it to think, write, and prioritize. Last year, with another senior leader in Quebec, I blocked from noon until one o'clock to take wellness walks. We would use the time to connect over lunch while we got some exercise. Interestingly, even on days when we were not able to connect, the block in my calendar would stand out as an important reminder not to work straight through. After many years into my professional career, having read countless articles and books about the value of locking in time for yourself, it took a pandemic for me to actually put it into practice."

Lunch is typically grab-and-go, but conscientious choices are now made to support her performance. When traveling for business, Lynn prefers to stop at a local grocery store and pick up a healthy salad or grab some sushi and head back to the office or hotel rather than go to a restaurant for a big meal. "My EA laughs at my fifteen-dollar grocery bill when I return home from a business trip and submit my travel food expenses."

"Every once and a while, I will sometimes relapse back into peanut butter and crackers for dinner. But for the most part, my food choices are nutrient-dense. I am consuming less meat, with greater emphasis on chickpeas, quinoa, and plant-based proteins." Wine is mostly restricted to weekends.

Lynn has adapted her routine to support her stability and balance when it comes to exercise and movement quality. A young fifty-nine, she has embraced yoga and, in doing so, has noticed a big difference in her morning mobility.

An annual, executive medical check-up allows her to compare her health metrics to years previous. She now looks for opportunities to reinforce positive trends or address concerns through formula adjustments. Achievement motivated, Lynn likes to know and track her numbers. A friend recently presented her with the physical challenge of sitting down on the floor and then standing back up without using her hands. It is harder than it sounds, but Lynn is determined to answer the call. She also enjoys keeping her approach to fitness fresh with thirty-day fitness challenges or new workouts on various fitness apps.

FINDING CALM AND PEACE OF MIND

The Maritimes is where Lynn goes to unplug and play with purpose. She is capable of tapping into a state of peace there unlike anywhere else. Returning regularly offers a renewal. The COVID-19 pandemic made working remotely from her happy place possible. Her best leisure day would include time with family and friends, a jump in the ocean after a long walk or run with her hot, sweaty running clothes still on, time to stretch in the shade on the front deck, a little gardening, and curling up with a good book and cup of decaf coffee. These days are now lived, not just dreamed about.

Lynn brings a discipline and commitment to her lifestyle choices that are impressive, but this alone could not compete with her pace. Her nature to push and give beyond her capacity would have continued to overpower her best intentions to live a healthy life and left her vulnerable. Abe's death brought Lynn to a crossroads, and she chose the path that required her to take a hard look at her priorities and adapt. The COVID-19 pandemic then broke her free from her old approach to work and further highlighted the value of time and playing with purpose. By embracing these life lessons, she has found her superpower: resiliency.

As Lynn worked through her **grief**, her approach shifted. Forced to become **acutely aware of the precious value of a minute**, she re-constructed **her formula to support the long game**. Possessing a heightened sensitivity to her specific individual needs resulted in a boost in performance, which opened doors to **exciting new opportunities**.

JANN ARDEN

Singer-Songwriter, Author, Actress

"*M*y mom really was funny, you know. She'd say, 'We don't care that you're a singer. It doesn't matter to us. We wouldn't care if you were a plumber, and as a matter of fact, we could use a plumber more than we could use a singer at this point in life.' I would ask my parents to come to shows, and Mom would say, 'Well, is it the same as the last show we saw? I don't know if we need to see that again. You give those tickets to somebody else.' It was never done in a hurtful way — it's just like, how many shows can the woman see? They were not stage parents at all, and they had shit to do. They had yards to clean up and chores to get done. Mom would say, 'It would be great if you could help Dad and me move the bird feeder when you are home after the show.'"

We were meeting virtually at her beautiful home in rural Springbank, Alberta, just west of Calgary. Jann showed me around her stunning fourteen-acre property. As you head out her back door, it is like walking into a Robert Bateman painting. After thirty-plus years on the road, she enjoys the solitude and intimacy with nature her home provides. At one point during our meeting, she went to let her dog out, and from the tree line just off her back deck emerged a doe and fawn. Jann greeted the pair like she would a neighbor dropping by to share a morning coffee.

Seeing Jann on the deck, the doe raised her head, tilting it to the side, and fixed her gaze as if to say hello. They shared a quick exchange; the deer, comforted by the sound of Jann's voice, returned to her grazing. "As you can see, I live in the trees in the country, out here by myself. I'll tell you, there is something special about being in nature in this way. My parents moved us out into the country when I was eight, and I loved it. I'm really not a city person. I don't do well in big cities. I don't feel good. I just don't — it's not for me. And so, I saved and said yes to jobs that I should never have done to be in this place and be prepared for whatever might come. I've worked hard, but I'm almost sixty years old, and at that age, you should be prepared."

Jann's talent and creativity are a gift that Canadians celebrate. As a singer, songwriter, broadcaster, author, and actor, her life has played out in the public eye. The multi-platinum, award-winning artist has received eight Juno Awards, the Queen's Diamond Jubilee

Medal, and a star on Canada's Walk of Fame. In 2017, she was appointed as a Member of the Order of Canada for her achievements as a singer-songwriter and broadcaster and her extensive charitable work. In 2020, she was inducted into the Canadian Music Hall of Fame. She is a best-selling author, continues to produce new music, and stars in a hit TV sitcom loosely based on her life titled *Jann*. At the age of sixty, she is celebrating five years of sobriety and offers a unique perspective on aging, success, and life-long learning.

A DECENT PERSON WAS LYING IN WAIT

Throughout our small talk, I could sense that Jann was curious but somewhat restrained. I described the book's intention and my curiosity about her secret sauce for success. As she became comfortable with our conversation, she welcomed me into her routine. Time with Jann is fun. She is happy, authentic, and kind, and has a wicked-sharp sense of humor. She shared that after a career of spending over 250 days a year on the road, the COVID-19 pandemic presented her with an opportunity to slow things down and take inventory of her life. Settling into a slower pace and developing a rhythm to her day appears to have given her a needed rest and has refueled her creativity. With humor, Jann openly shares her view of aging on her podcast and in her books. She believes that humans are genuinely incompetent and not self-sufficient until the age of forty. "I would never want to be young again, ever. There's nothing about it that's appealing to me." She celebrates and values her life experience and the "sureness" that it provides.

> **I hit the ditch enough times in my life. You have to be able to draw from that bucket and pull out a lesson learned if you are going to move forward. At twenty-five, or even thirty-five, the bucket isn't deep enough. You haven't made enough mistakes yet. At forty, you finally start fitting into yourself."**

She explains that she feels like a completely different person with every passing decade, her confidence growing exponentially with age. "I would never have done the TV show ten years ago. I have had earlier opportunities in television, but I didn't feel like I could do it."

Five years ago, after several health challenges, Jann found herself in the hospital with cardiac distress. This was a day that changed the direction of Jann's life. "My heart was pushing back from years of abusing alcohol and not eating right. My dad was an angry alcoholic — as a kid, I watched him drink morning, noon, and night. That was not me. I wasn't a person that drank every day, but I could drink two bottles of wine at dinner, no problem. I had tried to stop many, many times. I was just sick of the habit. Drinking is a young man's game, and my body no longer wanted to play."

It was clear that her health was in jeopardy. Seeing an opportunity for improved health, a compassionate nurse called out Jann's drinking. The nurse was kind but firm and challenged Jann to face her alcohol abuse. For whatever reason, Jann was granted clarity at that moment and decided that she would never have another drink. She has not. "When I sobered up, I realized how much I liked myself and that a decent person was lying in wait. I'm really grateful for whatever happened that day because my whole self was prepared to listen. It's amazing how the body can repair and carry on."

Positioning herself to heal became Jann's focus, and her formula for success started to emerge. "The small things in life all add up. You know, I am frequently asked what my big break was. People assume that I have had all these big things happen in my life to get me to where I am. Honestly, life is made of thousands of seemingly insignificant, benign events that, when added up, make a life." Applying this philosophy, Jann tweaked her day-to-day decisions, and her body began to heal.

With renewed energy, Jann has found another gear and continues to create. A few weeks before our discussion, she had just finished filming the third season of her TV show. "From the time I'm in pre-production to the time we finish eight episodes, it's about nine to ten weeks, five of which are spent filming. I swear to God, it is just giddy-up-and-go for sixteen- to seventeen-hour days when we are on set. I'm learning fifteen pages of dialogue a day, and drunk Jann or hungover Jann would never have seen the light of day to get this started." In addition to her TV career, her music career also continues. She would soon travel to Vancouver to record a new album, sharing that splendid voice that she says feels stronger than it ever has.

SELF-CARE REFLECTION #45

Have you experienced a time when, like Jann, you felt that somewhere within you "a decent person was lying in wait"? Do you perhaps feel that way now? If you were sitting down with Jann right now, what do you think her advice would be? Give yourself a few moments to reflect on that advice and write it down.

Jann's self-care formula is very Jann. She practices the 7 Wellness Rituals but does not hold herself to a rigid schedule. "If I feel like doing something, I do it, and if I don't, I don't. I'm not a planner. I don't have anything written in the calendar."

In getting sober, Jann found freedom. "When I quit drinking, I ended a relationship. With clarity, I asked, 'Oh my God, what am I doing with my life?' It just feels good not to have to answer to anybody. It's not to say that I'm not interested in ever being in a relationship again, but I don't know if that means living with anybody."

In her book *If I Knew Then: Finding Wisdom in Failure and Power in Aging* she describes herself as a "crone." She explains that, traditionally, a crone is a character in folklore and fairy tales who is usually somewhat disagreeable, can be malicious, and possesses supernatural, magical powers. Jann's version of the crone is a "kick-ass, take-no-prisoners, damn-the-torpedoes, own-your-own-crap, great kind of person to be." She is wise and unapologetic, fierce and forward-thinking — someone who is at the pinnacle of her own belonging. "I am a crone standing at the beginning of a new chapter in my life, and it is going to unfold exactly the way I want it to."

JANN'S FORMULA FOR HEALTH, STRENGTH & HOPE

Jann places a high priority on solitude and sleep. Time at home provides the solitude she craves. Jann is early to bed and very early to rise. Mornings are special to her. Recently, she started using a smart ring to track her sleep quality. The device measures temperature, heart rate, activity levels, and provides a sleep number that has become a reliable stake in the ground and helps her prioritize rest.

"Good sleep isn't always an option when you're on the road. You know, a different bed every night, but I'm still pretty good at making it a priority. And when I stopped drinking, I started sleeping eighty-five percent better and noticed a huge kick in my energy and improvement in my mood."

Jann is a vegan. "I came to this gradually. I haven't eaten red meat in almost twenty years but went full vegan almost five years ago." She feels more alert on this diet and mindful of what and when she eats. "I have a big garden and grow my own food. I'm still eating potatoes from last year." Self-taught, she turns to the internet for inspired vegan recipes.

Exercise is also a part of her every day. She enjoys her daily walks on the property — sometimes alone, sometimes in the company of friends. She also bikes and practices yoga. "I am not a fit-bitter or step-counter. I don't meditate."

In the basement of her home is a fully equipped gym that gets daily use. Pre-pandemic, a trainer would come to the house. This stopped during the lockdown. After a few sessions of virtual fitness instruction, she realized it was not for her and returned to training on her own. To pass the time while on the elliptical or bike, she watches TV or reads.

"I was an athlete growing up and played all kinds of sports. I remember my mom telling me I would have hip problems later in life from all the years of playing catcher on my baseball team."

Outside of the stiffness in the hips, Jann now lives pain-free. When asked if she does anything differently to maintain her mobility and flexibility at age fifty-nine that she was not doing a decade earlier at forty-nine, she said she walks more. "I'm fortunate. I've never had back or neck problems or any hand pain. You might think my hands would hurt with all the guitar playing over the years, but they aren't sore at all." Exercise makes her feel strong and healthy and seems to fuel her inner crone.

HAPPY TO BE SITTING ON AN APPLE CRATE

Jann has a tight inner circle of friends and family that also gives her strength. Her maternal grandmother, Clara, was one of the first crones she ever met. She shares in her recent book, "I was both enamored and a tiny bit afraid of her. I didn't know it then, but crones don't take crap from anyone, not even their own grandchildren." She would share stories with Jann about the wisdom afforded by time and tell Jann that she needed to wait to be wise.

Jann's mom, Joan, was her rock. Her mom used to tell her, "Your soul is your pilot; your body is your spaceship. If you can't be brave, be reckless." In late 2018, Joan passed away following a long battle with Alzheimer's disease. In life, she taught Jann about compassion, empathy, and forgiveness and helped Jann realize that good can come from bad. Joan would say, "The good thing about Alzheimer's is you forget to be afraid."

Jann misses her mom the most. And while her dad was a difficult man caught in his own battle with alcoholism, he loved her too, in his own way. When he passed away a few years before her mom, also from Alzheimer's disease, Jann went to clean out his beloved truck and found all eight CD slots filled with her records. "He would never have shared something like that with me, but the thought of him driving around in his pickup truck and listening to me sing, it still makes me kind of laugh."

> **66I really don't get stressed out. Ask anybody that knows me. I'm not really up; I'm not really down. I'm like my mom that way — just happy to be sitting on an apple crate."**

Jann enjoys sharing the harvest from her vegetable garden, long walks, and movie nights with good friends. She jokes with them that if her memory starts to fade, they had better "keep the pudding and cake coming because she will be a pain in the ass." Her friendships are a clear source of love and bring her great pleasure and joy. "I'm not happy and successful because of my accomplishments. I'm successful because of my friendships, because of the fine people that I have in my life."

Wired to be steady, her mental fitness appears resolute. Life has taught her to be mindful of her thoughts and keep her inner dialogue kind. "I really don't get stressed out. Ask anybody that knows me. I'm not really up; I'm not really down. I'm like my mom that way — just happy to be sitting on an apple crate."

Never bored a day in her life, her curiosity gives off an aura of youthful playfulness. She looks for opportunities to learn. "I can't sit idle. As soon as I finished taping the show, I went back to working on a novel I've been writing for the last ten years. And the funny part is, I've written three other books while working on the novel."

She is also very active with charity work. Recording cameo videos, she has raised over $175,000 for various charities. For weeks leading up to Mother's Day, she recorded about forty personalized versions of her award-winning song *Good Mother* each day, generating three to four thousand dollars a day for charity. "Every day, I pick a charity and send them 500 dollars. The cameos only take an hour or so, but it's so gratifying and amazing to be able to help people in this way. Finding a way to help has made such a difference in my life."

SELF-CARE REFLECTION #46

A theme that resonates throughout Jann's profile is gratitude. Gratitude for her creative talent, for the beauty of nature, for her family and friends. The "fine people she has in her life" sustain her. What are you most grateful for? How do you show up for the "fine people" in your life?

FINDING WISDOM IN OUR LONG CONVERSATION

Learning to treat herself with kindness has also allowed her to model the behavior for others. "I don't tolerate any kind of meanness or people speaking down to themselves or other people." She admits that it is sometimes hard for her to watch others figure out their journeys and must constantly remind herself that there is no shortcut in life. Everyone must put in the time and be allowed to make their own mistakes. We gain wisdom through what Jann calls the "long conversation."

She told me, "The longest conversation we have in life is the one we have with ourselves. Our inner dialogue, the focus of our thoughts, how we problem-solve are all part of an active conversation where key questions are asked and big decisions are made every day. When you realize the very discussion you have with yourself shapes how you navigate your life and that it is the real difference between failure and success, things change. Some people miss the value of this conversation or push it aside because it somehow seems too esoteric when really it is our most treasured possession. I mean, everything I've done in my life is based upon how I've encouraged myself. When I was younger, I didn't give myself the mental space to redirect or reevaluate my conversations. This limited me, and

I allowed it. Eventually, I realized that I'm the one that's creating 'this' or not creating 'that.' Our thoughts are real tangible things that have a big impact on how life plays out."

A champion of her gender, she says, "The whole narrative about women being marginalized as they age and hit some best-before date after the kids move out needs to change. Women waiting for the other shoe to drop — for a younger woman to come up and take over — is a mistake. Women should be wielding their knowledge, their wisdom, and their sage experience with confidence."

Jann celebrates who she is. She is not looking for the fountain of youth. She does not complain of aging or list the things that used to come easier. She keeps her thoughts focused on becoming the person she always hoped she would be — a crone. In *If I Knew Then*, she writes, "If I'm lucky, one day, a very old face will look back at me from the mirror, a face I once shied away from. I will love that old woman ferociously because she has finally figured out how to live a life of purpose — not in spite of, but because of, all her mistakes and failures."

"Women **waiting for the other shoe to drop** — for a younger woman to come up and take over — is a mistake. Women should be wielding their **knowledge**, their **wisdom**, and their **sage experience with confidence.**"

If **play brings us such joy** and is a positive healing force, why have so many of us forgotten how to do it? **Why are we so quick to dismiss it** as frivolous? At what age does it begin to feel **inaccessible, unproductive, or self-indulgent**?

NURTURE MENTAL FITNESS

7 WELLNESS RITUALS
FOR HEALTH, STRENGTH & HOPE

WELLNESS RITUAL #7: THE SCIENCE

> Play allows you to be creative while enhancing your imagination and emotional strength. Time spent in play provides an essential source of relaxation and has been shown to help relieve stress, improve brain function, and enhance relationships. Its regular practice also helps keep you young, develops critical social connections, and incentivizes additional healthy practices. All of our twenty-one mentors play hard and often do some of their best thinking when having fun.

When are you at your best? You might answer, "Well, Dwight, it's when I'm in 'the zone'" or "When I've had a good night's sleep" or "When I feel inspired by the people around me." All excellent answers. Here's what the research tells us. We put in our best effort when we are creative, playful, and trying new things. This was the belief of Friedrich Froebel, a German educator (1782–1852) who coined the word "kindergarten" and laid the foundation for early childhood education. Froebel considered play essential to human development, believing play helped children see how they connect with nature and the world around them.

He promoted early experimentation through play, arguing it was the best way to foster out-of-the-box thinkers primed to face life's challenges with a positive, creative mindset. Froebel wrote, "How a child plays is the forerunner of how they will work as an adult."[1] In the beginning, his kindergarten was thought by many to be a foolish waste of time where children played the day away on hillsides, planting gardens, playing with blocks, and looking after pets. Froebel pushed back, insisting that play requires a spirit of curiosity that engages the mind, body, and spirit. He believed play takes effort, imagination, dedication, patience, vision, and fortitude and is the truest expression of what is in a child's soul.[1]

Barbara Corbett, Ph.D., applied the teaching philosophy of Froebel for close to fifty years as director of the Froebel Education Centre in Mississauga, Ontario. In her book, *A Garden of Children,* she writes, "If we watch a child at play, we notice that although play requires a great deal of energy, it seems almost effortless. It flows easily and naturally. The playing child is happy, animated, and full of life. There is vitality in all she does, and at the very center of play is joyfulness."[2]

Joy through play is available to adults too.

When was the last time you truly let go and played for fun or were brought to tears of laughter in the company of others?

THE SCIENCE BEHIND "DON'T WORRY, BE HAPPY"

The field of positive psychology considers play foundational to our well-being. Psychologists now study that-which-makes-life-worth-living with the same keen interest they have had for despair for decades. The emphasis on all-things-fun marks a shift from traditional research on disorders and disease to the criteria that help our minds thrive. Experts are coming to realize that a working clinical understanding of mental illness does not qualify you as a happiness expert. Human happiness is complicated and follows a different set of parameters.

Martin Seligman and Mihaly Csikszentmihalyi, champions of positivity, define the joyfulness adults discover in play and the study of positive psychology this way:

> "It is about well-being, contentment, and satisfaction in the past; hope and optimism for the future; and flow and happiness in the present. At the individual level, it is about positive traits: the capacity for love and vocation, courage, interpersonal skill, aesthetic sensibility, perseverance, forgiveness, originality, future-mindedness, spirituality, high talent, and wisdom. At the group level, it is about the civic virtues and the institutions that move individuals toward better citizenship: responsibility, nurturance, altruism, civility, moderation, tolerance, and work ethic."[3]

While happiness is difficult to define and challenging to measure, the field of positive psychology shows us that happy people are more likely to be productive, creative, helpful, and enjoy good health. Happiness does not merely feel good; it also appears to benefit the health and ability of individuals and their communities.[4]

327

But if play brings us such joy and is a positive healing force, why have so many of us forgotten how to do it? Why are we so quick to dismiss it as frivolous? At what age does it begin to feel inaccessible, unproductive, or self-indulgent? When I presented a sample manuscript of this book to one publishing executive, he shared that while the evidence supporting the Wellness Rituals is well documented, he felt the mentors' "privileged lives" positioned the rituals out of reach for the average individual. The universal biological requirements for good health and the shared wisdom offered by the mentors were lost on him. The very idea that success controls our access to happiness or healing is not only tragically wrong; it is responsible for the reactive mindset that has contributed to our poor health. Needless to say, this was not the publishing house for my book. When did this type of limited thinking become so prevalent? The idea that once we reach adulthood, it is time for us to get down with the seriousness of life will stop us well short of our potential.

The research supporting adult play is strong, and to set the record straight, the health benefits of play are not dependent on a job title, professional influence, or bank balance. Play is accessible to everyone. It is nurturing. It is invigorating, and it eases our burden and renews our optimism. Studies have shown a direct link between play and improved creativity, imagination, energy levels, problem-solving ability, stress resiliency, cognitive function, mindfulness, and enhanced relationships.[3]

Play is not just for kids. Welcome to Wellness Ritual #7: Play with Purpose.

WHAT IS PLAY?

To answer this question, I turned to the happiness experts. *New York Times* bestselling author of *The Happiness Advantage* and *Big Potential*, psychologist Shawn Achor, believes happiness is not just a mood — it's a work ethic.[5,6] Considered one of the world's leading experts on human potential, his TED talk *The Happy Secret to Better Work* has over 16,000,000 views. Watch it if you haven't seen it. Watch it again if you have. Stories of "Amy the Unicorn" and "Bobo" will bring a smile to your face, and Shawn's delivery will inspire action. When asked for his definition of happiness, Shawn describes it as "the joy you feel when you are moving toward your potential. It is the belief that change is possible."[7] This is the essence of playing with purpose.

Sitting down with Oprah to record a *Super Soul Sunday* episode, Shawn shared that "we can use our brain to change how we process the world, and that in turn changes how we react to it."[7] He explains that we are taught to believe that we are what happens to us, but this is not the case. We are much more than the sum of our genetics and our environment. Research shows that happiness is a choice that profoundly affects our health, even when life is difficult. The forces of nature versus nurture may establish an initial happiness baseline. Still, with a few small positive changes, Achor states that you can significantly shift happiness and optimism at any age and elevate the quality of your sleep, energy, and overall well-being. He says, "When we are happy — when our mindset and mood are positive — we are smarter, more motivated, and thus more successful. Happiness is the center, and success revolves around it."[5] More on this theme to come.

Dr. Stuart Brown, psychiatrist, founder of the National Institute for Play, and bestselling author of *Play: How it Shapes the Brain, Opens the Imagination, and Invigorates the Soul*, writes, "Play is a state of mind that one has when absorbed in an activity that provides enjoyment and a suspension of sense of time. It is self-motivated, so you want to do it again and again."[8] He defines play as a process, not a thing or a particular action. Having studied play for years, he sees it as time spent "without" purpose and emphasizes the experience of play.

Brené Brown, research professor, lecturer, podcast host, and author of 6 #1 *New York Times* bestsellers, including *Atlas of the Heart*, *Dare to Lead*, *Daring Greatly*, and *The Gifts of Imperfection*, considers play essential to wholehearted living. She writes, "Play — doing things just because they're fun and not because they'll help achieve a goal — is vital to human development."[9] She too defines play as time spent without purpose and adds that it is doing something you don't want to end that leads to a loss of self-consciousness. Like Froebel, Brown believes play is at the very core of creativity and innovation.

Deepak Chopra calls on us to awaken our inner child to the joys of play. He writes, "Your inner child isn't just a memory. It is the aspect of your awareness that wants to feel joy, innocence, and freedom."[10] He believes that when we experience true play, there is a strong desire to want to stay in that amazing state of freedom and fearlessness that play allows. To bring playfulness back into your life, Chopra encourages adults to return to the source of their awareness of the human need for this joy. He says, "On the surface of the mind is a constant stream of thoughts, feelings, sensations, and images. This stream of consciousness is distracting and demanding. It never stops; it never ends in its demands. Yet, at a deeper level, what really matters isn't mind-made. All the qualities that make life worthwhile spring from a deeper source."[10]

Wayne Dyer's description of play and our struggle to prioritize it in adulthood may be my favorite. He wrote, "It is never too late to have a happy childhood."[11] As an internationally renowned author and speaker in the fields of self-development and spiritual growth, Wayne spent much of his career encouraging adults to continue to explore the wonders of the world with the curiosity of a child. He believed that we don't have to give up being an adult to be more childlike and that the fully integrated person can simultaneously be both. "When you dance, your purpose is not to get to a certain place on the floor. It's to enjoy each step along the way," he shared.[12]

Play means something different to everyone. Some people love walking barefoot in the grass, some love a Sunday morning crossword puzzle, and some love to sing in the shower. I was recently at a friend's home for a weekend barbeque when my friend's three-year-old son, Gavin, grabbed my hand and said, "Let me show you the potato bugs." I knew Gavin to be a thoughtful, happy, inquisitive little boy through stories his father had shared with me, but I hadn't seen him since he was still learning to walk. The fact that I was a stranger didn't seem to matter to him. I was a friend of his dad's, which was good enough for him. Fearlessly, he approached a group of adults gathered in his backyard, took my hand and guided me down a wood-chipped path. Near its edge, he proudly lifted a stone to show me the little creatures. I'm not sure if it was our discovery of three potato bugs and a slug hiding under that rock or his opportunity to share the backyard potato bug secret with me, but his amazement of the world he revealed was spectacular. Our shared moment still brings a smile to my face.

There isn't a right or a wrong way to play. The only requirement, in my opinion, is the intention or "purpose" to leave enough time for it to happen. Had I narrowed my focus to the conversation I was having with the other adults in my friend's backyard, I would have missed out on the gift Gavin gave me that afternoon. Play experts universally agree that play is best experienced "without purpose." But if we are to prioritize the experience as adults and give ourselves permission to rediscover our childhood sense of wonder, we must be purposeful in our commitment to play, and then let it unfold without expectation.

PLEASURE VS. HAPPINESS

When looking to bring more play into our lives, it is important to understand the difference between activities that generate momentary pleasure from those that develop long-term happiness. I appreciate that this might seem like I'm splitting hairs at a quick glance, but biologically, there is a significant difference between the two. How we play matters.

To simplify the neuroscience, play has a biological ripple effect. Every time you play, your body releases chemicals that interact with pleasure and pain receptors in your brain. The experience of "runner's high" or the euphoric state that follows a particularly good workout happens because of how endorphins affect our brain following active play. The altered chemical state can lead to a more positive outlook, improve immune response, and reduce stress levels. It has been shown to help block sources of pain.

Quick experiences of pleasure that trigger our dopamine reward centers tell our brains that we want more and to repeat whatever activity just happened.[14] Our brains are brilliant at quickly linking feelings of enjoyment with a pleasurable activity to encourage repetition of a rewarding behavior. Dopamine is now thought to play a significant role in encoding the memories associated with a reward to ensure we know how to achieve the experience again.[14] Like any other biological process, this trigger must be kept in check if we are to continue to enjoy good health.

To help ease the burden of stress and routine, we need the release that pleasurable experiences provide; in moderation, they are essential to healthy psychological function and well-being.[15] However, if highly arousing, quick pleasure activities are our only source of play, we risk overstimulating our dopamine reward pathways, which can result in addictive behaviors and self-destructive habits. Overindulging in tasty foods, video games, pornography, social media, or illicit drugs all trigger our dopamine reward circuitry. Making healthy choices and practicing self-control with our play is imperative to maintaining good health. Over time, if our bodies become reliant on higher levels of dopamine to experience the rewarding feeling our brains have come to expect, we can put our health at risk and push our happiness out of reach. This dopamine dominance can be a slippery slope. In addition to its link to addiction, it has been shown to decrease our serotonin levels.[14,16]

Serotonin is our contentment neurotransmitter. It tells our brain our needs are met and is associated with feelings of happiness and fulfillment. It also plays a vital role in supporting our memory, learning, body temperature, sleep, sexual behavior, and hunger. Lack of serotonin is thought to play a role in depression, anxiety, and other mental health conditions.[17] By consuming foods containing tryptophan (the amino acid used to make serotonin), like salmon, eggs, turkey, tofu, pineapples, nuts, and seeds, you can increase your serotonin. Ten to fifteen minutes of daily exposure to direct sunlight and engaging in regular active play also help to boost and balance our body's serotonin levels.

Many of the mentor profiles highlight the essential value of adversity and showcase how life's struggles often unlock our greatest accomplishments and most profound feelings of joy and happiness. This raises an important point. Not all activities that result in high levels of enjoyment are fun. Marriage, parenting a child, training for a marathon, losing weight, rehabbing an injury, learning a new language, completing a degree, launching a business, and volunteering all take effort and are certainly not always a good time. When we push our physical limits and challenge our minds through profound experiences like these, we often stumble across the most meaningful moments of our lives. Fear, uncertainty, pain, or feelings of vulnerability can trap us in the exclusive pursuit of short-term, pleasure-seeking behaviors and rob us of the increased health and happiness achieved through more meaningful commitments. If the next dopamine release must be as strong or stronger than the previous one, we can chemically compromise our ability to feel happiness.[15] Watching television may allow you to unwind and relax from a challenging day, which on some days, is a welcomed reward, but is it a habit that adds to your level of happiness?

Nine out of ten Canadian adults spend an average of twenty-one hours per week watching TV or video content on a screen or device.[18] What happiness or health benefits can be claimed from this use of time?

I have worked with many athletes who have battled through tremendous hardship to find their way back to the starting line-up and compete again. On the day they return to play, the gratitude they express for their body's ability to heal and the opportunity for a second shot elevates their love for the game they play to a level often unknown to them prior to their injury.

On a more personal note, I have completed the Bataan Memorial Death March Marathon twice. The race is held annually in the high desert terrain of the White Sands Missile Range in New Mexico and commemorates the heroic service members who defended the Philippine Islands during World War II. Given the spirit of the race, it is appropriately brutal and sets a high bar in its test of participants' physical and mental capacity. The training for this event is punishing, and the race is grueling, but the experience of crossing the finish line is one of the highlights of my life. Despite the suffering, not only did I return a second time, but I have recently begun considering running it again. If I may again quote Milhay Cskiszentmihalyi, "The best moments in our lives are not the passive, receptive, relaxing times — although such experiences can also be enjoyable if we have worked hard to attain them. The best moments usually occur when a person's body or mind is stretched to its limits in a voluntary effort to accomplish something difficult and worthwhile."

Dr. Robert Lustig, author of *The Hacking of the American Mind: The Science Behind the Corporate Takeover of our Bodies and Brains,* defines the following seven fundamental differences between pleasure-seeking dopamine and happiness-promoting serotonin.[19,20]

1. Pleasure is short-lived; happiness is long-lived.
2. Pleasure is visceral; happiness is ethereal.
3. Pleasure is taking; happiness is giving.
4. Pleasure can be achieved with substances; happiness cannot.
5. Pleasure is often experienced alone; happiness is often experienced in social groups.
6. Extremes of pleasure lead to addiction, whether they be substances or behaviors. There is no such thing as being addicted to too much happiness.
7. Pleasure is tied to dopamine; happiness is tied to serotonin.

FINDING FLOW IN PLAY

There is no mistaking the experience of "flow." Think of it as your sweet spot — when you are so immersed in an activity that nothing else matters, time no longer holds any meaning, fear of failure falls away, and distractions fade into the background. In this state, self-consciousness disappears as you strike a balance between your unique personal challenges and skills.

Cskiszentmihalyi describes the essence of flow as removing the interference of the thinking mind.[13] When NBA superstar Stephen Curry releases a three-pointer in the heat of a game, he is not questioning his ability to make the shot or considering his elbow angle. When Vladimir Guerrero Jr. hits a baseball 467 ft. that explodes off his bat at 118 mph, he is not thinking about weight transfer or bat speed. On my Bataan race day, I wasn't thinking of my running mechanics. In flow, the stepping stones of skill development and self-doubt are left behind.

Csikszentmihalyi offers the following five ways to create more flow in life:[13]

Flow is a dynamic balance between anxiety, where the difficulty is too high for your skill level, and boredom, where the difficulty is too low. The enjoyment experienced in flow inspires people to face more complex challenges and push their personal development. The need for Jim Leech to narrow his focus to the safe placement of his next step in the final stretch of his expedition to the North Pole or Silken Laumann's remarkable recovery to return to the Barcelona Olympics are perfect examples of these five strategies in action.

Our brains can only process so much information at a time. Csikszentmihalyi points out that while in flow, nearly all of the brain's available inputs are devoted to one activity. This is why the perception of time changes, discomfort goes unnoticed, and random negative thoughts don't enter the mind.[13] The brain is too busy focusing on one thing to keep track of anything else. The practice of mindfulness or the mental energy encouraged during meditation or yoga provides a similar escape.

SET GOALS THAT HAVE CLEAR
AND IMMEDIATE FEEDBACK.

BECOME IMMERSED IN THE
PARTICULAR ACTIVITY.

PAY ATTENTION TO WHAT IS
HAPPENING IN THE MOMENT.

LEARN TO ENJOY THE
IMMEDIATE EXPERIENCE.

PROPORTION YOUR SKILLS TO
THE CHALLENGE AT HAND.

PLAY FOR LIFE

Many studies demonstrate that happy people experience better health.[21-25] Positive emotions are associated with more robust immune system responses to infection,[24,26] healthier levels of heart rate variability, and reduced cardiovascular disease.[25,27] Negative emotions have been shown to harm cardiovascular, immune, and endocrine systems.[4,21] Depressed individuals are more likely to be obese, twice as likely to smoke, and tend to exercise less.[4] But what is the underlying physiological mechanism between our subjective well-being and our health?

One prominent theory is that people who play are happier and healthier because they are more likely to practice healthy behaviors. Another theory is that play is strongly linked to positive, fulfilling social relationships, which accounts for the bump in health that accompanies the ritual of playing with purpose.

It appears both are true. Playful, happy people are more likely to eat well, get enough sleep, and stay active while cultivating a sense of belonging and commitment to a social network, which is also vital to good health.

Social connections and meaningful relationships both cause happiness and are formed from happiness as play increases sociability and improves the quality of our social interactions. Mentor Michael Richardson's cycling crew is an excellent example of this social advantage. Dr. Robyne Hanley-Dafoe's work discussed in Wellness Ritual #6 highlights the impact belonging has on resiliency. There is no doubt that the presence of meaningful, supportive relationships in our lives, even just one or two, boosts our health. But this still doesn't answer the question of how.

Can our mindset elevate our health, or is it the other way around? While more research is needed here, positive psychologists have shown a strong causal link between happiness and health. Joy is associated with lower heart rates, lower cortisol levels, reduced inflammation, improved heart and immune function, and even slow disease progression.[28-30] Another study found that levels of optimism could be used to predict future health outcomes, such as mortality and cancer fatality.[31] Adding strength to this evidence are studies showing how positive emotions can undo the ill-effects of negativity by speeding physiological recovery.[28-30] Not only do negative emotions predict mortality, but positive emotions predict longevity. In short, the higher your life satisfaction, the greater your life expectancy.[28-30]

335

Shawn Achor explains that negative emotions narrow our focus and action down to our triggered fight or flight response, whereas positive emotions broaden the number of possibilities we process, making us more thoughtful, creative, and open to new ideas.[5] Research shows that individuals primed to experience joy or contentment are capable of thinking a wider array of thoughts and ideas than individuals primed to feel either anxiety or anger.[32] By broadening our cognition and behavior, positive emotions make us more creative and help us build more intellectual, social, and physical resources that we can call on down the road. Achor calls this broadening effect a "real biological chemical advantage" over negative thinkers. As our brains become flooded with dopamine and serotonin, we feel good, but we also level up our brains' learning centers, allowing us to organize new information, keep that information in the brain longer, and retrieve it faster later on.[5]

Playfulness also appears to elevate the mood of those around us. Mirror neurons in our brains activate when seeing someone else having fun, laughing, or smiling. Even if we are not feeling happy or have been explicitly told not to smile ourselves, it is practically impossible to hold back a smile when another directs kindness and a smile in our direction. Achor calls smiles contagious and explains that our brains are designed to be connected through mirror neurons, allowing us to co-process the world and share our emotional response.[5] This wireless connection operates at lightning speed. Studies show that our brains can identify emotion in another person's facial expression within thirty-three milliseconds and respond the same way just as quickly.[33] When three strangers enter a room, the most emotionally expressive person has been shown to transmit their mood non-verbally to the others within just two minutes.[34]

HOW TO INTEGRATE PLAY

According to play expert Dr. Stuart Brown, "if we stop play, our behavior becomes fixed."[8] Here are some strategies he recommends to incorporate more play into your life and prevent that from happening.

1. **Reframe the idea of play.** Give yourself permission to play every day. Play can mean simply talking to your dog, dancing in your home, or listening to your

favorite album. Any time you think play is a waste, remember that it offers serious health benefits for you and others. He calls play "the purest expression of love."

2. **Record a play history.** Brown suggests we mine our past for play memories. What did you do as a child that excited you? Did you engage in those activities alone, with others, or both? How can you recreate that today?

3. **Surround yourself with playful people.** Choose to spend time with friends and family members who are playful. Positive people are not necessarily happy all the time, but their outlook tends to lean toward the glass being half full, not half empty. Their positive energy and smile will help elevate your mood and make it easier for you to stay focused on the practice of this Wellness Ritual.

4. **Play with little ones.** Through play, children learn to express themselves verbally and non-verbally in creative and imaginative ways. They are fearless, open, curious, and creative when allowed to play without structure. Getting on the floor and playing with a child is one of the best ways to connect with your playful inner spirit.

CHAPIN CLINICAL CORNER

"Play is not trivial, it is highly serious and of deep significance."
– Friedrich Froebel

If your most important personal relationships feel more like obligatory job sharing, you need to sit down with your loved ones and figure out how to introduce more play into your lives. Play is one of the most effective ways to keep relationships fresh and exciting. Playing together brings joy, vitality, and resilience to your relationships. Play can also help heal resentments, disagreements, and hurt feelings. Regular play teaches us to trust one another and feel safe, enabling us to work together, open ourselves to intimacy, and try new things.[35] By consciously incorporating more humor and play into your daily interactions, you can improve the quality of your romantic relationships and your connections with co-workers, family members, and friends.[35]

To help my patients burdened by the weight of their responsibilities or pain rediscover joy, I encourage them to follow Shawn Achor's recommended daily happiness exercises. Having tested his claim that these exercises are proven to make anyone, from a four-year-old to an eighty-four-year-old happier, I can confirm their effectiveness. "Scientifically, happiness is a choice," Achor says. He explains that research has shown you can rewire your brain to make yourself happy by practicing these six simple happiness exercises every day for three weeks.[7]

ACHOR'S SIX DAILY HAPPINESS EXERCISES

1. **Gratitude Exercises.** Write down three things you're grateful for that occurred over the last twenty-four hours. They don't have to be profound. It could be a beautiful sunrise or catching every green light on the way to work, but you must

choose three different things every day and be very specific in your description. If you write, "I am grateful for my partner," it doesn't work. But if you write, "I am grateful for my partner because he or she gave me a kiss as I left the house, and this means I'm loved," you can begin to shift the brain's pattern of thinking. This practice trains your brain to scan the world in a new way as you search for and recognize positive experiences instead of steeping in threats and negativity all day. Achor calls this practice the fastest way of teaching optimism. By being thankful for our health, loved ones, and the beauty found in nature, including potato bugs, we give birth to delight and curiosity and open ourselves to a willingness to be surprised. This is the spirit of play. After twenty-one days, the actual practice of this gratitude exercise seems to matter less than the fact that you have dedicated time every day to look for happiness.

2. **The Happiness Doubler.** Take one positive experience from the past twenty-four hours and spend two minutes writing down every detail about that experience that you can remember. As you relive this moment, your brain labels it as meaningful, deepening the event's imprint and positive ripple effect. Our brains can't tell the difference between visualization and actual experience, so this practice allows you to multiply the positive biological response to the best part of your day.

3. **The Fun Fifteen.** Do fifteen minutes of cardiovascular activity, like walking around the block daily with a friend, neighbor, or dog. This shouldn't be difficult if you are practicing Wellness Ritual #4: Move to Stay Young. In an interview with the *Washington Post*, Achor states this practice is "equivalent to taking antidepressants for the first six months, but with a 30% lower relapse rate over the next two years."[36] This is not a repudiation of antidepressants, but rather a testament to the positive impact exercise has on our mental health.

4. **Meditation.** Every day, take two minutes to stop whatever you're doing and concentrate on slow, deep, rhythmic breathing. A short mid-day mindfulness break like this can result in a calmer, happier outlook. Achor did this at Google and had employees back away from their computers for two minutes a day and simply

watch their breath go in and out. The practice raised accuracy rates, improved reported levels of happiness, and reduced daily stress.[36]

5. **Conscious Acts of Kindness.** At the start of every day, send a short positive email or text praising or thanking one person you know. Our brains become addicted to feeling good by making others feel good. Reach out to old friends, mentors, teachers, coaches, and colleagues and thank them for their influence on your life. The added bonus of this practice is that your inbox will start filling up with positivity as your community responds to your kindness.

6. **Deepen Social Connections.** Spend time with family and friends. Our social connections are among the best predictors of long-term health and life expectancy. Carve out time daily to connect with those who matter most to you and give them your full attention.

If you are stuck in a fight or flight response, you are constantly training your brain to be on the lookout for threats. Over time, this focus limits your thinking and perspective to the negativity in your life and leaves little room for optimism or play. Practicing the six exercises above for the next three weeks can break a pattern of heightened negativity.

RITUAL ACTIVATION

"Be miserable. Or motivate yourself. Whatever has to be done, it's always your choice."
– Wayne Dyer

RITUAL TARGET

1. **Explore your play history.** How did you play as a kid? What games, activities, or places gave you pleasure in your youth? How can you recreate a similar experience now? As a child, I spent a fair bit of time in the summer on the beaches of Lake Huron. Days were spent playing in the sand and battling waves with my siblings to exhaustion. The sound of a seagull, an orange sky at sunset, and the feel of sand between my toes still remind me of those happy childhood memories. When I return to the Great Lake beaches now as an adult, I experience an instant connection to that time in my life. It is my happy place.

2. **Look for opportunities to be playful and spread joy.** Smile and say hello to at least five strangers today. Thanks to the dominant action of our mirror neurons, all five are likely to smile back. I like to think of this as a smile wave (similar to the "wave" baseball fans start at a park — a great example of young and old at play). If you come across a friend who needs an emotional boost, surprise them with their favorite drink from the local coffee shop or mail them a funny card. Receiving personal mail by post stands out in today's world. Remember to laugh as much as possible.

3. **Give yourself permission to have fun.** Once a week, put your phone down, turn off the TV, and give yourself the time and permission to do something that

341

makes you happy. Be spontaneous with your use of this time, set aside your inhibitions, and try something fun. Look for opportunities to change your pace. Go to the park with a friend, child, or grandchild to throw a Frisbee, fly a kite, or take a ride on the swing set. Call up a friend and catch a movie or local band. Host a game night with friends or neighbors. The point is to be silly and carefree.

4. **Get active.** Practice Wellness Ritual #4.

5. **Just play.** Other than your commitment to play, there are no rules. The more unstructured and spontaneous your play, the better.

IN SUMMARY

We often give up play as adults for more serious pursuits. Reclaim your childish wonder and playful spirit, and you will unlock a long list of far-reaching health benefits, including stress reduction, improved immune response and cardiovascular health, and a boost in memory, creativity, and problem-solving ability. Play nurtures our personal happiness and enhances the quality of our relationships and connections to our community. Discovering happiness through play is an indication that you are moving toward your biological potential. This practice is a choice you can make even when life is hard.

AFTERWORD

MY LESSONS LEARNED

The space provided to record your family medical history on most clinical intake forms is often too small. My family's genetic vulnerability is a mixed bag of tricks that features many of the frequent flyers, including heart disease, diabetes, high cholesterol, stroke, chronic gall-bladder disease, cancer, macular degeneration, depression, attention-deficit disorder, dyslexia, obesity, osteoarthritis, and Alzheimer's disease. Sadly, when you examine the ailments your relatives bring to the table, I'm guessing your list isn't much different.

Determined to push the health, performance, and longevity marks established by the Chapins before me, I prioritize my health and keep an eye on trouble spots. Given the nature of my work, how could I look a patient in the eye and hold them accountable if I couldn't demonstrate an ability to take good care of myself?

At fifty years old, I am within five pounds of the weight I was when I graduated from university over twenty-five years ago. I eat well, exercise daily, and for the most part, approach each day with a sense of curiosity and excitement. My mother likes to remind me that my sense of wonder was fostered during my early Froebelian education. They say mothers know best. In my case, it is hard to argue with that logic; my mother was also my senior kindergarten teacher. I trust her theory that early encouragement to play helped shape my positive outlook and believe my playfulness makes me a better husband, father, and clinician. Gray hair and wrinkles at the corners of my eyes reflect the years I've lived, but I still feel as healthy and strong today as I did at thirty-five.

Outside of the odd common cold or sports injury, I enjoyed good health for the better part of my thirties and forties. Confident I had crafted a winning formula, I made an appointment for a comprehensive executive health exam a month before my forty-ninth birthday. The timing of this appointment was important to me and had been circled on my calendar for over two decades.

In my mid-twenties, I went home one weekend to visit my parents and catch one of my brother's baseball games. While my father was hitting fly balls to the boys before the game, he started to experience sudden and severe chest and left arm pain. The widowmaker, a name given to the blockage in one of the major blood pipelines to the heart, had also decided to catch the ball game that particular day, and it was knocking at my dad's front door for a ticket. A few days later, my father lay in a hospital bed recovering from an angioplasty and stent in his left anterior descending coronary artery. At fifty years old, he had narrowly escaped an early death from a heart that had reached its breaking point.

My father is not a smoker or drinker. He lives an active life and has kept his weight in check, knowing his genetic predisposition to high cholesterol. Stress was his vice, and it had a hold of him. Seeing him in the hospital was the first chink in his armor I had ever witnessed, and his vulnerability and the thought of losing him rocked my world.

On the day of his surgery, I remember thinking how lucky we were. He had cheated death, and I was given a twenty-five-year head start on ensuring I didn't end up with the same ill-tempered visitor at my front door. Shortly after, I set a course to reverse engineer his experience, determined to keep my heart healthy and stress in check. This master plan included scheduling a full cardiac review thirteen months ahead of my half-century milestone birthday.

With borderline arrogance, I went to this appointment expecting to be told I was in excellent health. I was putting in the work and felt I deserved a healthy score card that revealed a widening gap between my chronological and biological age. Unfortunately, that was not the case.

Even though I was practicing what I believed at the time to be a healthy lifestyle, I had become complacent in my habits and lost track of my health metrics.

With cholesterol levels at an alarmingly high level, I was quickly referred for a stress echocardiogram, a test done to assess how well the heart works under stress, and a cardiac CT calcium score to assess the amount of calcified plaque in my heart. Optimal total cholesterol values are below 5.2 mmol/L, with LDL cholesterol below 2.0 mmol/L.[1] My numbers were 7.4 and 5.6 respectively. Thankfully, the coronary artery disease that often accompanies high cholesterol levels was minimal, and given my lifestyle, I was considered a decent candidate for primary prevention.

At this point, my work on this book had already begun, so I shared its premise with my cardiologist and family doctor as we met to discuss my blood work and cardiac test scores. Together we agreed to attack my risk profile with a very low dose of statin and the practice of the mentors' 7 Wellness Rituals and re-evaluate my progress in six months. By spring 2021, my total cholesterol was down to 4.0 mmol/L and LDL to 2.5 mmol/L. By early 2022, I had reduced my cardiac risk from the highest to the lowest category. My total cholesterol was 3.4 mmol/L and my LDL was 1.9 mmol/L.

> ❝ **I needed to go all in if I was to avoid heart disease and live a long life, which meant I had to break my formula down and rebuild it from the ground up.**

I'll never forget when my cardiologist called with the good news. Initially, he wanted me on a much higher dose of statins. He had agreed to support my desire to treat my condition with the aggressive practice of the Wellness Rituals and a very conservative statin dose if I could demonstrate the ability to get my LDL levels below 2.0 mmol/L. When I did, he shared that I had rejuvenated his enthusiasm for primary prevention and the value of healthy lifestyle practices. He admitted that our conversation stood out as an anomaly in his world. He had become accustomed to delivering bad news or increasing patients' medications. Learning this made me even more determined to bring this book to you.

I needed to go all in if I was to avoid heart disease and live a long life, which meant I had to break my formula down and rebuild it from the ground up.

Drawing from the mentors' formulas and the science behind their excellence, I identified seven key issues with my lifestyle and made the following changes:

KEY ISSUE #1:
I needed to recognize the emotional toll working as a primary care practitioner during the pandemic had on my health. I was tired, stressed, unhappy, and uncertain about my future.

FORMULA TWEAKS:

By limiting alcohol consumption to the occasional glass of wine with dinner, reducing my coffee consumption and limiting it to the morning, and practicing a consistent pre-sleep ritual, my sleep quality improved dramatically. Jim Treliving warned me of the dangers that lay waiting if I did not prioritize the importance of rest. Claudette McGowan, Jim Leech, and Pattie Lovett-Reid helped me establish the structure my recovery practice was lacking. I now get seven to eight hours of sleep seven days a week, even if it means I'm teased for being the first to bed in our family or for cutting social engagements short. Like Claudette, I no longer need an alarm clock. Inspired by Greg Wells' practice of cold water immersion, I now spend the last thirty seconds of my morning shower standing under cold water and once again feel renewed, ready to answer Jim's challenge to bring my "A-game" to the day.

I begin to prepare for bed an hour before I want to be asleep. Most nights, this is 10 p.m., but when it isn't, Dr. Robyne has helped me adapt and recalibrate to a three-day average. My pre-bed ritual includes connecting with my wife and sons, reading, watching sports, and completing a ten-minute meditation. I no longer check work email after 7 p.m. or watch the late-night news.

KEY ISSUE #2:
I needed to change what and when I was eating to achieve my cholesterol targets.

FORMULA TWEAKS:

At first, this realization came as a surprise. I thought my diet was heart healthy, but after meeting with a registered dietitian, I quickly realized where further improvements could be made. Jen Sygo's story inspired me to face this challenge with a sense of adventure. It encouraged me to embrace variety in my diet by experimenting with new fruits, vegetables, and food preparation techniques. I have significantly reduced my red meat consumption, have made an effort to eat fish once or twice a week, and consume a rainbow of fruits and vegetables every day. I have also started eating a vegetarian diet one day a week. If I crave a dessert, it is now fruit or, occasionally, a small bowl of frozen yogurt. I dropped lunch meat, bacon, white rice, cheese, and fast food on the fly.

My breakfast is usually oatmeal with cinnamon, walnuts, and a little honey or an egg-white omelet with a mix of chopped veggies. Dr. Greg Wells reminded me of the value of healthy snacking between meals, and I now have fuel stashes in my car, briefcase, and office. Mid-morning, I'll have a handful of nuts and berries or one of Jeffrey Latimer's protein-rich, antioxidant power shakes.

I pack a lunch, which is always leftovers from the night before or a power salad with protein, and try to finish dinner before 7:30 p.m. to extend the time before my next meal to eleven hours.

KEY ISSUE #3:
I needed to learn how to manage my energy differently to meet the elevated demands of my day.

FORMULA TWEAKS:
During the first year of the pandemic, days in the clinic were emotionally charged. Patients were scared and had limited access to care, which triggered their pain and anxiety. To keep up with the pace in the clinic, I had developed a bad habit of eating breakfast around 6:30 a.m. and then not eating again until 1:30 or 2 in the afternoon. By the time I took a break to have lunch, I was starving, had very low energy, and was not in the best of moods. After a ten-minute meal at my desk, I'd jump back into patient care. Looking back on this pattern, I can't believe I didn't recognize its negative impact on my performance, leadership, mood, creativity, and productivity. In serving others, I had forgotten to take care of myself.

Khamica Bingham and Pattie Lovett-Reid's disciplined focus on the fine detail of their self-care helped me recognize my mistakes. After speaking with Francois Olivier, I began searching for areas I could bring more balance and energy to my day. I was living the negative stress spiral he described, bouncing from one crisis to the next. His ability to press pause and intentionally slow his pace long enough to reset left a lasting impression on me.

When I asked him how he did it, he simply said, "At the end of the day, I know I've done my best. I go to sleep and start over again tomorrow. Every day has an end." This advice helped me bring my day to a controlled end too, and with practice, I've gotten quite good at it. Michael Grange's description of knowing when to let go of the rope also helped. I now enjoy greater satisfaction in my work.

KEY ISSUE #4:
I needed to introduce greater variety into my physical movement.

FORMULA TWEAKS:

On a typical week, I'll run twenty to twenty-five kilometers. Jogging helps me clear my mind and sharpen my problem-solving skills. I love the post-run euphoria, and I'm drawn to the simplicity and freedom running provides — no class schedules, no travel to the gym, and no equipment needed. Given my family cholesterol and cardiac issues, I now have another reason to run.

Drawing from Dr. Greg Wells and Silken Laumann's formula, I varied my runs and started experimenting with HIIT. My VO2 max scores (the amount of oxygen my body is able to utilize) quickly improved to levels considered above average for a man ten years younger.

As exciting as this trend was, I also found that my lower back and hamstrings were feeling tight and sore at the end of a long day in the clinic or a more strenuous workout. Turning to Dr. Andy Smith and Phillip Crawley's approach, I adapted my training and began investing more time in my flexibility. I may feel thirty-five, but the reality is that I am fifty.

Andy shared, "I am not obsessed with staying young, turning gray, or the passing of the clock. I am not motivated by trying to hold onto my youth or some idea of it. I live life with an intentional purpose to bring life to my years." With his voice echoing in my ear, I now practice a morning mobility routine, use a foam roller, schedule regular chiropractic and massage treatments, apply greater discipline to my pre-run dynamic warm up, and complete a longer, slower cool down. As a result, my muscle soreness and functional range of motion have improved.

I also started to take calls and meetings while walking. If Dr. Andy Smith can lead one of Canada's largest academic health institutions using this technique, my leadership would surely be better for it too.

KEY ISSUE #5
I needed to re-introduce resistance training into my 150 minutes of weekly activity.

FORMULA TWEAKS:

This one was harder for me. Growing up playing team sports, I've never been particularly drawn to lifting weights. I consider my 150 minutes of weekly activity non-negotiable, but my commitment to resistance training has always been a little soft. Knowing that, my cardiologist and exercise physiologist made a point of reminding me that resistance training helps the heart. I've set a recurring reminder that pops up on my phone every Friday morning to hold my focus. It reads, "Studies show resistance training for less than an hour a week is associated with roughly 40–70% decreased risk of cardiovascular disease and all-cause mortality, independent of aerobic exercise."[2]

Herbie Kuhn's passionate commitment to his running streak and Michael Grange's advice on how to kindly re-introduce exercise helped me pick up the weights again. Michael "Pinball" Clemons taught me how to weave it into my day with a smile. If the practice was going to stick, it had to be accessible and fun. After my morning mobility routine and every run, I now complete twenty-five push-ups. I have a set of free weights in my garage and a chin-up bar. When I get home from work, I'll complete at least five pull-ups or chin-ups before entering the house. When in and out of the garage doing chores on the weekend or between patients at the clinic, I practice my squat, lunge, hinge, push, pull, and carry with resistance. Without disruption, I've found a way to add resistance training to my week and feel stronger for it.

ISSUE #6:
I needed to be present.

FORMULA TWEAKS:

I was flirting with caregiver burnout and had developed an unhealthy focus on the threat waiting around the next corner. I was missing the present moment far too often, and I knew it, but I continued to struggle with breaking free from my routine and the busyness of my mind. With my fight or flight stress response in overdrive, I set normalizing my sleep routine as the first step. Alison Dantas' story helped me realize the importance of this. Everything feels heavier and harder in fatigue.

Meeting with a mental health expert helped me appreciate the value of establishing boundaries and creating time for myself. At first, "me-time" felt uncomfortable. If I wasn't busy doing something I perceived to be productive, it was hard for me to relax, and this would sometimes seed a feeling of anxiety. Randy Lennox helped me ride through this temporary storm with the practice of quiet solitude. Lynn Langrock showed me how to block time in my schedule as another tool to manage pace. I make sure some of this time is spent alone in nature and some is spent in prayer, meditation, and reflection. Now back on the left side of my stress response curve, the practice of Dr. Robyne's five pillars of resiliency keep me there. A trail not far from our home follows a small creek for miles. My mental fitness is stronger when I visit this creek at least once a week.

ISSUE #7:
I needed to have more fun.

FORMULA TWEAKS:

My life had become too serious, and I was missing my friends, sports, and travel. After speaking with Jann Arden, I was immediately drawn to her ability to find joy in life's everyday experiences and just be happy sitting on an apple crate. Life has taught her to be mindful of her thoughts and keep her inner dialogue kind. With so much to be grateful for, I intentionally changed the track playing in my head and started a daily gratitude practice. Suddenly, I was experiencing more "potato bug" moments. Riding the ripple effect of this joy, I discovered Shawn Achor's work and put his happiness exercises into action. I try to start a "smile wave" with my patients every day.

Michael Richardson and Lynn Langrock reminded me of the importance of our social connections and scheduling time for play and travel. I now make sure I always have at least one event with a good friend or family member scheduled in the near future. The planning and anticipation of these gatherings can be just as fun as the events themselves.

It took eighteen months to restore my health to the point where a performance formula could maintain it. I now possess the awareness and discipline to call on the biological power found within it. Implementing the 7 Wellness Rituals has given me a healthy heart despite the genetic hand I was dealt. This was my journey, and to test the merits of this book, I explored and pushed my comfort level within each of the 7 Wellness Rituals.

Your own journey to better health may have already begun, or maybe this book is the catalyst. I encourage you to apply each ritual in your day, as all of them are equally important in supporting your health and well-being; however, you do not need to place the same emphasis on all seven simultaneously. Weigh the outcomes of the rituals against your most pressing health challenges as a way to sequence them. Above all, be patient with yourself, practice self-care, and stay positive.

Regardless of where you start, you will benefit from the momentum generated by the simple choice to live a healthier life. This choice is the greatest gift you could give yourself. It is not bound by age or circumstance and is the first step you must take as you finish this book. The next step is to ask for help. Engage your existing healthcare team or begin building a new one that will support you in your journey. Empower this group to help you craft a formula built on the 7 Wellness Rituals that aligns with your current state of health, life stage, and performance goals.

The anticipation and acceptance of a decline in health as some sort of pre-programmed and inevitable part of aging is a common and closely held belief that must be left behind. Sure there are physical and mental realities associated with getting older, but these changes do not need to hold you back.

> 66 **Blaming pain, weight gain, disease, and dysfunction on age or a busy schedule while refusing to adapt is a heavy burden to carry and limits your potential.**

Our bodies are continuously repairing, rebuilding, and renewing. Our DNA is hard-wired to respond to the practice of the rituals shared in this book. Do not make the mistake I did and get locked into a routine that no longer serves your goals out of habit. Do not let your age or current health challenges prevent you from making healthier choices. It is never too late to improve your health and live life with joy and expectancy. Put the 7 Wellness Rituals to work, and your body's response will amaze you.

Take good care,

Dwight Chapin

SELF-CARE REFLECTION #47

For this last exercise, consider your current daily routine and commitment to self-care. In your journal, write down one Ritual Activation recommendation you are willing to implement immediately for each of the 7 Wellness Rituals. Post this list on your bathroom mirror and share your intention to put the evidence presented in this book to work with a loved one and your healthcare team. Take this step, and you will be on your way to a healthier, happier life.

_____

_____

_____

_____

_____

_____

_____

_____

_____

ACKNOWLEDGMENTS

I have heard it said by musicians that they did not choose the song that became their signature tune, but rather the song chose them. I think back on how this book came to be, and in a real sense, it chose me as its author in answer to a call that became louder every day as we emerged from the COVID-19 pandemic, and I witnessed my patients' fight to stay healthy in its aftermath. I understood my role in helping patients in clinical practice and had done enough writing to know that conveying advice on wellness in a book would take me into uncharted waters. I would have to go on a learning journey, manage my calendar with precision, embrace criticism, and double down on resilience. It would take support.

When I sat down with my wife, Stephanie, to explain this calling, she wrapped me in a warm embrace and told me that I'd best get started. There was no hesitation, no questioning, but only love in her response.

Before speaking with Stephanie, I had decided that I would move forward only if I had her complete support. My wife has always provided space in our relationship for my big ideas while keeping me tethered to the ground with her kind heart. Knowing the project would be all-consuming, I was mindful of the sacrifice I was asking her to make by giving me her blessing. Truthfully, I also needed to hear that she thought I could do it. Her love gave me the courage to begin writing the book and the confidence to see it through to completion. Without it, the book would not exist. After twenty-five years of marriage, three kids, a professional practice, two Grey Cup rings, and now a book, she continues to inspire me to reach for the stars.

With Stephanie's blessing, I shared my plan with our three sons, Liam, Ethan, and Aidan; my parents, Ross and Cathy Chapin; my siblings, Sperry Bilyea and Robert Chapin; my in-laws, Charles Wilson and Luz-Maria Alvarez-Wilson and Jack and Clare Harris; and my dear aunt, Dr. Barbara Galloway. This group of extraordinary humans completes my inner circle. They bring meaning and purpose to my life, and their unwavering encouragement over the last few years made the days, when the research and writing felt hard, feel lighter.

I was fortunate to be raised in a loving family with parents that inspired accountability, hard work, and big ideas. My mother and father continue to show me the way through their mentorship, and their impact on my skill set as a husband, father, and healthcare provider are immeasurable.

Growing up in a family that loves books leaves a mark. My grandmother opened a bookshop in the west end of Toronto in 1964 called The Book Mark, and when she sold it in the late 1990s, it was one of the country's oldest independently owned and operated bookstores. My father and Aunt Barb were also in the book business; for many years, my dad owned a Canadian book wholesaler business and my aunt owned and operated the second Book Mark from Atlantic Beach, Florida. I have fond memories of unpacking books and carefully shelving them at all three locations. As such, given a choice, I still prefer the feel of a book in my hand over a device. Books surrounded me in my youth and fueled my curiosity.

Before sharing my work outside my inner circle, my Aunt Barb and my mom pored over hours of video, interview transcripts, and early drafts of the mentor profiles. These exchanges greatly impacted how I structured the book and presented the mentors' stories. Having worked with many local authors, my Aunt Barb's guidance and support were especially helpful. Her belief and conviction in seeing this book in print made it possible.

Drs. Ian Dawe and Michael Odlozinski, two of my best friends, did the work only best friends can do. Their interest, encouragement, contribution, distraction, kindness, and humor ensured I came up for air and, without a doubt, made this book better.

I knew early on that the mentors' stories would be the heartbeat of *Take Good Care*. Their honest, sobering, and inspiring experiences would reach readers in ways a clinical study could not and bring the 7 Wellness Rituals to life. As the group of mentors came together, my excitement grew. I was overwhelmed by their genuine support, trust, transparency, and shared sense of urgency for my call to action. I do not know how to adequately thank them for their time and willingness to join me in this project. They chose to pay it forward; your improved health is their reward. I will forever treasure our time together and the valuable life lessons I learned from them.

The first mentor to agree to participate was Phillip Crawley. Other than my immediate family, clinic staff, and patients, I hadn't shared a face-to-face conversation with another human in months on the day I met with Phillip to pitch my book. With everyone working from home due to the pandemic, the downtown core lay utterly silent, as did *The Globe and Mail* editorial floor on the day I walked into Phillip's office. I entered this meeting with an idea and left with an action plan. This is one of Phillip's many talents. With Phillip's endorsement, Francois Olivier, Andy Smith, and Jim Leech agreed to come aboard within a few weeks, and I was off and running. I hold tremendous gratitude for Phillip's willingness to put his influence behind my vision.

John Danson, an old friend, introduced me to Jim Treliving and Jeffrey Latimer. Stephanie introduced me to Randy Lennox and Pattie Lovett-Reid. Randy then called Jann Arden, and Jeffrey called Silken Laumann, and as spring of 2021 approached, I had close to ten mentors ready to go. To recruit the rest of the group, I leaned into my network.

Along the way, I was extremely fortunate to receive coaching from many others. Gifted writers Josh O'Kane and Cathal Kelly reviewed early manuscripts and helped guide me through various publishing options. I also turned to writer Kristine Laco for advice on numerous occasions. Having access to experienced professional writers of this caliber was invaluable. Their advice was always spot on, and they have become trusted advisors.

Pattie Lovett-Reid and her husband, Jim, also deserve a special thank you. Pattie introduced me to Jim when I was ready to begin my search for a publisher. Having just completed and successfully launched his first book, *Leading to Greatness*, Jim offered to introduce me to his editor, who had helped him prepare his manuscript and book plan for prospective publishers. This is when Don Loney and I first met.

There are rare occurrences in life, perhaps only a handful, when your paths cross with someone new, and it is as if you've known one another for decades. This was the case when I first met Don. With over forty-five years of experience in publishing, Don has seen it all, and with his guidance, my manuscript and book plan were quickly ready to be shared. Don's patience, wisdom, talent, and keen respect for my voice showed up every time we met. He is an extraordinary editor and a very special person. I will forever be grateful to Jim for this introduction and consider my new-found friendship with Don a great blessing.

In short order, Don led me to Tabitha Rose and her team at Life to Paper Publishing, and I knew my book had found its home. Tabitha and Jennifer Goulden, her business partner and right-hand, are gifted, talented, creative storytellers. They both love books and work tirelessly for their authors. The experience of bringing this book to life with them has been a pleasure. A special thank you to the Life to Paper crew, especially Monty Langford and Katrina de Liberato, for their work behind the scenes and creative influence on the finished product.

I must also thank a team of clinicians for reviewing my work and sharing their clinical wisdom: registered dietitian Nazima Qureshi, Drs. Patrick Welsh and Noah Litvak, and Ian Dawe and Michael Odlozinski again are deserving of acknowledgment. Two of my professional mentors, Drs. Bruce Fligg and Peter Diakow, also deserve my deepest gratitude. I am the clinician I am today largely due to their investment in my growth and development.

To complete this book while maintaining a full caseload of patients, I needed to lean on Dr. Emily Danson, my business partner, and the rest of our High Point Wellness Centre team in a big way and fiercely protect the pockets of time I had dedicated to the book. They took to this challenge without hesitation and allowed me the freedom to write without distraction. I am extremely grateful for their unwavering support and encouragement.

One of the advantages of my role as Team Chiropractor for the Toronto Argonauts Football Club is the opportunity to get to know the men outside of the game of football. I have worked with some of the best to play for the Canadian Football League (CFL), including Michael "Pinball" Clemons, Ricky Ray, Chad Owens, S.J. Green, Trevor Harris, Chris Van Zeyl, Shawn Lemon, Henoc Muamba, Andrew Harris, and McLeod Bethel-Thompson. These men have pushed my skill and opened my eyes to the human body's performance limits and healing potential.

On McLeod's lower ribcage is a tattoo that reads, "The reward for hard work is more hard work." He lives this truth day in and day out. Watching these men work has motivated me to reach higher. As the years pass and the fine details of the Toronto Argonauts' thrilling come-from-behind 2022 Grey Cup victory fade, my memory of supporting McLeod that season will last a lifetime. His determination, kindness, competitive spirit, and sharp intellect elevate those in the room with him. I am very grateful for our shared journey, friendship, and his willingness to help bring some of my recommendations to life.

In the early days, I knew Chinaka Hodge was the person I wanted to write the foreword. Chinaka is an award-winning and masterful storyteller, making her an easy selection, but as a patient of mine, she could also speak to the value of the Ritual Activations offered in the book. Her excitement for my journey as a new author made me want to work even harder.

Lastly, to my patients, as I stated in the dedication, your trust in me is the inspiration behind this book. The stories and strategies I have shared hold power to add quality years to your lives. I offer this work as a collection of my clinical skill set and the current leading research in hopes that it will motivate you to do the work. Thank you for trusting me with your health.

REFERENCES

Chapter 1: Wellness Ritual #1: Prioritize Sleep, Rest, and Recovery

1. Eva Bianconi et al., "An Estimation of the Number of Cells in the Human Body," Human Biology 40, no. 6 (Winter 2013): 463–71, https://doi.org/10.3109/03014460.2013.807878.

2. Liu Y. et al., "Prevalence of Healthy Sleep Duration Among Adults – United States, 2014," Morbidity and Mortality Weekly Report 65, no. 6 (February 2016): 137–41, https://doi.org/10.15585/mmwr.mm6506a1.

3. Geraldine S. Perry, Susheel P. Patil, and Letitia R. Presley-Cantrell, "Raising Awareness of Sleep as a Healthy Behavior," Preventing Chronic Disease 10, no. 130081 (August 2013), http://dx.doi.org/10.5888/pcd10.130081.

4. American Academy of Sleep Medicine, International Classification of Sleep Disorders, 3rd ed. (Darien, IL: American Academy of Sleep Medicine, 2014).

5. Michael J. Sateia, "International Classification of Sleep Disorders – Third Edition: Highlights and Modifications," Chest 146, no. 5 (November 2014): 1387–94, https://doi.org/10.1378/chest.14-0970.

6. Harneet K. Walia and Reena Mehra, "Overview of Common Sleep Disorders and Intersection with Dermatologic Conditions," International Journal of Molecular Sciences 17, no. 5 (May 2016): 654, https://doi.org/10.3390/ijms17050654.

7. Vijay Kumar Chattu et al., "Insufficient Sleep Syndrome: Is It Time to Classify It as a Major Noncommunicable Disease?" Sleep Science 11, no. 2 (Spring 2018): 56–64, https://doi.org/10.5935/1984-0063.20180013.

8. Laila Aldabal and Ahmed S. Bahammam, "Metabolic, Endocrine, and Immune Consequences of Sleep Deprivation," Open Respiratory Medicine Journal 5, no. 1 (2011): 31–43, https://doi.org/10.2174/1874306401105010031.

9. Michael A. Grandner et al., "Mortality Associated with Short Sleep Duration: The Evidence, the Possible Mechanisms, and the Future," Sleep Medicine Reviews 14, no. 3 (2010): 191–203, https://doi.org/10.1016/j.smrv.2009.07.006.

10. Alexandros N. Vgontzas et al., "Insomnia with Short Sleep Duration and Mortality: The Penn State Cohort," Sleep 33, no. 9 (September 2010): 1159–64, https://doi.org/10.1093/sleep/33.9.1159.

11. Érico Castro-Costa et al., "Association Between Sleep Duration and All-Cause Mortality in Old Age: 9-Year Follow-Up of the Bambui Cohort Study, Brazil," Journal of Sleep Research 20, no. 2 (September 2011): 303–10, https://doi.org/10.1111/j.1365-2869.2010.00884.x.

12. Carla S. Moller-Levet et al., "Effects of Insufficient Sleep on Circadian Rhythmicity and Expression Amplitude of the Human Blood Transcriptome," Proceedings of the National Academy of Sciences of the United States of America 110, no. 12 (February 2013): E1132–41, https://doi.org/10.1073/pnas.1217154110.

13. Jean-Philippe Chaput, Suzy L. Wong, and Isabelle Michaud, "Duration and Quality of Sleep Among Canadians Aged 18 to 79," Statistics Canada, https://www150.statcan.gc.ca/n1/pub/82-003-x/2017009/article/54857-eng.htm.

14. Danice K. Eaton et al., "Youth Risk Behavior Surveillance – United States, 2009," Morbidity and Mortality Weekly Report 59, no. 5 (June 2010): 1–142, Europe PMC.

15. Centers for Disease Control and Prevention (CDC), "Perceived Insufficient Rest or Sleep Among Adults – United States, 2008," Morbidity and Mortality Weekly Report 58, no. 42 (October 2009): 1175–9, Pub Med.

16. Patrick M. Krueger and Elliot M. Friedman, "Sleep Duration in the United States: A Cross-Sectional Population-Based Study," American Journal of Epidemiology 169, no. 9 (May 2009): 1052–63, https://doi.org/10.1093/aje/kwp023.

17. Roah A. Merdad, Akil Hammam, and Siraj Omar Wali, "Sleepiness in Adolescents," Sleep Medicine Clinics 12, no. 3 (September 2017): 415–28, https://doi.org/10.1016/j.jsmc.2017.03.014.

18. Stephanie Corkett, "2020 Sleep in America Poll Shows Alarming Levels of Sleepiness and Low Levels of Action," National Sleep Foundation, March 9, 2020, https://www.thensf.org/2020-sleep-in-america-poll-shows-alarming-level-of-sleepiness/.

19. "Brain Basics: Understanding Sleep," National Institute of Neurological Disorders and Stroke, last modified September 26, 2022, https://www.ninds.nih.gov/health-information/public-education/brain-basics/brain-basics-understanding-sleep.

20. Shalini Paruthi et al., "Recommended Amount of Sleep for Pediatric Populations: A Consensus Statement of the American Academy of Sleep Medicine," Journal of Clinical Sleep Medicine 12, no. 6 (2016): 785–6, https://doi.org/10.5664/jcsm.5866.

21. Nathaniel F. Watson et al., "Recommended Amount of Sleep for a Healthy Adult: A Joint Consensus Statement of the American Academy of Sleep Medicine and Sleep Research Society," Sleep 38, no. 6 (June 2015): 843–4, https://doi.org/10.5665/sleep.4716

22. Danielle Pacheco and Anis Rehman, "The Bedroom Environment: An In-Depth Look at How Each Aspect of Your Bedroom Setting Influences How Well You Sleep," National Sleep Foundation, last modified June 17, 2022, https://sleepfoundation.org/sleep-polls-data/other-polls/2013-international-bedroom-poll.

23. Jennifer Robinson, "What Are REM and Non-REM Sleep?" WebMD, last modified November 16, 2022, https://www.webmd.com/sleep-disorders/sleep-101.

24. James E. Gangwisch et al., "Short Sleep Duration as a Risk Factor for Hypertension: Analyses of the First National Health and Nutrition Examination Survey," Hypertension 47, no. 5 (May 2006): 833–9, https://doi.org/10.1161/01.HYP.0000217362.34748.e0.

Oliver Cameron Reddy and Ysbrand D. van der Werf, "The Sleeping Brain: Harnessing the Power of the Glymphatic System through Lifestyle Choices," Brain Sciences 10, no.11 (November 2020): 868, https://doi.org/10.3390/brainsci10110868.

26. "Brain Basics: Understanding Sleep," National Institute of Neurological Disorders and Stroke, last modified September 26, 2022, https://www.ninds.nih.gov/health-information/patient-caregiver-education/brain-basics-understanding-sleep.

27. Alina Masters et al., "Melatonin, the Hormone of Darkness: From Sleep Promotion to Ebola Treatment," Brain Disorders and Therapy 4, no. 1 (2014): 1000151, https://doi.org/10.4172/2168-975X.1000151.

28. Christopher Drake et al., "Caffeine Effects on Sleep taken 0, 3, or 6 Hours Before Going to Bed," Journal of Clinical Sleep Medicine 9, no.11 (November 2013): 1195–200, https://doi.org/10.5664/jcsm.3170.

29. "Effects of Light on Circadian Rhythms," Centers for Disease Control and Prevention, last modified April 1, 2020, https://www.cdc.gov/niosh/emres/longhourstraining/light.html.

30. Rachel R. Markwald, Imran Iftikhar, and Shawn D. Youngstedt, "Behavioral Strategies, Including Exercise, for Addressing Insomnia," ACSM's Health and Fitness Journal 22, no. 2 (Spring 2018): 23–9, https://doi.org/10.1249/FIT.0000000000000375.

Chapter 2: Wellness Ritual #2: Consume Healthy Fuel

1. Ashkan Afshin et al., "Health Effects of Dietary Risks in 195 Countries, 1990–2017: A Systematic Analysis for the Global Burden of Disease Study 2017," The Lancet 393, no. 10184 (May 2019): 1958–72, https://doi.org/10.1016/S0140-6736(19)30041-8.

2. "Overweight and Obese Adults," Statistics Canada, last modified June 25, 2019, https://www150.statcan.gc.ca/n1/pub/82-625-x/2019001/article/00005-eng.htm.

3. "Obesity," Government of Canada, last modified December 15, 2006, https://www.canada.ca/en/health-canada/services/healthy-living/your-health/lifestyles/obesity.html.

4. "Obesity in Canada," Obesity Canada, 2022, https://obesitycanada.ca/obesity-in-canada/.

5. "What Is an Inflammation?" National Center for Biotechnology Information, last modified February 22, 2018, https://www.ncbi.nlm.nih.gov/pubmedhealth/PMH0072482/.

6. "Foods That Fight Inflammation," Harvard Health Publishing, November 16, 2021, https://www.health.harvard.edu/staying-healthy/foods-that-fight-inflammation.

7. "Quick-Start Guide to an Anti-Inflammation Diet," Harvard Health Publishing, May 1, 2020, https://www.health.harvard.edu/staying-healthy/quick-start-guide-to-an-antiinflammation-diet.

8. David Sinclair and Matthew D. LaPlante, Lifespan: Why We Age — And Why We Don't Have To (New York: Simon & Schuster/Atria Books, 2019).

9. "Ultra-Processed Food Consumption in Canada," Louis Bonduelle Foundation, January 8, 2018, https://www.fondation-louisbonduelle.org/en/2018/01/08/ultra-processed-food-canada/.

10. Jean-Claude Moubarac, Ultra-Processed Foods in Canada: Consumption, Impact on Diet Quality and Policy Implications (Montreal: TRANSNUT, 2017), https://www.heartandstroke.ca/-/media/pdf-files/canada/media-centre/hs-report-upp-moubarac-dec-5-2017.ashx.

11. "Can Diet Heal Chronic Pain?" Harvard Health Publishing, February 15, 2021, https://www.health.harvard.edu/pain/can-diet-heal-chronic-pain.

12. Anette Christ, Mario Lauterbach, and Eicke Latz, "Western Diet and the Immune System: An Inflammatory Connection," Immunity 51, no. 5 (November 2019): 794–811, https://doi.org/10.1016/j.immuni.2019.09.020.

13. Christine Mikstas, "Healthy Foods High in Polyphenols," Nourish, November 23, 2022, https://www.webmd.com/diet/foods-high-in-polyphenols#1.

14. "Are All Processed Meats Equally Bad for Health?" Harvard School of Public Health, 2019, https://www.hsph.harvard.edu/news/hsph-in-the-news/are-all-processed-meats-equally-bad-for-health/.

15. Nick Paumgarten, "Energy, And How To Get It," New Yorker, November 1, 2021, https://www.newyorker.com/magazine/2021/11/08/energy-and-how-to-get-it.

16. Govind Warrier and Michael A. Incze, "I Want to Lose Weight: Which Diet is Best?" JAMA Internal Medicine 181, no. 9 (July 2021): 1268, https://doi.org/10.1001/jamainternmed.2021.3342.

17. "Energy Drinks," National Center for Complementary and Integrative Health, last modified July 2018, https://www.nccih.nih.gov/health/energy-drinks.

18. "The Health Benefits of 3 Herbal Teas," Harvard Health Publishing, October 21, 2021, https://www.health.harvard.edu/nutrition/the-health-benefits-of-3-herbal-teas.

19. "The Microbiome," Harvard School of Public Health, https://www.hsph.harvard.edu/nutritionsource/microbiome/.

20. Judson A. Brewer et al., "Can Mindfulness Address Maladaptive Eating Behaviors? Why Traditional Diet Plans Fail and How New Mechanistic Insights May Lead to Novel Interventions," Frontiers in Psychology 9, no. 1 (2018): 1418, https://doi.org/10.3389/fpsyg.2018.01418.

21. Prashant Regmi and Leonie K. Heilbronn, "Time-Restricted Eating: Benefits, Mechanisms, and Challenges in Translation," iScience 23, no. 6 (June 2020): 101161, https://doi.org/10.1016/j. isci.2020.101161.

22. Jeff Rothschild et al., "Time-Restricted Feeding and Risk of Metabolic Disease: A Review of Human and Animal Studies," Nutrition Reviews 72, no. 5 (May 2014): 308–18, https://doi.org/10.1111/nure.12104.

23. Emily N. C. Manoogian , Amandine Chaix, and Satchidananda Panda, "When to Eat: The Importance of Eating Patterns in Health and Disease," Journal of Biological Rhythms 34, no. 6 (December 2019): 579–81, https://doi.org/10.1177/0748730419892105.

24. Amandine Chaix et al., "Time-Restricted Eating to Prevent and Manage Chronic Metabolic Diseases," Annual Review of Nutrition 39, no. 1 (August 2019): 291–315, https://doi.org/10.1146/annurev-nutr-082018-124320.

25. Rangan Chatterjee, Feel Great, Lose Weight: Simple Habits for Lasting and Sustainable Weight Loss (Dallas, TX: BenBella Books, 2020).

Chapter 3: Wellness Ritual #3: Fight For Your Waistline

1. "Overweight and Obese Adults, 2018," Statistics Canada, June 25, 2019, https://www150.statcan.gc.ca/n1/pub/82-625-x/2019001/article/00005-eng.htm.

2. "Almost Half of Canadians' Daily Calories Come From Ultra-Processed Foods," Statistics Canada, November 18, 2020, https://www150.statcan.gc.ca/n1/daily-quotidien/201118/dq201118g-eng.htm.

3. Kirsty L. Spalding et al., "Dynamics of Fat Cell Turnover in Humans," Nature 453, no. 1 (2008): 783–7, https://doi.org/10.1038/nature06902.

4. Elise Jeffery et al., "Rapid Depot-Specific Activation of Adipocyte Precursor Cells at the Onset of Obesity," Nature Cell Biology 17, no. 1 (March 2015): 376–85, https://doi.org/10.1038/ncb3122.

5. "Why People Become Overweight," Harvard Health Publishing, June 24, 2019, https://www.health.harvard.edu/staying-healthy/why-people-become-overweight.

6. "Carbohydrates and Blood Sugar," Harvard School of Public Health, https://www.hsph.harvard.edu/nutritionsource/carbohydrates/carbohydrates-and-blood-sugar/.

7. James W. Anderson et al., "Carbohydrate and Fiber Recommendations for Individuals with Diabetes: A Quantitative Assessment and Meta-Analysis of the Evidence," American Journal of Clinical Nutrition 23, no. 1 (February 2004): 5–17, https://doi.org/10.1080/07315724.2004.10719338.

8. Cara B. Ebbeling et al., "Effects of a Low-Glycemic Load vs Low-Fat Diet in Obese Young Adults: A Randomized Trial," Journal of the American Medical Association 297, no. 19 (May 2007): 2092–102, https://doi.org10.1001/jama.297.19.2092.

9. "Facts About Saturated Fats," Medline Plus, last modified December 2020, https://medlineplus.gov/ency/patientinstructions/000838.htm.

10. "The Facts on Trans Fats," Heart and Stroke, https://www.heartandstroke.ca/healthy-living/healthy-eating/the-facts-on-trans-fats#:~:text=Health%20Canada%20has%20banned%20artificial,removed%20from%20the%20food%20supply.

11. "Saturated Fats," Heart and Stroke Symptoms, last modified November 1, 2021, https://www.heart.org/en/healthy-living/healthy-eating/eat-smart/fats/saturated-fats.

12. Bob Murray and Christine Rosenblume, "Fundamentals of Glycogen Metabolism for Coaches and Athletes," Nutrition Reviews 76, no.4 (April 2018): 243–59, https://doi.org/10.1093/nutrit/nuy001.

13. "Taking Aim at Belly Fat," Harvard Health Publishing, April 12, 2021, https://www.health.harvard.edu/staying-healthy/taking-aim-at-belly-fat.

14. Herman Pontzer et al., "Daily Energy Expenditure through the Human Life Course," Science 373, no. 6556 (August 2021): 808–12, https://doi.org/10.1126/science.abe5017.

15. "Metabolism and Weight Loss: How You Burn Calories," Mayo Clinic, October 8, 2022, https://www.mayoclinic.org/healthy-lifestyle/weight-loss/in-depth/metabolism/art-20046508#:~:text=Men%20usually%20have%20less%20body,means%20men%20burn%20more%20calories.

16. Olga Spadaro et al., "Caloric Restriction in Humans Reveals Immunometabolic Regulators of Health Span," Science 375, no. 6581 (February 2022): 671–7, https://doi.org/10.1126/science.abg7292.

17. Jayanthi Raman, Evelyn Smith, and Phillipa Hay, "The Clinical Obesity Maintenance Model: An Integration of Psychological Constructs Including Mood, Emotional Regulation, Disordered Overeating, Habitual Cluster Behaviours, Health Literacy and Cognitive Function," Journal of Obesity 240128, no. 1 (2013), https://doi.org/10.1155/2013/240128.

18. Miguel Alonso Alonso et al., "Food Reward System: Current Perspectives and Future Research Needs," Nutrition Reviews 73, no. 5 (May 2015): 296–307, https://doi.org/10.1093/nutrit/nuv002.

Chapter 4: Wellness Ritual #4: Move To Stay Young

1. Aviroop Biswas et al., "Sedentary Time and Its Association with Risk for Disease Incidence, Mortality, and Hospitalization in Adults: A Systematic Review and Meta-Analysis," Annals of Internal Medicine 162, no. 2 (January 2015): 123–32, https://doi.org/10.7326/M14-1651.

2. Stephanie A. Prince et al., "Daily Physical Activity and Sedentary Behaviour Across Occupational Classifications in Canadian Adults," Statistics Canada, September 16, 2020, https://www150.statcan.gc.ca/n1/pub/82-003-x/2020009/article/00002-eng.htm.

3. Ekelund et al., "Does Physical Activity Attenuate," 1302–10.

4. Charles E. Matthews et al., "Amount of Time Spent in Sedentary Behaviors in the United States, 2003–2004," American Journal of Epidemiology 167, no. 7 (April 2008): 875–81, https://doi.org/10.1093/aje/kwm390.

5. David W. Dunstan et al., "Associations of TV Viewing and Physical Activity with the Metabolic Syndrome in Australian Adults," Diabetologia 48, no. 1 (November 2005): 2254–61, https://doi.org/10.1007/s00125-005-1963-4.

6. Frank B. Hu et al., "Physical Activity and Television Watching in Relation to Risk for Type 2 Diabetes Mellitus in Men," Archives of Internal Medicine 161, no. 12 (June 2001): 1542–8, https://doi.org/10.1001/archinte.161.12.1542.

7. Marc T. Hamilton, Deborah G. Hamilton, and Theodore W. Zderic, "Role of Low Energy Expenditure and Sitting in Obesity, Metabolic Syndrome, Type 2 Diabetes, and Cardiovascular Disease," Diabetes 56, no. 11 (November 2007): 2655–67, https://doi.org/10.2337/db07-0882.

8. Karen I. Proper et al., "Sedentary Behaviors and Health Outcomes Among Adults: A Systematic Review of Prospective Studies," American Journal of Preventive Medicine 40, no. 2 (February 2011): 174–82, https://doi.org/10.1016/j.amepre.2010.10.015.

9. Sophie Carter et al., "Sedentary Behavior and Cardiovascular Disease Risk: Mediating Mechanisms," Exercise and Sport Sciences Reviews 45, no. 2 (April 2017): 80–6, https://doi.org/10.1249/JES.0000000000000106.

10. I-Min Lee et al., "Effect of Physical Inactivity on Major Non-Communicable Diseases Worldwide: An Analysis of Burden of Disease and Life Expectancy," Lancet 380, no. 9838, (July 2012): 219–29, https://doi.org/10.1016/S0140-6736(12)61031-9.

11. Lewis Smith et al., "The Association Between Objectively Measured Sitting and Standing with Body Composition: A Pilot Study Using MRI," BMJ Open 4, no. 6 (June 2014): e005476, https://doi.org/10.1136/bmjopen-2014-005476.

12. Anders Grøntved and Frank B. Hu, "Television Viewing and Risk of Type 2 Diabetes, Cardiovascular Disease, and All-Cause Mortality: A Meta-Analysis," JAMA 305, no. 23 (June 2011): 2448–55, https://doi.org/10.1001/jama.2011.812.

13. Sebastien F. M. Chastin et al., "Associations Between Objectively-Measured Sedentary Behaviour and Physical Activity with Bone Mineral Density in Adults and Older Adults, the NHANES Study," Bone 64, no. 1 (July 2014): 254–62, https://doi.org/10.1016/j.bone.2014.04.009.

14. Martin J. O'Donnell et al., "Risk Factors for Ischaemic and Intracerebral Haemorrhagic Stroke in 22 Countries (The INTERSTROKE Study): A Case-Control Study," The Lancet 376, no. 9735 (July 2010): 112–23, https://doi.org/10.1016/S0140-6736(10)60834-3.

15. Susan C. Gilchrist et al., "Association of Sedentary Behavior with Cancer Mortality in Middle-Aged and Older US Adults," JAMA Oncology 6, no. 8 (2020): 1210–7, https://doi.org/10.1001/jamaoncol.2020.2045.

16. Preetha Anand et al., "Cancer Is a Preventable Disease That Requires Major Lifestyle Changes," Pharmaceutical Research 25, no. 9 (July 2008): 2097–116, https://doi:10.1007/s11095-008-9661-9.

17. Steven C. Moore et al., "Association of Leisure-Time Physical Activity with Risk of 26 Types of Cancer in 1.44 Million Adults," JAMA Internal Medicine 176, no. 6 (June 2016): 816–25, https://doi.org/10.1001/jamainternmed.2016.1548.

18. Charles E. Matthews et al., "Amount of Time Spent in Sedentary Behaviors and Cause-Specific Mortality in US Adults," The American Journal of Clinical Nutrition 95, no. 2 (February 2012): 437–45, https://doi.org/10.3945/ajcn.111.019620.

19. Mark Hamer, Ngaire Coombs, and Emmanuel Stamatakis, "Associations Between Objectively Assessed and Self-Reported Sedentary Time with Mental Health in Adults: An Analysis of Data from the Health Survey for England," BMJ Open 4, no. 3 (2014): e004580, https://doi.org/10.1136/bmjopen-2013-004580.

20. Jeff K. Vallance et al., "Associations of Objectively-Assessed Physical Activity and Sedentary Time with Depression: NHANES (2005–2006)," Preventive Medicine 53, no. 4–5 (October 2011): 284–8, https://doi.org/10.1016/j.ypmed.2011.07.013.

21. Darren M. Roffey et al., "Causal Assessment of Occupational Standing or Walking and Low Back Pain: Results of a Systematic Review," The Spine Journal 10, no. 3 (2010): 262–72, https://doi.org/10.1016/j.spinee.2009.12.023.

22. Charles E. Mathews et al., "Mortality Benefits for Replacing Sitting Time with Different Physical Activities," Medicine and Science in Sports and Exercise 47, no. 9 (September 2015): 1833–40, https://doi.org/10.1249/MSS.0000000000000621.

23. Hunter Hsu and Ryan M. Siwiec, "Knee Osteoarthritis," StatPearls, last modified September 4, 2022, https://www.ncbi.nlm.nih.gov/books/NBK507884.

24. Kamile E. Barbour et al., "Vital Signs: Prevalence of Doctor-Diagnosed Arthritis and Arthritis-Attributable Activity Limitation — United States, 2013–2015," Morbidity and Mortality Weekly Report 66, no. 9 (March 2017): 246–53, http://dx.doi.org/10.15585/mmwr.mm6609e1.

25. "2017 Canadian Opioid Prescribing Guideline," Canadian Centre on Substance Use and Addiction, https://www.cfpc.ca/CFPC/media/Resources/Pain-Management/Opioid-poster_CFP_ENG.pdf.

26. "More Evidence That Exercise Can Boost Mood," Harvard Health Publishing, May 1, 2019, https://www.health.harvard.edu/mind-and-mood/more-evidence-that-exercise-can-boost-mood.

27. "Weight Training May Boost Brain Power," Harvard Health Publishing, January 1, 2017, https://www.health.harvard.edu/mind-and-mood/weight-training-may-boost-brain-power?utm_source=delivra&utm_medium=email&utm_campaign=wr20170106-walking&utm_id=356213&dlv-ga-memberid=11189015&mid=11189015&ml=356213.

28. Larry A. Tucker, "Physical Activity and Telomere Length in U.S. Men and Women: An NHANES Investigation," Preventive Medicine 100, no. 1 (July 2017): 145–51, https://doi.org/10.1016/j.ypmed.2017.04.027.

29. Abdullah Alansare et al., "The Effects of High-Intensity Interval Training vs. Moderate-Intensity Continuous Training on Heart Rate Variability in Physically Inactive Adults," International Journal of Environmental Research and Public Health 15, no. 7 (July 2018): 1508, https://doi.org/10.3390/ijerph15071508.

30. Paul H. Falcone et al., "Caloric Expenditure of Aerobic, Resistance, or Combined High-Intensity Interval Training Using a Hydraulic Resistance System in Healthy Men," Journal of Strength and Conditioning Research 29, no. 3 (March 2015): 779–85, https://doi.org/10.1519/JSC.0000000000000661.

31. Hailee L. Wingfield et al., "The Acute Effect of Exercise Modality and Nutrition Manipulations on Post-Exercise Resting Energy Expenditure and Respiratory Exchange Ratio in Women: A Randomized Trial," Sports Medicine Open 1, no. 1 (December 2015): 11, https://doi.org/10.1186/s40798-015-0010-3.

32. Michael A. Wewege et al., "The Effects of High-Intensity Interval Training vs. Moderate-Intensity Continuous Training on Body Composition in Overweight and Obese Adults: A Systematic Review and Meta-Analysis," Obesity Reviews 18, no. 6 (June 2017): 635–46, https://doi.org/10.1111/obr.12532.

33. Romeo B. Batacan Jr. et al., "Effects of High-Intensity Interval Training on Cardiometabolic Health: A Systematic Review and Meta-Analysis of Intervention Studies," British Journal of Sports Medicine 51, no. 6 (February 2017): 494–503, https://dx.doi.org/10.1136/bjsports-2015-095841.

34. Matthew M. Robinson et al., "Enhanced Protein Translation Underlies Improved Metabolic and Physical Adaptations to Different Exercise Training Modes in Young and Old Humans," Cell Metabolism 25, no. 3 (March 2017): 581–92, https://doi.org/10.1016/j.cmet.2017.02.009.

35. Darren E. R. et al., "Evidence-Based Risk Assessment and Recommendations for Physical Activity Clearance: An Introduction," Applied Physiology, Nutrition, and Metabolism 36, no. 1 (July 2011): S1–2, https://doi.org/10.1139/h11-060.

36. "The Physical Activity Readiness Questionnaire for Everyone: The International Standard for Preparticipation Screening," PAR-Q+, http://eparmedx.com/?page_id=79.

Chapter 5: Wellness Ritual #5: Protect Your Strength

1. Elhuyar Fundazioa, "Study on 90-Year-Olds Reveals the Benefits of Strength Training," ScienceDaily, September 27, 2013, www.sciencedaily.com/releases/2013/09/130927092350.htm.

2. Andrew P. Wroblewski et al., "Chronic Exercise Preserves Lean Muscle Mass in Masters Athletes," The Physician and Sportsmedicine 39, no. 3 (September 2011): 172–8, https://doi.org/10.3810/psm.2011.09.1933.

3. Darren G. Candow and Philip D. Chilibeck, "Differences in Size, Strength, and Power of Upper and Lower Body Muscle Groups in Young and Older Men," The Journals of Gerontology: Series A Biological Sciences and Medical Sciences 60, no. 2 (February 2005): 148–56, https://doi.org/10.1093/gerona/60.2.148.

4. Wroblewski et al., "Chronic Exercise Preserves," 172–8.

5. Tommy Cederholm, Alfonso J. Cruz-Jentoft, and Stefania Maggi, "Sarcopenia and Fragility Fractures," European Journal of Physical and Rehabilitation Medicine 49, no. 1 (February 2013): 111–7, PubMed.

6. Richard Matthew Dodds et al., "The Epidemiology of Sarcopenia," Journal of Clinical Densitometry 18, no. 4 (Fall 2015): 461–6, https://doi.org/10.1016/j.jocd.2015.04.012.

7. Kristen E. Bell et al., "Muscle Disuse as a Pivotal Problem in Sarcopenia-Related Muscle Loss and Dysfunction," Journal of Frailty and Aging 5, no. 1 (2016): 33–41, https://doi.org/10.14283/jfa.2016.78.

8. Hidekatsu Yanai, "Nutrition for Sarcopenia," Journal of Clinical Medicine Research 7, no. 12 (December 2015): 926–31, https://doi,org/10.14740/jocmr2361w.

9. Giulia Bano et al., "Inflammation and Sarcopenia: A Systematic Review and Meta-Analysis," Maturitas 96, no. 1 (February 2017): 10–5, https://doi.org/10.1016/j.maturitas.2016.11.006.

10. Si-Jin Meng and Long-Jiang Yu, "Oxidative Stress, Molecular Inflammation and Sarcopenia," International Journal of Molecular Sciences 11, no. 4 (April 2010): 1509–26, https://doi.org/10.3390/ijms11041509.

11. Frank Mayer et al., "The Intensity and Effects of Strength Training in the Elderly," Deutsches Ärzteblatt International 108, no. 21 (May 2011): 359–64, https://doi.org/10.3238/arztebl.2011.0359.

12. Gary R. Hunter et al., "Sarcopenia and Its Implications for Metabolic Health," Journal of Obesity 2019, no. 8031705 (March 2019), https://doi.org/10.1155/2019/8031705.

13. Kristen M. Beavers et al., "Effect of Exercise Type During Intentional Weight Loss on Body Composition in Older Adults with Obesity," Obesity (Silver Spring) 25, no. 11 (November 2017): 1823–9, https://doi.org/10.1002/oby.21977.

14. Michael H. Thomas and Steve P. Burns, "Increasing Lean Mass and Strength: A Comparison of High Frequency Strength Training to Lower Frequency Strength Training," International Journal of Exercise Science 9, no. 2 (April 2016): 159–67, PubMed.

15. Robert G. McMurray et al., "Examining Variations of Resting Metabolic Rate of Adults: A Public Health Perspective," Medicine and Science in Sports and Exercise 46, no. 7 (July 2014): 1352–8, https://doi.org/10.1249/MSS.0000000000000232.

16. Renée de Mutsert et al., "Associations of Abdominal Subcutaneous and Visceral Fat with Insulin Resistance and Secretion Differ Between Men and Women: The Netherlands Epidemiology of Obesity Study," Metabolic Syndrome and Related Disorders 16, no. 1 (February 2018): 54–63, https://doi.org/10.1089/met.2017.0128.

17. Maria Grazia Benedetti et al., "The Effectiveness of Physical Exercise on Bone Density in Osteoporotic Patients," BioMed Research International 2018, no. 4840531 (2018), https://doi.org/10.1155/2018/4840531.

18. Jung-Hoon Choi, Da-Eun Kim, and Heon-Seock Cynn, "Comparison of Trunk Muscle Activity Between Traditional Plank Exercise and Plank Exercise With Isometric Contraction of Ankle Muscles in Subjects with Chronic Low Back Pain," Journal of Strength and Conditioning Research 35, no. 9 (September 2021): 2407–13, https://doi.org/10.1519/JSC.0000000000003188.

19. de Mutsert et al., "Associations of Abdominal Subcutaneous," 54–63.

20. Jonathan C. Mcleod, Tanner Stokes, and Stuart M. Phillips, "Resistance Exercise Training as a Primary Countermeasure to Age-Related Chronic Disease," Frontiers in Physiology 10, no. 1 (June 2019): 645, https://doi.org10.3389/fphys.2019.00645.

21. Bong-Sup Park et al., "Effects of Elastic Band Resistance Training on Glucose Control, Body Composition, and Physical Function in Women With Short- vs. Long-Duration Type-2 Diabetes," Journal of Strength and Conditioning Research 30, no. 6 (June 2016): 1688–99, https://doi.org/10.1519/JSC.0000000000001256.

22. Thalita B. Leite et al., "Effects of Different Number of Sets of Resistance Training on Flexibility," International Journal of Exercise Science 10, no. 3 (September 2017): 354–64, PubMed.

23. Seyed Hojjat Zamani Sani et al., "Physical Activity and Self-Esteem: Testing Direct and Indirect Relationships Associated with Psychological and Physical Mechanisms," Neuropsychiatric Disease and Treatment 12, no. 1 (October 2016): 2617–25, https://doi.org/10.2147/NDT.S11681.

24. Paul Rowe, Adam Koller, and Sandeep Sharma, "Physiology, Bone Remodeling," StatPearls, last modified January 27, 2022, https://www.ncbi.nlm.nih.gov/books/NBK499863/.

25. Dok Hyun Yoon, Jun-Young Lee, and Wook Song, "Effects of Resistance Exercise Training on Cognitive Function and Physical Performance in Cognitive Frailty: A Randomized Controlled Trial,"

Journal of Nutrition, Health, and Aging 22, no. 8 (August 2018): 944–51, https://doi.org/10.1007/s12603-018-1090-9.

26. Brett R. Gordon et al., "The Effects of Resistance Exercise Training on Anxiety: A Meta-Analysis and Meta-Regression Analysis of Randomized Controlled Trials," Sports Medicine 47, no. 12 (December 2017): 2521–32, https://doi.org/10.1007/s40279-017-0769-0.

27. Hugo Luca Corrêa et al., "Resistance Training Improves Sleep Quality, Redox Balance and Inflammatory Profile in Maintenance Hemodialysis Patients: A Randomized Controlled Trial," Scientific Reports 10, no. 11708 (July 2020), https://doi.org/10.1038/s41598-020-68602-1.

28. Nicholas Ratamess and Brent A. Alvar, "Progression Models in Resistance Training for Healthy Adults," Medicine and Science in Sports and Exercise 41, no. 1 (January 2009): 687–708, https://doi.org/10.1249/MSS.0b013e3181915670.

29. Christoph Centner et al., "Low-Load Blood Flow Restriction Training Induces Similar Morphological and Mechanical Achilles Tendon Adaptations Compared with High-Load Resistance Training," Journal of Applied Physiology 127, no. 6 (December 2019): 1660–7, https://doi.org/10.1152/japplphysiol.00602.2019.

30. Helmi Chaabene et al., "Acute Effects of Static Stretching on Muscle Strength and Power: An Attempt to Clarify Previous Caveats," Frontiers in Physiology 10, no. 1468 (November 2019), https://doi.org/10.3389/fphys.2019.01468.

31. "2017 JUNO Awards Gala Tribute to Randy Lennox," YouTube, April 18, 2017, https://www.youtube.com/watch?v=1f9XKPcS7EM.

32. "Randy Lennox: The Exit Interview," FYI Music News, January 3, 2021, https://www.fyimusicnews.ca/articles/2021/01/03/randy-lennox-exit-interview.

Chapter 6: Wellness Ritual #6: Nurture Mental Fitness

1. Paul Smetanin et al., "The Life and Economic Impact of Major Mental Illnesses in Canada," RiskAnalytica, on behalf of the Mental Health Commission of Canada, December 2011, https://www.mentalhealthcommission.ca/wp-content/uploads/drupal/MHCC_Report_Base_Case_FINAL_ENG_0_0.pdf.

2. Sylvia Ann Hewlett and Carolyn Buck Luce, "Extreme Jobs: The Dangerous Allure of the 70-Hour Workweek," Harvard Business Review, December 2006, https://hbr.org/2006/12/extreme-jobs-the-dangerous-allure-of-the-70-hour-workweek.

3. "COVID-19 Pandemic Triggers 25% Increase in Prevelance of Anxiety and Depression Worldwide," World Health Organization, March 2, 2022, https://www.who.int/news/

item/02-03-2022-covid-19-pandemic-triggers-25-increase-in-prevalence-of-anxiety-and-depression-worldwide.

4. "Experiences of Health Care Workers During the Covid-19 Pandemic, September to November 2021," Statistics Canada, June 3, 2022, https://www150.statcan.gc.ca/n1/daily-quotidien/220603/dq220603a-eng.htm.

5. Joseph Fuller and William Kerr, "The Great Resignation Didn't Start with the Pandemic," Harvard Business Review, March 23, 2022, https://hbr.org/2022/03/the-great-resignation-didnt-start-with-the-pandemic.

6. Viv Groskop, "Workplace Anxiety — and How to Overcome It," Financial Times, April 25, 2022, https://www.ft.com/content/0239be22-a04a-4d80-9490-180484f4f9cf.

7. "Women in the Workplace 2022," Lean In, https://womenintheworkplace.com/.

8. Rita Trichur, "Amplify: Taking a 'Momcation' — a Holiday without My Husband and Kids Saved — My Sanity," The Globe and Mail, June 3, 2022, https://www.theglobeandmail.com/canada/article-amplify-taking-a-momcation-a-holiday-without-my-husband-and-kids-saved/.

9. "Almost Half of Mothers in Canada Are 'Reaching Their Breaking Point,'" Canadian Women's Foundation, May 5, 2021, https://canadianwomen.org/blog/almost-half-of-mothers-in-canada-are-reaching-their-breaking-point/.

10. Lauren M. Webb and Christina Y. Chen, "The COVID-19 Pandemic's Impact on Older Adults' Mental Health: Contributing Factors, Coping Strategies, and Opportunities for Improvement," International Journal of Geriatratric Psychiatry 37, no. 1 (January 2022), https://doi.org/10.1002/gps.5647.

11. Wendy Hudson de Alencar Fontes et al., "Impacts of the SARS-CoV-2 Pandemic on the Mental Health of the Elderly," Frontiers in Psychiatry 11, no. 1 (August 2020): 841, https://doi.org/10.3389/fpsyt.2020.00841.

12. Alia Crum and Thomas Crum, "Stress Can Be a Good Thing If You Know How to Use It," Harvard Business Review, September 3, 2015, https://hbr.org/2015/09/stress-can-be-a-good-thing-if-you-know-how-to-use-it.

13. Siang Yong Tan and Angela Yip, "Hans Selye (1907–1982): Founder of the Stress Theory," Singapore Medical Journal 59, no. 4 (April 2018): 170–1, https://doi.org/10.11622/smedj.2018043.

14. "Dehydration Headache," Cleveland Clinic, last modified December 3, 2021, https://my.clevelandclinic.org/health/diseases/21517-dehydration-headache#:~:text=When%20you're%20dehydrated%2C%20your,can%20lead%20to%20a%20headache.

15. "Medication Overuse Headaches," Mayo Clinic, last modified December 8, 2020, https://www.mayoclinic.org/diseases-conditions/medication-overuse-headache/symptoms-causes/

syc-20377083#:~:text=Medication%20overuse%20headaches%20or%20 rebound,may%20trigger%20 medication%20overuse%20headaches.

16. Ann Pietrangelo and Marney A. White, "What the Yerkes-Dodson Law Says About Stress and Performance," healthline, October 22, 2020, https://www.healthline.com/health/yerkes-dodson-law.

17. Amy F. T. Arnsten et al., "The Effects of Stress Exposure on Prefrontal Cortex: Translating Basic Research into Successful Treatments for Post-Traumatic Stress Disorder," Neurobiology of Stress 1, no. 1 (January 2015): 89–99, https://doi.org/10.1016/j.ynstr.2014.10.002.

18. Eric Anderssen, "Can a Community Reach Zero Youth Suicide? In Peel, That is Exactly What They're Trying to Do," The Globe and Mail, December 17, 2020, https://www.theglobeandmail.com/canada/ article-can-a-community-reach-zero-youth-suicide-in-peel-that-is-exactly-what/.

19. Irvan Sam Schonfeld, Renzo Bianchi, and Stefano Palazzi, "What is the Difference between Depression and Burnout? An Ongoing Debate," Rivista de Psichiatria 53, no. 4 (Summer 2018): 218–9, https://doi.org/10.1708/2954.29699.

20. Panagiota Koutsimani, Anthony Montgomery, and Katerina Georganta, "The Relationship between Burnout, Depression, and Anxiety: A Systematic Review and Meta-Analysis," Frontiers in Psychology 10, no. 1 (March 2019): 284, https://doi.org/10.3389/fpsyg.2019.00284.

21. Moïra Mikolajczak and Isabelle Roskam, "Parental Burnout: Moving the Focus from Children to Parents," New Directions for Child and Adolescent Development 2020, no. 174 (November 2020): 7–13, https://doi.org/ 10.1002/cad.20376.

22. Dene Moore, "Worker Burnout is Becoming Endemic and It's Everyone's Job to Treat It," The Globe and Mail, February 7, 2022, https://www.theglobeandmail.com/business/careers/future-of-work/ article-worker-burnout-is-becoming-endemic-and-its-everyones-job-to-treat-it/.

23. Kathleen Brewer-Smyth and Harold G. Koenig, "Could Spirituality and Religion Promote Stress Resilience in Survivors of Childhood Trauma?" Issues in Mental Health Nursing 35, no. 4 (April 2014): 251–6, https://doi.org/ 10.3109/01612840.2013.873101.

24. Andrew Harris, "Radical Acceptance in a Time of Uncertainty," HopeWay, June 8, 2022, https:// hopeway.org/blog/radical-acceptance.

25. Betty-Ann Heggie, "The Healing Power of Laughter," Journal of Hospital Medicine 15, no. 5 (May 2019): 320, https://doi.org/10.12788/jhm.3205.

26. Arlnjot Flaa et al., "Personality May Influence Reactivity to Stress," BioPsychoSocial Medicine 1, no. 5 (March 2007), https://doi.org/10.1186/1751-0759-1-5.

27. Train Your Brain Like an Olympian: Gold Medal Techniques to Unleash Your Potential at Work. Jean Francois Menard. 2020. ECW Press. page 84

Chapter 7: Wellness Ritual #7: Play with Purpose

1. "The Power of Play," Froebel Trust, froebel.org.uk/about-us/the-power-of-play.

2. Barbara E. Corbett, A Garden of Children (Mississauga, ON: Uncle Goose Toys, 1980).

3. Martin E. P. Seligman and Mihaly Csikszentmihalyi, "Positive Psychology: An Introduction," in Flow and the Foundations of Positive Psychology (New York: Springer, 2014), 279–98.

4. Ed Diener and Louis Tay, "A Scientific Review of the Remarkable Benefits of Happiness for Successful and Healthy Living," in Happiness: Transforming the Development Landscape (Thimphu, Bhutan: Centre for Bhutan Studies and GNH, 2017), 90–117, https://www.bhutanstudies.org.bt/ publicationFiles/OccasionalPublications/Transforming%20Happiness/Chapter%206%20A%20 Scientific%20Review.pdf.

5. Achor, The Happiness Advantage.

6. Shawn Achor, Big Potential: How Transforming the Pursuit of Success Raises Our Achievement, Happiness, and Well-Being (New York: Crown, 2018).

7. Shawn Achor, "Oprah Super Soul Session with Shawn Achor" Videos, Shawn Achor, 2019, shawnachor.com/media/.

8. Stuart Brown, Play: How It Shapes the Brain, Opens the Imagination, and Invigorates the Soul (New York: Penguin, 2010).

9. Brené Brown, The Power of Vulnerability: Teachings on Authenticity, Connection, and Courage (Louisville, CO: Sounds True, 2012).

10. Brooke Diaz, "Awaken Your Inner Child to the Joys of Play," Chopra, June 6, 2022, chopra.com/ articles/awaken-your-inner-child-to-the-joys-of-play.

11. Wayne W. Dyer, "It's Never Too Late to Have a Happy Childhood," Facebook, December 24, 2013, facebook.com/drwaynedyer/photos/its-never-too-late-to-have-a-happy-childhood-when-you-watch-children-playing-not/10152082973181030/.

12. "Wayne Dyer Quotes," BrainyQuote, brainyquote.com/quotes/wayne_dyer_173500.

13. "Mihaly Csikszentmihalyi & Flow," Pursuit of Happiness, pursuit-of-happiness.org/ history-of-happiness/mihaly-csikszentmihalyi/.

14. Olivia Guy-Evans, "Brain Reward System," Simply Psychology, July 8, 2021, simplypsychology.org/ brain-reward-system.html.

15. Kent C. Berridge and Morten L. Kringelbach, "Pleasure Systems in the Brain," Neuron 86, no. 3 (May 2015): 646–64, https://doi.org/10.1016/j.neuron.2015.02.018.

16. "Serotonin," Cleveland Clinic, last modified March 18, 2022, my.clevelandclinic.org/health/articles/22572-serotonin.

17. Patti Summerfield, "Canadians Spend 21 Hours a Week Watching TV and Video Content," Media in Canada, February 11, 2022, mediaincanada.com/2022/02/11/canadians-spend-21-hours-a-week-watching-tv-and-video-content/.

18. Robert Lustig, The Hacking of the American Mind, (New York: Avery, 2018).

19. "The Hacking of the American Mind with Robert Lustig," University of California Television, YouTube, September 6, 2017, youtube.com/watch?v=EKkUtrL6B18&t=71s.

20. Yoichi Chida and Andrew Steptoe, "Positive Psychological Well-Being and Mortality: A Quantitative Review of Prospective Observational Studies," Psychosomatic Medicine 70, no. 7 (September 2008): 741–56, https://doi.org/10.1097/PSY.0b013e31818105ba.

21. Ed Diener and Micaela Y. Chan, "Happy People Live Longer: Subjective Well-Being Contributes to Health and Longevity," Applied Psychology: Health and Well-Being 3, no. 1 (January 2011), 1–43, https://doi.org/10.1111/j.1758-0854.2010.01045.x.

22. Ryan T. Howell, Margaret L. Kern, and Sonja Lyubomirsky, "Health Benefits: Meta-Analytically Determining the Impact of Well-Being on Objective Health Outcomes," Health Psychology Review 1, no. 1 (July 2007): 83–136, https://doi.org/10.1080/17437190701492486.

23. Sheldon Cohen et al., "Emotional Style and Susceptibility to the Common Cold," Psychosomatic Medicine 65, no. 4 (Summer 2003): 652–7, https://doi.org/10.1097/01.psy.0000077508.57784.da.

24. Mimi R. Bhattacharyya et al., "Depressed Mood, Positive Affect, and Heart Rate Variability in Patients with Suspected Coronary Artery Disease," Psychosomatic Medicine 70, no. 9 (November 2008): 1020–7, https://doi.org/10.1097/PSY.0b013e318189afcc.

25. Janice K. Kiecolt-Glaser et al., "Psychoneuroimmunology: Psychological Influences on Immune Function and Health," Journal of Consulting and Clinical Psychology 70, no. 3 (June 2002): 537–47, https://doi.org/10.1037//0022-006x.70.3.537.

26. Julia K. Boehm et al., "A Prospective Study of Positive Psychological Well-Being and Coronary Heart Disease," Health Psychology 30, no. 3 (May 2011): 259–67, https://doi.org/10.1037/a0023124.

27. Heather N. Rasmussen, Michael F. Scheier, and Joel B. Greenhouse, "Optimism and Physical Health: A Meta-Analytic Review," Annals of Behavioural Medicine 37, no. 3 (June 2009): 239–56, https://doi.org/ 10.1007/s12160-009-9111-x.

28. Barbara L. Fredrickson, "The Role of Positive Emotions in Positive Psychology: The Broaden-and-Build Theory of Positive Emotions," American Psychologist 56, no. 3 (March 2001): 218–26, https://doi.org/10.1037//0003-066x.56.3.218.

29. Nicole M. Lawless and Richard E. Lucas, "Predictors of Regional Well-Being: A County Level Analysis," Social Indicators Research 101, no. 3 (July 2010): 341–57, https://doi.org/10.1007/s11205-010-9667-7.

30. Eric S. Kim et al., "Optimism and Cause-Specific Mortality: A Prospective Cohort Study," American Journal of Epidemiol 185, no. 1 (January 2017): 21–9, https://doi.org/10.1093/aje/kww182.

31. Barbara L. Fredrickson and Christine Branigan, "Positive Emotions Broaden the Scope of Attention and Thought-Action Repertoires," Cognition and Emotion 19, no. 3 (May 2005): 313–32, https://doi.org/10.1080/02699930441000238.

32. Goleman, Daniel, Social Intelligence (New York: Bantam, 2006).

33. Howard S. Friedman and Ronald E. Riggio, "Effect of Individual Differences in Nonverbal Expressiveness on Transmission of Emotion," Journal of Nonverbal Behavior 6, no. 2 (December 1981): 96–104, SpringerLink.

34. Lawrence Robinson et al., "The Benefits of Play for Adults," HelpGuide, last modified December 5, 2022, https://www.helpguide.org/articles/mental-health/benefits-of-play-for-adults.htm.

35. Brigid Schulte, "Do These Exercises for Two Minutes a Day and You'll Immediately Feel Happier, Researchers Says," The Washington Post, June 29, 2015, washingtonpost.com/news/inspired-life/wp/2015/06/29/do-these-exercises-for-two-minutes-a-day-and-youll-immediately-feel-happier-researchers-say/.

Afterword: My Lessons Learned

1. "High Cholesterol," Mayo Clinic, last modified January 11, 2023, https://www.mayoclinic.org/diseases-conditions/high-blood-cholesterol/diagnosis-treatment/drc-20350806.

2. Yanghui Liu et al., "Associations of Resistance Exercise with Cardiovascular Disease Morbidity and Mortality," Medicine and Science in Sports and Exercise 51, no. 3 (March 2019): 499–508, https://doi.org/10.1249/MSS.0000000000001822.

DR. DWIGHT CHAPIN

INDEX